PHARMACOLOGY - RESEARCH, SAFETY TESTING AND REGULATION

CISPLATIN

PHARMACOLOGY, CLINICAL USES AND ADVERSE EFFECTS

PHARMACOLOGY - RESEARCH, SAFETY TESTING AND REGULATION

Additional books in this series can be found on Nova's website under the Series tab.

Additional E-books in this series can be found on Nova's website under the E-book tab.

CANCER ETIOLOGY, DIAGNOSIS AND TREATMENTS

Additional books in this series can be found on Nova's website under the Series tab.

Additional E-books in this series can be found on Nova's website under the E-book tab.

PHARMACOLOGY - RESEARCH, SAFETY TESTING AND REGULATION

CISPLATIN

PHARMACOLOGY, CLINICAL USES AND ADVERSE EFFECTS

TOSHIKO KOJIMA
AND
YOKO MORITA
EDITORS

Nova Science Publishers, Inc.
New York

For permission to use material from this book please contact us:
Telephone 631-231-7269; Fax 631-231-8175
Web Site: http://www.novapublishers.com

Additional color graphics may be available in the e-book version of this book.

Library of Congress Cataloging-in-Publication Data

ISBN: 978-1-61942-359-6

Published by Nova Science Publishers, Inc. †New York

CONTENTS

PREFACE

Cisplatin is a platinum-based anticancer drug and widely used for the treatment of human testicular, ovarian, bladder, cervical, head and neck, and small cell lung cancers. Its anticancer activity results from the modification of DNA through covalent cross-linkings or platinum (Pt)-DNA adducts. This book presents topical research in the study of the pharmacology, clinical uses and adverse effects of cisplatin therapy.

Chapter I - Cisplatin [*cis*-diamminedichloroplatinum(II)], a platinum-based anticancer drug, is widely used for the treatment of cancers, in particular : human testicular, ovarian, bladder, cervical, head and neck, and small cell lung cancers. Its anticancer activity results from the modification of DNA through covalent cross-linkings or platinum (Pt)-DNA adducts. The DNA adducts interfere with transcription, translation and lead to apoptosis. However, many patients relapse with cisplatin resistance. This review focuses on current knowledge on the cellular responses to cisplatin, including those involved in adducts formation and characterization, cellular accumulation, enhanced DNA repair and apoptosis. In addition, newer and novel strategies to overcome cellular resistance to cisplatin are described. This information provides powerful tools for the rational design for the development of more effective platinum-based drugs for future cancer treatment.

Chapter II - Although administration of anti-cancer drugs in high doses results in serious side effects due to their strong toxicity, many kinds of chemical compounds and recombinant proteins are used against various types of cancer. It would be more beneficial for cancer patients if they could take an effective dose without unexpected and unwanted side effects. Cisplatin (CDDP) is one example. It is one of the most effective anti-cancer agents. It requires an appropriate drug delivery system (DDS). Encapsulation of drug molecules into liposomes is one typical DDS strategy, but it is still necessary to improve the combination of drug and lipids to obtain the best efficiency of incorporation. The authors' first approach was to establish a highly-efficient method to prepare liposomes incorporating CDDP. The authors exploited cis-diamminedinitratoplatinum (CDDP3), which is highly soluble in water and labile in the presence of chloride ions converting into CDDP, to prepare liposomes containing CDDP at high concentration, because the insolubility of CDDP in water considerably inhibits incorporation. As expected, the loading efficiency of CDDP into liposomes was dramatically improved with CDDP3 in chloride-ion-free conditions, compared with CDDP used by itself.

Furthermore, the liposomes were conferred with the ability to target a specific locus of tumor *in vivo*, being conjugated with Sialyl Lewis X (SLX) on the surface. The SLX liposome (SLX-Lip) is considered to mimic leucocyte accumulating in the inflammatory region of arthritis and tumors with high affinity to E-selectin expressed on the vascular endothelial cells. CDDP encapsulated into SLX-Lip (CDDP-SLX-Lip) was then evaluated *in vivo* as a sophisticated active targeting DDS.

The acute toxicity of CDDP was markedly reduced by the use of liposome. Intravenous administration of CDDP-SLX-Lip at doses of 18 and 25 mg CDDP/kg weight to normal mice showed a survival rate of 75 % even at 14 days after injection, while CDDP at the same doses showed survival rates of 25 and 0 %. Decrease of body weight was 20 to 25 % for 3 days after administration of these liposomes, but recovered in a couple of days within the loss of 10 %. Histologically, no abnormality was observed in the kidney, spleen or liver of normal mice after administration of CDDP-SLX-Lip at a dose of 25 mg CDDP/kg weight.

The anti-tumor effect of CDDP-SLX-Lip or CDDP-Lip administered via tail veins was evaluated in tumor-bearing mice. The amount of CDDP accumulated in tumors at 48 h after injection was 6 times more when CDDP-SLX-Lip was administered than with CDDP-Lip. The anti-tumor effect at the dose of 25 mg/kg weight in lung carcinoma-bearing mice was shown to be significant when CDDP was actively directed to tumors suppressing the growth.

Thus, CDDP at high doses was demonstrated to be incorporated into liposome and specifically directed to tumors *in vivo*, showing a practical anti-tumor effect. It may be worth doing further evaluation for a clinical study.

Chapter III - Cisplatin, cis-diamminedichloroplatium, was firstly discovered of its antitumor activity during a study on the effects of electric current on bacterial growth in 1965 (1) and was later developed to be the cornerstone of modern chemotherapy in early 1970s. Cisplatin plays an important role as one of the most widely used and the most effective chemotherapy for various epithelial cancers. Cisplatin-based chemotherapy is responsible for high cure rate of germ cell tumor, high response and remission rate of ovarian cancer. It is capable of stabilizing various cancers, including non-small cell lung cancer, small cell lung cancer as well as other cancers: head and neck, bladder, stomach, anal and cervix. Cisplatin, when use concurrently with radiotherapy, is a potent radiation sensitizer, therefore, it has been widely used to improve local control in head and neck, lung, cervix, esophagus and anal cancer. The clinical use of cisplatin, however, has been impeded by several adverse effects, such as renal toxicity, electrolyte imbalance, severe nausea with vomiting, neuropathy and ototoxicity. All these unfavorable effects can be minimized by applying some strategies as will be mentioned later. This review article covers cisplatin application on various aspects: pharmacology, current evidence-based clinical use, side effects and prevention.

Chapter IV - Cisplatin, (cis- diamminedichloroplatinum, CDDP)), has been widely used over the last 30 years for chemotherapy of various solid tumors, including testicular and ovarian, bladder, oral, head and neck and small cell lung and bladder cancers.[1-3] It has been thought for long time that the formation of intra-stranded and inter-stranded crosslinked DNA adducts triggers apoptosis signaling by high mobility group box 1 (HMGB1) protein recognition and the consequent blocking of nucleotide excision repair (NER).[4-7] However, both *in vivo* and *in vitro* researches have suggested that only a very modest fraction of the administered cisplatin reacts with nuclear DNA and produces cytotoxic lesions, and the largest amount reacts with various types of proteins outside and inside of cells *via* coordinating to cysteine, methionine, histidine and tyrosine residues.[8,9] For instance, following intravenous administration cisplatin can bind extensively to serum proteins[9-11] such as albumin,[10,12] transferrin8,[13] and hemoglobin;[11,14,15] and transport proteins such as the organic cation transporters (OCTs)[16] and the copper transporters Ctr1.[17] And inside cells cisplatin can also bind to various polypeptides and proteins, including Cu-transporting ATPases ATP7B and ATP7A,[18] the copper chaperone Atox1,[19-21] insulin,[22] metallothioniens,[15,23-25] cytochrome *c*,[15,26-29] superoxide dismutase,[29-32] ubiquitin,[29,33] and etc. Such interactions may have a crucial effect on the bioavailability, transport and metabolism of cisplatin, and some are thought to be associated with undesired side effects and acquired resistance of the drug.[9]

On the other hand, a number of cellular proteins and enzymes are implicated in the cellular responses to the formation of platinated DNA adducts, in particular, inter-stranded crosslinked DNA adducts, including those involved in regulating the signaling of DNA damage, cell-cycle checkpoints and arrest, DNA repair and cell death.[5,7] However, this chapter is mainly focused on highlighting the update advances on the research of directly interactions between cisplatin and proteins which are thought to be associated with the cellular uptake, transport, efflux and distribution of cisplatin, looking to future directions of development of platinum-based anticancer agents.

Chapter V - Cisplatin [cis-diamminedichloroplatinum (II)] is one of several platinum containing compounds used for the treatment of a variety of malignancies. It is generally accepted that cisplatin initiates cell death primarily through the formation of intrastrand cross-links, the majority of which involve neighboring purine bases. Subsequently, cisplatin has been placed as one of the pivotal chemotherapeutic agents in the treatment of gastric and esophageal cancers by combining with fluorouracil, irinotecan, and taxane. During the progress of advanced gastric cancer treatment, cisplatin has usually gained a constituent of several doublet or triplet regimens such as CS (cisplatin and S-1), ECF (epirubicin, cisplatin, and fluorouracil), and DCF (docetaxel, cisplatin, and fluorouracil). In particular, survivals of gastric cancer patients that received CS have been proved to be superior to, or at least equal to, those of the control regimens of S-1 monotherapy (in Japan) or CF (cisplatin and fluorouracil) (in the United States). In esophageal cancer, CF has been recognized as an active regimen in an adjuvant or neoadjuvant setting, or as a powerful partner of radiotherapy (chemoradiation).

Although cisplatin is widely used and promising, a great individual variability in both outcomes and toxicities hamper the wide therapeutic window. Response to platinum is influenced by the detoxification capacity of platinum-DNA adducts. One of the responsible factors relevant to platinum detoxification is glutathione S-transferases (GSTs), and there are interindividual and interethnic variabilities of GSTs activity that are determined by genetic polymorphism of the gene. This chapter highlights the current achievement of gastric and esophageal cancer treatment incorporating cisplatin, as well as current knowledge on molecular differences in pharmacologically relevant genes involved in the metabolism of cisplatin. This knowledge will contribute towards optimizing therapy selection on an individual basis with an anticipation of superior efficacy with a minimal chance of toxicity, and ultimately allowing treatment to be individualized which realizes the maximum patient benefit of the current exciting cisplatin-based regimen.

Chapter VI - It is known that cisplatin is one of the most effective and widely used cytotoxic agents in the treatment of a variety of malignancies, in both childish and adult patients. Cisplatin cytotoxicity originates from its binding to DNA that causes significant distortion of helical structure and results in the inhibition of DNA replication and transcription. Although its effectiveness, the continued clinical use of cisplatinum is limited by the onset of severe side effects (e.g. nephrotoxicity, ototoxicity and neurotoxicity) and drug resistance.

Bcl-2 and Bax are apoptotic regulating proteins belonging to Bcl-2 family. The first one is an anti-apoptotic member, involved in a cellular pro-survival function. Recent findings show that Bcl-2 plays an important role in the regulation of mitochondrial fusion, phenomenon noticed during cisplatin-resistance. Bax, a pro-apoptotic factor, provokes after death stimulus the perturbation of mitochondrial membrane potential with the externalization of apoptotic factors such as cytochrome c and AIF (Apoptosis Inducing Factor). Consequently, both Bcl-2 and Bax are involved in the mitochondrial apoptotic caspase-dependent and -independent pathway. The purpose of this work is to summarize the authors' recent results about cisplatin treatment both *in vivo* and *in vitro*.

In vivo studies were carried out on postnatally developing rat cerebellum and hippocampus, after a single injection of 5 μg/g or 10 μg/g b.w.; the attention was focused on immunocytochemical changes of pro-apoptotic and antiapoptotic proteins.

In vitro, 20/48h 40μM cisplatin is used on B50 neuroblastoma rat cells in order to investigate the activation of mitochondrial apoptotic pathways by means of immunolabelling and western blotting of cytochrome c and AIF and the apoptotic regulation through immunocytochemical analysis of the Bcl-2 and Bax opposite function.

Chapter VII - This article focuses primarly on the thermal properties of the anti-cancer drug cisplatin and shows that information on its thermal properties provide positive impact in a broad range of applications in addition to extending the authors' understanding of the basic science of coordination chemistry and pharmaceutical chemistry. Studies on the thermal properties of cisplatin include: i) The bond energies (Pt–NH_3, Pt–Cl) and proton affinity of cisplatin are calculated by means of the density functional theory. Comparison of the calculated bond energies with the experimental values that are derived from enthalpy changes are also given. ii) Temperature-resolved thermal analysis with the use of evolved gas analysis-electron impact ionization mass spectrometry (EGA-EIMS) and ion attachment mass spectrometry (IAMS) techniques. iii) Thermal decomposition kinetics for cisplatin in nitrogen by using EGA-IAMS. Activation energy and pre-exponential factor of cisplatin obtained via EGA-IAMS are reported. iv) Mass spectrometric analysis of cisplatin by the conventional EIMS and the newly developed novel Li^+-IAMS in connection with a quadrupole mass analyzer are also described.

Chapter VIII - The discovery of cisplatin can be traced back to the 1960s, when a physical chemist named Rosenberg discovered it while working in a small laboratory in Michigan. He noted that when an electric current passed between two platinum electrodes within a bacterial culture, the growth of Escherichia coli was inhibited due to the formation of inorganic platinum compounds, provided that ammonium and chloride ions were present. This was due to the action of a compound in the environment, Peyronie´s chloride, which was described in 1845 as cis-diaminocloroplatinum.

Chapter IX - The environment of the earth has changed consistently since primitive life was born on the earth hundreds of millions of years before 40. The change of the external environment for hundreds of millions of years brought the evolution of the creature, and the straight foundation that was not able to support a change of the external environment perished.

Chapter X - Neoplasm is a well-established risk factor for suffering a thrombotic vascular event. However, the relationship of chemotherapic agents with these events, particularly with cerebral infarction has not been well established yet. Some publications have related to cisplatin with a slight increase in the probability of suffering a stroke, but the underlying mechanism implicated remains still unknown.

In: Cisplatin: Pharmacology, Clinical Uses and Adverse Effects ISBN: 978-1-61942-359-6
Editors: Toshiko Kojima and Yoko Morita

Chapter I

NEW INSIGHTS INTO CELLULAR RESPONSES TO CISPLATIN

Adisorn Ratanaphan*
Laboratory of Pharmaceutical Biotechnology
Department of Pharmaceutical Chemistry,
Faculty of Pharmaceutical Sciences
Prince of Songkla University, Hat-Yai, Songkhla, Thailand

ABSTRACT

Cisplatin [*cis*-diamminedichloroplatinum(II)], a platinum-based anticancer drug, is widely used for the treatment of cancers, in particular : human testicular, ovarian, bladder, cervical, head and neck, and small cell lung cancers. Its anticancer activity results from the modification of DNA through covalent cross-linkings or platinum (Pt)-DNA adducts. The DNA adducts interfere with transcription, translation and lead to apoptosis. However, many patients relapse with cisplatin resistance. This review focuses on current knowledge on the cellular responses to cisplatin, including those involved in adducts formation and characterization, cellular accumulation, enhanced DNA repair and apoptosis. In addition, newer and novel strategies to overcome cellular resistance to cisplatin are described. This information provides powerful tools for the rational design for the development of more effective platinum-based drugs for future cancer treatment.

INTRODUCTION

Cisplatin [(*cis*-diamminedichloroplatinum(II)] (Figure 1), an alkylating agent and anticancer drug, is widely used for the treatment of human testicular cancer, bladder cancer and head and neck cancer (Loehrer and Einhorn, 1984; Pratt et al, 1994 Zwelling & Korn, 1982). The activity of cisplatin was found in the early sixties (Rosenberg et al., 1965, 1967, 1969) and was approved for use as an anticancer drug in 1978.

---

* Tel.: 66-7428-8867; Fax: 66-7442-8239; E-mail: adisorn.r@psu.ac.th.

Following intravenous injection of cisplatin, the neutral, relatively unreactive complex is spread in the serum and when uncharged diffuses passively across cell membranes. Activation of cisplatin then occurs by hydrolysis and loss of the chloride ions to form a cationic species that reacts with DNA, proteins, and other intracellular components (Coley & Martin, 1973). In the blood plasma, the high chloride concentration at approximately 100 mM keeps cisplatin predominately in the uncharged and relatively unreactive dichloro form. This form may react to some degree with the sulfhydryl groups of plasma proteins. The free dichloro form enters cells by passive diffusion. Cisplatin is a highly polar molecule that does not readily diffuse across lipid membranes (Hall et al., 2008). Although several lines of evidence have addressed the uptake of cisplatin through ion pumps and transporters (Hall et al., 2008), the copper influx transporter or copper transporter 1 (CTR1) has currently been shown to control the entry to cells of platinum-containing cancer drugs including cisplatin (Figure 2)(Holzer and Howell, 2006; Holzer et al., 2004a, 2004b, 2006a, 2006b; Howell et al., 2010; Jandial et al., 2009; Larson et al., 2009; Pabla et al., 2009; Safaei, 2006; Safaei et al., 2004, 2008; Wu et al., 2009).

In the cytoplasm, the relatively low chloride concentration of approximately 2-30 mM would favor the aquation reaction.

The aquation reaction is driven by the high concentration of water and low concentration of chloride in the tissues. The rate constant for the hydrolytic replacement of the first chloro ligand at 37°C is 7x 10^{-3} min^{-1} and this corresponds to a half-life of 2 h (Coley & Martin, 1973). The hydrolysis of the first chloro group is about twice as fast as for the second chloro group (Cubo et al., 2009). The aquated platinum complex can then react rapidly with a variety of strong binding sites (Pratt et al., 1994).

The cytotoxicity of cisplatin to the cancer cells is directly related to how much drug enters the cell, and its cellular accumulation. It is generally accepted that the cytotoxicity of cisplatin results from the interaction of the drug with DNA through forming a covalent bond between a platinum atom and guanine or adenine.

DNA is attacked by an activated platinum(II) complex at the guanine residues in position N7, in double stranded DNA from the side of the major groove. The attack is apparently preceeded by an electrostatic attraction between the positively charged platinum(II) complex and the negatively charged phosphodeoxyribose DNA backbone and facilitated by a bidirectional diffusion along the backbone (Holler, 1993). The initial attack of DNA by activated cisplatin is followed by the replacement of the remaining chloro ligand before the DNA adduct performs an intramolecular attack on a second purine residue (either guanine or adenine)(Bernges & Holler, 1991).

The formation of crosslinks is followed by a local, partial unwinding of double stranded DNA together with a second wave of crosslink formation. The formation of the crosslinks can be separated from the release of the second chloro group by employing the diaqua complex of cisplatin.

Formation and Characterization of Cisplatin-DNA Adducts

The distribution of bifunctional adducts formed by cisplatin has been studied extensively by mapping with restriction endonucleases and exonucleases (Cohen et al., 1980; Kelman & Buchbinder, 1978; Royer-Pokora et al., 1981; Tullius & Lippard, 1981), by replication mapping with prokaryotic and eukaryotic DNA polymerases (Fichtinger-Schepman et al., 1982; Hemminki & Thilly, 1988; Pinto & Lippard, 1985; Villani et al., 1988), by enzymatic digestion analysis (Eastman, 1983, 1986, 1987; Fichtinger-Schepman et al., 1985, 1987a, 1987b) and by NMR spectroscopic studies of platinated oligonucleotides (Berners-Price et al., 1992; Sherman & Lippard, 1987).

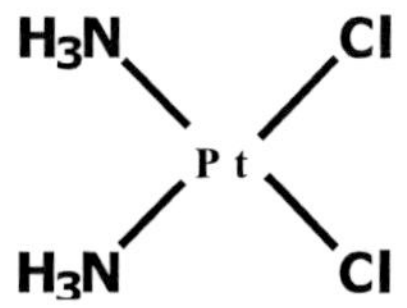

Figure 1. Structure of *cis*-diamminedichloroplatinum(II) or cisplatin.

The predominant adducts formed by cisplatin on DNA *in vitro* are 1,2-intrastrand crosslinks between the purine N7 positions in d(GpG) (>65% of the total adducts) and d(ApG) sequences (20%-25%), while longer range intrastrand adducts and interstrand crosslinks are minor products (~4%) (Fichtinger-Schepman et al., 1985).

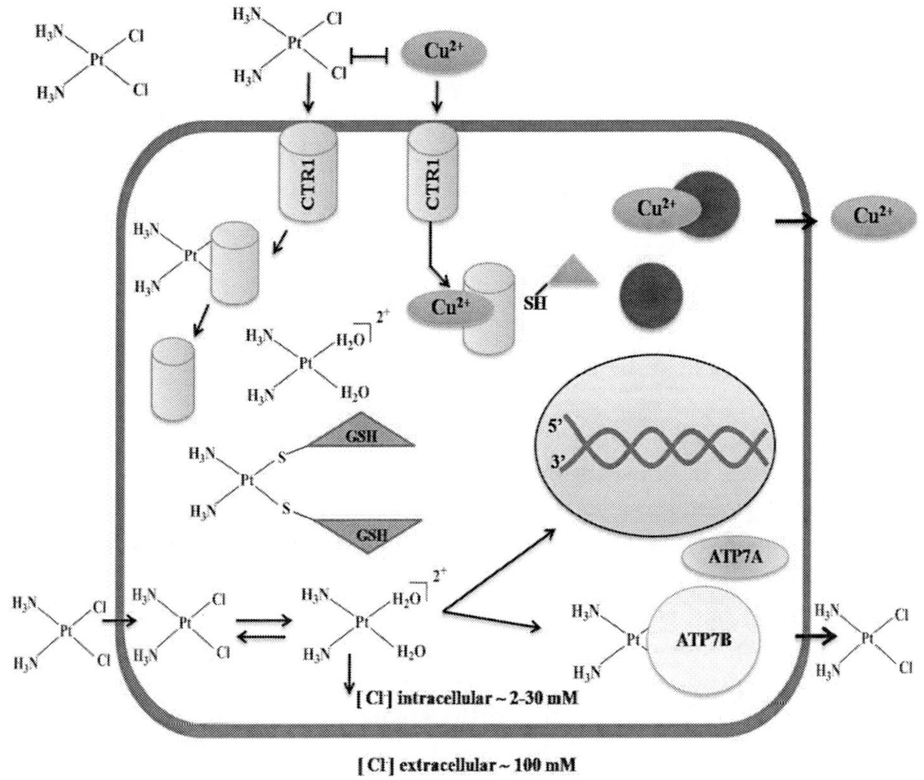

Figure 2. Schematic representation of the cellular uptake, accumulation and efflux of cisplatin in a mammalian cell. The free, neutral dichloro form of cisplatin can enter the cell by passive diffusion across the lipid bilayer or the copper influx transporter, copper transporter 1 (CTR1). In the cell, cisplatin can be inactivated by binding to glutathione (GSH), thiol- containing molecules in the cytoplasm or nuclear DNA. Cisplatin can be effluxed from the cell through the copper exporters ATP7B (copper-transporting ATPase β) or ATP7A (copper-transporting ATPase α).

Immunochemical detection of adducts (Bedford et al., 1988) has been employed to show that the intrastrand d(GpG) crosslink represents 50%-75% of the total platinum-DNA adducts formed in human cells in culture, as well as being the predominant adduct detected in the white blood cells of cancer patients undergoing cisplatin chemotherapy.

The presence of d(GpG) adducts in the white blood cells of patients is associated with a favorable response to chemotherapy (Reed et al., 1987), leading researchers to seek a correlation between a tumor response and the cellular removal of such adducts.

Although the interstrand crosslinks represent a minor portion and are generally regarded as too rare to account for the cytotoxicity of cisplatin, DNA interstrand crosslinks occur predominantly between two guanine N7 atoms on opposite strands (Eastman, 1987). A distance of ~3 angstrom is required for the cisplatin crosslinking reaction. Thus, two adjacent guanine residues on the opposite strands, either in the 5'-CG-3' or 5'-GC-3' sequences, are the most probable reaction sites on DNA.

However, in both cases, formation of the crosslink in the B-DNA implies a large distortion of the double helix since the two N7 atoms in d(CG) and d(GC) sequences are separated by about 9 and 7 angstrom, respectively. Manipulation of three-dimensional molecular models inferred that the d(CG) sequence is more able to match the interstrand cross-linking requirement (Eastman, 1987). An *in vitro* study has shown that RNA synthesis by a bacteriophage RNA polymerase acting on platinated DNA is blocked at the level of the adducts. The ability of adducts to terminate transcription has been used to map the cisplatin binding sites on a double-stranded DNA. Analysis of the modification patterns shows that the interstrand crosslinks are preferentially formed at the d(GC) sequences. This has been confirmed by a chemical study of the interstrand adduct within the d(CGAGC) sequence. The guanine residues at the d(GC) site are not reactive with DMS, which indicates that platination occurs at the N7 position of these residues (Lemaire et al., 1991).

Interaction of Cisplatin with Proteins

The interaction of cisplatin with proteins is of particular significance, and it is believed to play an important role in the distribution of the drug and inactivation responsible for determining its efficacy and toxicity (Casini et al., 2008; Sun et al., 2009; Timerbaev et al., 2006). It has been reported that albumin is not the major binding partner of cisplatin and that other proteins also have important roles in the pharmacokinetics of the drug (Timerbaev et al., 2006). It is intriguing, that protein adducts affect some crucial aspects of protein structures and functions (Table 1).

For instance, the platination of human serum albumin caused the partial unfolding of protein structure at a high drug concentration, and induced intermolecular crosslinks possibly at Cys34 and/or Met298 via bifunctional adducts or via NH_3 release (Ivanov et al., 1998; Neault & Tajmir-Riahi, 1998). Myoglobin, a small protein, that contains a heme group necessary for oxygen transport in skeletal muscles and myocardial cells, intramolecularly formed mono- and bi-functional adducts with cisplatin. Its putative platinum-binding sites were His116 and His119 (Zhao & King, 2010). A number of intramolecular crosslinks also occurred in ubiquitin adducts (Casini et al., 2009). The loss of activity by protein aggregation and prevention of the C-terminal heat shock protein 90 was reported as the consequence of cisplatin binding but the protein did not exhibit any conformational change (Ishidaa et al., 2008).

Again it is intriguing that cisplatin can cause a structural perturbation of a synthetic peptide containing a Zn^{2+} finger domain. The platinum links to the Zn^{2+}-binding sites by ejection of the Zn^{2+} and this led to a subsequent loss of the protein tertiary structure, and implied the inhibition of critical biological functions regulated by the Zn^{2+} finger protein. Such a mechanism has been discussed for the apoptosis process mediated by the interaction of cisplatin and other platinum-based compounds with the Zn^{2+} finger transcriptional factors (Bose et al., 2005).

Table 1. Some consequences of protein adducts by cisplatin

Protein	Consequences
BRCA1 (Atipairin et al., 2011)	Conformational change of the apo-form of the RING
hCtr1 (Crider et al., 2010)	Intramolecular crosslinks through replacing all platinum
Ubiquitin (Casini et al., 2009)	Four distinct adducts: $[Pt(Ub)(NH_3)_2Cl]$,
Cytochrome *c* (Zhao & King,	Monoadduct at Met 65
Hsp90 (Ishidaa et al., 2008)	Dimer formation, inhibition of aggregation prevention of
Lysozyme (Casini et al., 2007)	Monofunctional adduct at His 15
C4 zinc-finger module (Bose et al.,	Structural perturbation of a synthetic peptide containing
Na, K-ATPase (Neault et al.,	Binding constant $1.93x10^4$ M^{-1}, led to secondary
Transferrin (Cox et al., 1999)	Monofunctional adduct at Met 256
Urease (Du et al., 1999)	Secondary structural change,
Albumin (Neault & Tajmir-Riahi,	Binding constant $8.52x10^2$ M^{-1},
γ-Globulin (Chen et al., 1994)	12.4 mol platinum per protein molecule

Likewise, the nucleocapsid Zn^{2+} finger NCp7 protein, a protein required for the recognition and packaging of viral RNA, became attached to some platinum compounds that inhibited its nucleic acid binding and prevented viral infectivity (de Paula et al., 2009; Musah, 2004). The Zn^{2+} finger protein, therefore, is a potential target for platinum compounds in medicinal applications. Recently, the interaction of cisplatin with the BRCA1 DNA repair protein has been studied. It revealed that the apo-form, not the holo-form, of BRCA1 underwent more folded structural rearrangement upon cisplatin binding at His 117, and this inactivated an E3 ubiquitin ligase activity (Atipairin et al., 2010; 2011a).

Effects of Cisplatin on Transcription

Cisplatin-DNA adducts formed at d(ApG) or d(GpG) sites do not cause an absolute block to the formation of a single phosphodiester bond by either an *E.coli* RNA polymerase or a wheat germ RNA polymerase II (Corda et al., 1992, 1993). The transcription is impeded more by bifunctional than monofunctional adducts. The GpTpG intrastrand crosslink and GpC/CpG interstrand crosslinks are blocked at several nucleotides before the elongation reaches the interstrand crosslink (Corda et al., 1993). In the eukaryotic RNA polymerase, the transcription is completely blocked on the strand carrying the metal complex, whereas transcription elongation is not blocked on the complementary strand but showed a slight inhibition (Corda et al., 1991). The effect of cisplatin damage on RNA pol II elongation was investigated using site-specifically-placed cisplatin adducts. The GTG adduct produces an effective block to RNA pol II elongation, inhibiting the polymerase by 80%. In contrast, RNA pol II completely bypassed the cisplatin GG intrastrand adduct. These studies indicate that the inhibition of RNA pol II transcription observed following the treatment of cells with cisplatin is likely to reflect the combined effects of DNA damage at the level of both transcription initiation and elongation (Cullinane et al., 1999). This result differs from the effect of site-specifically platinated DNA templates on T7 RNA polymerase. An elongation complex is strongly blocked by a cisplatin 1,2-intrastrand d(GpG) and a 1,3-intrastrand d(GpTpG) cross-link located on the template strand (Jung & Lippard, 2003). Recently, *in vitro* interactions of the anticancer platinum drugs with the *BRCA1* gene and its encoded protein have been investigated (Ratanaphan et al., 2005, 2009). The cisplatin-modified *BRCA1* protected a cleavage by some restriction endonucleases, implying that cisplatin preferentially produces the 1,2-intrastrand d(GpG) crosslinks. The transcriptional transactivation activity of the BRCA1 protein is dramatically diminished in the presence of multiple cisplatin-damaged *BRCA1* sites, and a repair-mediated transcriptional transactivation of cisplatin-damaged *BRCA1* appeared to be associated with increased DNA interstrand crosslinks and altered its thermal stability (Ratanaphan et al., 2009). Cisplatin treatment also triggers ubiquitylation-mediated RNA pol II degradation in HeLa cells. The ubiquitylated polymerase was mostly unbound or only loosely associated with chromatin. This altered polymerase is rapidly destroyed by proteosomes (Jung & Lippard, 2006).

The transcription factor IIH (TFIIH) activity is modified by a cisplatin-DNA adduct. It plays a role both in initiation of basal transcription and in DNA repair, and several inherited human disorders are associated with mutations in the TFIIH subunits (Araújo et al., 2000).

The presence of DNA damage leads to inhibition of the transcription mechanism (Vichi et al., 1997). Disruption of chromatin remodeling is another mechanism by which a cisplatin adduct could interfere with transcription. Cisplatin inhibited transcription by altering the native nucleosomal organization, and limiting the nucleosomal sliding that protected an access of the RNA polymerase to the DNA template, and exhibited a significant decrease in the heat-induced mobility (Ober & Lippard, 2008; Wu et al., 2008).

Effect of Cisplatin on Protein Translation

The effect of cisplatin on *in vitro* translation has been studied using guinea pigs and rabbit reticulocyte. The peptide synthesis is inhibited in a concentration and time dependent manner. The translation inhibition is nearly maximal after a 30-min exposure. Translation is inhibited by cisplatin at concentrations that have been found after the administration of therapeutic doses. The suppression of peptide synthesis is due to an interaction between cisplatin and mRNA. Large peptide products are inhibited to a greater extent than products with faster electrophoretic mobility (Rosenberg & Sato, 1988). The decrease of protein synthesis started from the inhibition of polyribosome formation in *in vitro* translation. The inhibition is first on the initial step of protein synthesis. Cisplatin causes an accumulation of 48S particles accompanied by a decreased amount of completed 80S initiation complexes. The cisplatin blocks the initiation of translation by preventing the joining of the 60S ribosomal subunit to the 48S preinitiation subunit (Rosenberg & Sato, 1993). The mean inhibition concentration (IC_{50}) of cisplatin for inhibition of translation is 23 μM (Sato et al., 1996). It has been shown that mRNA and rRNA in rabbit reticulocyte lysates were crosslinked to form high molecular weight adducts after the extraction of RNA from polyribosomes of cisplatin-treated reactions. The arrest of elongation by cisplatin appeared to be due to the accumulation of cisplatin-RNA adducts at the damage sites. The intramolecular mRNA crosslinks within the hairpin loops or other secondary structures at the 5'-untranslated region or the open-reading frame may be the important events that inhibited the translocation ability of the ribosomes (Hostetter et al., 2009).

Cisplatin-Induced Apoptosis

Apoptosis, also known as programmed cell death, is a process in which the cell plays an active role in its own death. Apoptosis is characterized by specific changes to morphology: its structure shrinks, chromatin condenses, blebbing of the plasma membrane occurs and marginates at the nuclear membrane and cells fragment into apoptotic bodies. The apoptotic bodies are phagocytosed and degraded within by macrophages. Cisplatin-induced DNA damage causes a fall in the mitochondrial permeability transition (MPT) (Custódio et al., 2009). The altered MPT produce factors that facilitate the rupture of mitochondria such as reactive oxygen species, Bax, and Ca^{2+}, and result in the releases of cytochrome *c* and procaspase-9 (Kroemer et al., 1997). Those two proteins bind to cytosolic Apaf-1 and ATP in an apoptosome complex, leading to the activation of caspase-9. Activated caspase-9 causes the activation of caspase-3, -6, and -7 with the subsequent cleavage of key substrates (Reed, 2002). The final outcome is the formation of the apoptotic bodies. In addition, cleavage and activation of apoptosis-related regulators such as caspase-3, -8, and -9, and p53, were found in human bladder cancer cells treated with cisplatin (Konstantakou et al., 2009). The cells underwent cisplatin-induced apoptosis by the up-regulation of pro-apoptotic genes, and the down-regulation of anti-apoptotic genes in p53-dependent and p53-independent responses. Cisplatin-induced apoptosis may be initiated by damage to the phospholipid layer of the cell membrane, which triggers the sphingomyelin-ceramide signaling system of cell death (Noda et al., 2001). Moreover, cisplatin also induces apoptosis through death receptors by which the drug increases the expression of the Fas receptor and ligand (Mansouri et al., 2003). The Fas-associated death domain (FADD) can form an apoptosome complex with procaspase-8 that activates caspase-8. The active caspase-8 subsequently activates the caspase-3, -6, and -7 that cleaves key substrates and finally leads to the digestion of the cell. Caspase-8 may activate the proapoptotic protein Bid that triggers the apoptotic cell death through the mitochondrial pathway.

Cisplatin can induce two major distinct apoptotic pathways, i.e., the p53-dependent mitochondrial apoptosis and the Fas/Fas ligand-dependent caspase-8-induced apoptotic cascade (Mansouri et al., 2003). Induction of the JNK/p38 signaling pathway in response to cisplatin induced apoptosis via Fas ligand induction in ovarian cancer cells. However, the function of the JNK signaling pathway in apoptosis induced by cisplatin also remains unclear (Mansouri et al., 2003).

Cellular Resistance to Cisplatin: How do Cancer Cells Become Resistant to Cisplatin?

Since its introduction in clinical practice, cisplatin has become one of the most important drugs for treating cancer patients. Some patients whose cancers initially respond well to cisplatin-based chemotherapy become refractory to subsequent treatments. Cellular resistance to cisplatin is caused by a wide variety of mechanisms. Postulated mechanisms include decreased drug accumulation, increased levels of the intracellular thiols, and increased DNA repair (Kartalou & Essigmann 2001). In addition, when exposed to cisplatin, some ovarian cancer cells develop secondary mutations on their BRCA2 gene that restore the gene's ability to repair DNA. This restoration of gene function then makes the cancer cells resistant to cisplatin chemotherapy (Swisher et al., 2008).

Decreased Drug Accumulation

The development of cisplatin resistance is associated with a decrease in intracellular accumulation of the drug. Decreased cisplatin accumulation has been extensively demonstrated in many cisplatin-resistant cell lines (Andrews et al., 1990; Hromas et al., 1987; Kraker & Moore, 1988; Mann et al., 1988, 1990, 1991; Waud, 1987). Recent studies have shown that the development of resistance to cisplatin is associated with reduced intracellular accumulation of the drug in resistant colon adenocarcinoma (Oldenburg et al., 1994), the testis tumor, and the bladder tumor cell lines (Koeberle et al., 1996). The decreased drug accumulation could be attributed to decreased influx, decreased intracellular binding, or an increased efflux (Figure 3).

The precise mechanism of cisplatin uptake remains unknown. However, the process is believed to occur through a combination of passive diffusion and carrier-mediated transport processes (Gately & Howell, 1993). Two membrane proteins that may be involved in the uptake and efflux have been identified in cisplatin-resistant cells, i.e., a 48-kDa protein with a decreased expression and a 200-kDa glycoprotein with an increased expression (Kawai et al., 1990), respectively. Both proteins are distinct from the membrane drug-efflux pump encoded by the multidrug resistance gene (MDR), which is not involved in cisplatin resistance. Cisplatin resistance associated with reduced uptake can be overcome in vitro by co-administration of a calmodulin antagonist.

Recently, the high- affinity copper transporter CTR1 has been implicated in cisplatin transport in non-renal cells (Ishida et al., 2002; Kuo et al., 2007; Lin et al., 2002). Several lines of evidence derived from cell models have indicated that CTR1 regulates the cytotoxicity of cisplatin by affecting drug uptake (Holzer & Howell, 2006; Lin et al., 2002; Safaei et al., 2009) and that the copper exporters ATP7A (copper-transporting ATPase α) and ATP7B (copper-transporting ATPase β) are involved in cisplatin resistance by promoting efflux (Katano et al., 2002, 2003, 2004; Safaei et al., 2004, 2008; Samimi & Howell, 2006; Samimi et al., 2003, 2004). Knockdown of CTR1 reduces cisplatin uptake by 80% (Ishida et al., 2002; Lin et al., 2002) and renders mammalian and yeast cells resistant to cisplatin and some other platinum drugs (Larson et al., 2009; Lin et al., 2002).

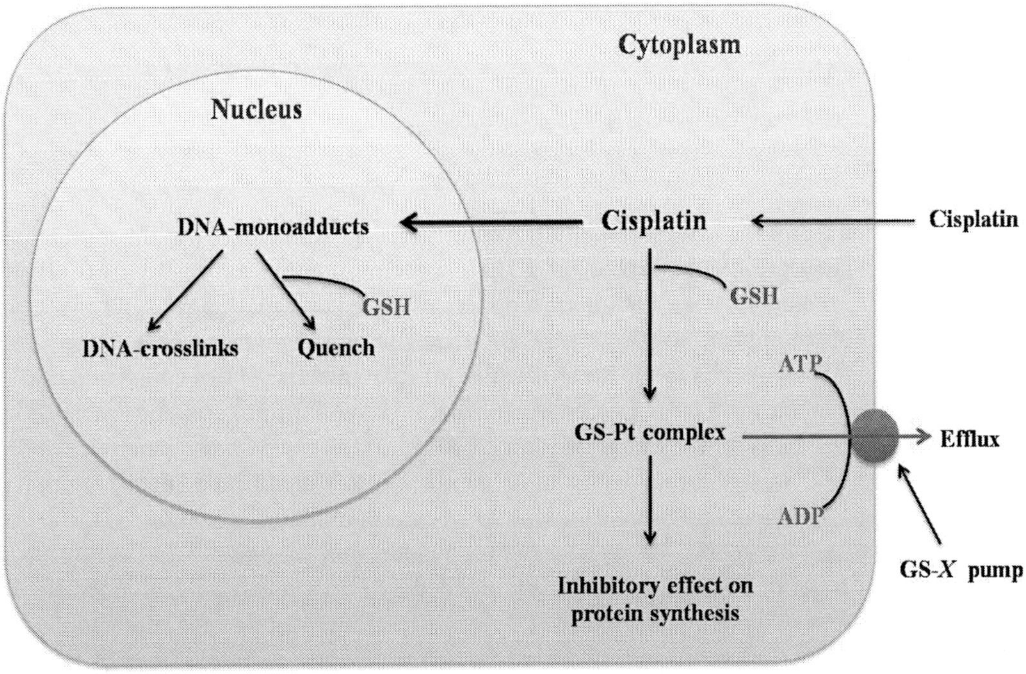

Figure 3. Schematic representation of the mechanism of cellular resistance to cisplatin, including increased detoxification and DNA repair by GSH and efflux from the cell via the GS-X pump.

Glutathione

Glutathione (GSH) is a tripeptide thiol, γ-glutamylcysteinylglycine. GSH is the major cellular non-protein thiol and has a variety of physiologically important functions in cellular defense and metabolism, such as modulation of the thiol-disulfide status of cellular proteins, protection of cells from oxidative stress, and detoxication of electrophilic compounds, (Ishikawa, 1992). Cisplatin resistance is found to be closely associated with an increased intracellular level of GSH (Godwin et al., 1992). GSH forms a GSH-cisplatin complex in a 2:1 molar ratio. The GSH-platinum complex is then eliminated from cancer cells by an ATP-dependent glutathione S-conjugate export pump (Ishikawa, 1992; Ishikawa & Ali-Osman, 1993)(Figure 3). Elimination of the GSH-platinum complex from cancer cells may represent an important mechanism that reduces the intracellular accumulation of the platinum complex. GSH may protect cells by intercepting reactive platinum complexes before they can react with DNA. GSH also protects cells by participating in DNA repair, possibly by stabilizing the repair enzymes such as DNA polymerase. Resistant cell lines with high levels of glutathione-S-transferase (GST) have been reported (Teicher et al., 1987). This enzyme catalyzes a conjugation between GSH and electrophilic molecules such as cisplatin, leading to the formation of an inactive product. Elevated glutathione S-transferase P1-1 (GSTP1-1) expression has been associated with resistance to cisplatin-based chemotherapy and with cellular resistance to cisplatin cytotoxicity in many experimental systems. In addition, it has been shown that variants of GSTP1-1 can confer low-level resistance to cisplatin in some cell lines. However, the rates of GSTP1-1-mediated catalysis are extremely slow, suggesting that alternative mechanisms are needed to explain GSTP1-1-associated resistance to cisplatin (Peklak-Scott et al., 2008).

Metallothionein

Metallothionein proteins (MT) constitute a family of low molecular weight intracellular metalloproteins. They are characterized by a high cysteine content and a high affinity for heavy metal ions, including zinc, cadmium, copper, mercury and platinum (Andrews et al., 1987). Metallothionein appears to play a physiological role in the metabolism and storage of essential trace metals as well as in the detoxification of toxic metals. MT is composed of 30% cysteine and can account for a large percentage of the intracellular thiol content. Because it is rich in thiol groups, MT is a likely target for an electrophilic agent such as cisplatin. Another possible role for MT was reported when transfection of nontransformed mouse mammary C127 cells with a bovine papillomavirus shuttle vector containing a human MT-IIa gene conferred resistance to cisplatin as well as to melphalan and chlorambucil (Kelley et al., 1988). Transcription of the MT gene is strongly induced by heavy metal ions, glucocorticoids, interferon, and stress. Cisplatin binds to MT with 10 platinum atoms per molecule. Upon binding, it loses its amine ligands and displaces heavy metal ions. Multiple lines of evidence have shown that tumor cell lines with acquired resistance to cisplatin overexpress metallothionein. They have demonstrated the induction of metallothionein by cisplatin in subcutaneously inoculated tumors. These data indicate that cisplatin resistance can be prevented or reversed by the modulation of metallothionein synthesis. Propargylglycine, an inhibitor of g-cystathionase, specifically inhibits the cystathionine pathway and decreases the intracellular pool of free cysteine, thereby decreasing metallothionein and glutathione synthesis. It has been reported that an increase in antitumor activity can be obtained by a therapy that combines cisplatin and propargylglycine (Saga et al., 2004).

Increased DNA Repair

DNA repair pathways play an important role in cisplatin resistance. They have been extensively studied for many years both in the preclinical and clinical settings. The DNA repair processes are the cellular responses associated with the restoration of the normal nucleotide sequence of DNA after damage (Bohr et al., 1987). Evidence for the importance of DNA repair pathways comes most directly from the rare, inherited human disorders, in which defects in DNA repair mechanisms are associated with hypersensitivity to radiation and DNA damaging drugs. Cisplatin-based chemotherapy is the standard treatment in the initial therapy of advanced-stage ovarian cancer. Although up to 80% of patients have an early favorable response to therapy, less than 20% of individuals experience long-term disease-free survival (Young et al., 1989). As a result of the primary or acquired resistance, most ovarian cancer patients eventually relapse from cisplatin-resistant disease (Berek & Hacker, 1990). Cisplatin-resistant cell lines show increased levels of DNA repair, as measured by the loss of platinum adducts, DNA repair synthesis, and reactivation of cisplatin-damaged plasmid DNA. Platinum-DNA adduct formation and repair have been investigated in cisplatin-sensitive and -resistant human ovarian cancer cell lines (Zhen et al., 1992). In the overall genome, the initial frequency of both cisplatin lesions was higher in the parental than in the resistant cells. Resistant and parental cells had similar initial frequencies of intrastrand and interstrand crosslinks in the dihydrofolate reductase (*DHFR*) gene after cisplatin treatment of the cells. There was no increase in the repair efficiency of intrastrand crosslinks in the *DHFR* gene in the resistant cells compared with the parental cells. However, interstrand crosslinks were removed much faster in the resistant cells. The results indicate that acquired cellular resistance to cisplatin may be associated with an increased gene-specific DNA repair efficiency of a specific lesion, the interstrand crosslink, without marked changes in the overall genome repair. The human excision repair cross complementing gene 1 (*ERCC1*), the first cloned human excision repair gene, has been shown to be transcribed at increased levels in cells from some patients after cisplatin-based therapy (Parker et al., 1990). Preferential repair of genes may be related to the openness or accessibility of the chromatin in actively transcribed genomic regions (Bohr et al., 1987; Reeves, 1984; Wilkins & Hart, 1974). These results strengthen the conception that DNA repair at the gene level may be an important resistance mechanism to cisplatin treatment.

Cisplatin is an effective chemotherapeutic agent for the treatment of testicular cancer and is used in combination regimines for a variety of other tumors. Although many patients initially respond to treatment, a common problem is acquired resistance. The intrinsic resistance observed in some patients is multifactorial in nature and includes contributions from differential drug uptake, cellular detoxification systems, and DNA repair mechanism (Reed et al., 1996; Zamble & Lippard, 1995; Zamble et al., 1995). The loss of DNA mismatch repair activity enhanced sensitivity to cisplatin (Fink et al., 1996). Nucleotide excision repair is also a major mechanism contributing to cisplatin resistance. The global genome repair and transcription-coupled repair are the major mechanisms for repair of nucleotide excision. In the non-actively transcriped strands of gene, the adduction of cisplatin is first recognized by the XP (Xeroderma pigmentosum) protein that initiates the process of GGR, which simply means repair anywhere in the genome. However, the repair of adducts on transcriped strands uses TCR that is more rapid than GGR (Hartman & Ford, 2003). The cell lines from patients with XP mutations are highly sensitive to cisplatin by about 4-fold more than in normal cells (Dijt et al., 1988).

Cisplatin resistance could be caused by enhanced expression of other proteins involved in repair. DNA polymerase beta (Polβ) is reported to be the only polymerase that will efficiently bypass a cisplatin 1,2-d(GpG) intrastrand crosslink This indicates that higher expression levels of this protein will increase replicative bypass (Hoffmann et al., 1995). The *ERCC1* is one of the essential components of the mammalian nucleotide excision repair (NER) pathway. When the relative expressions of the genes encoding for ERCC1 was monitored in tumor tissue from human ovarian patients, the mRNA levels were significantly higher in tissue from patients who were clinically resistant to cisplatin therapy when compared with the tissue of patients who respond favorably to treatment (Selvakumaran et al., 2003). The proliferating cell nuclear antigen (PCNA) is another protein that is required for the NER pathway to function and this protein was also found to be overexpressed in cell lines that showed resistance to cisplatin exposure (Lyakhovich & Shekhar, 2004). C-fos and C-myc are both proto-oncogenes that have been correlated with cisplatin resistance following drug exposure. Activating the transcription of these genes may lead to a cascade of gene expressions that, in turn, stimulates the activity of proteins having a direct role in DNA repair (Kashini-Sabet et al., 1990). A tumor suppressor gene product, p53, has been linked to the ability of DNA repair mechanisms. Disruption of the gene encoding for p53 in human breast cancer cells increased their sensitivity to cisplatin, possibly because of a decrease in DNA repair (Fan et al., 1995). Recently, there is emerging evidence of the role of the tumor suppressor protein BRCA1 in the DNA repair pathways that strongly indicates that it is involved in mediating the response to chemotherapeutic treatment of cancer through HR during the repair of DSBs (Quinn et al., 2003). Inhibition of the BRCA/Fanconi anemia pathway enhances sensitivity to cisplatin in cancer cells. In contrast, cancer cells that are defective in this pathway confer cisplatin resistance.

Epigenetics in Resistance to Cisplatin

Epigenetics is defined as heritable changes in gene expression that are not due to any alteration in the DNA sequence (Holliday, 1987). The best-known epigenetics is DNA methylation and then, more recently, the discovery of the inactivation of microRNA (miRNA) genes by DNA methylation (Lujambio et al., 2007; Pogribny et al., 2010; Saito et al., 2006). DNA methylation is currently found in post-translational modifications to histones. Hypermethylation of the CpG islands in the promoter regions of the tumor suppressor genes is a major event in the origin of many cancers. It can affect genes involved in the cell cycle, DNA repair, the metabolism of carcinogens, apoptosis, all of which are involved in the progression of cancer (Esteller, 2007; Herman & Baylin, 2003). The emerging evidence has indicated that epigenetics can be involved in the development of cisplatin resistance in non-small cell lung cancer (NSCLC) (O'Byrne et al., 2011). In addition, inhibition of DNA methyltransferase reverses cisplatin-induced drug resistanc in murine neuroblastoma cells (Qiu et al., 2005).

Other Mechanisms of Cellular Resistance to Cisplatin

Based on the above results, factors including decreased drug accumulation, intracellular thiol contents, and DNA repair capacity, can affect the sensitivity of human cells to cisplatin. However, no clear-cut dominant mechanism of resistance to cisplatin has been identified in human cancer cells. Cisplatin resistance of a particular cell may be due to several possible mechanisms. Moreover, a given cell may use more than one mechanism or can develop simultaneously several mechanisms of resistance. There are other mechanisms that may be involved in cellular resistance to cisplatin, such as altered folate metabolism (Scanlon et al., 1989), changes in oncogene expression (Basu & Cline, 1995; Sklar, 1988), modulation by protein kinases (Dhar & Basu, 2008; Folbergrova et al., 1987; Hofmann et al., 1988; Kharbanda et al., 1995; Nehme et al., 1997), and loss of DNA mismatch repair (Aebi et al., 1996; Drummond et al., 1996; Fink et al., 1997; Nehme et al., 1997). In addition, an increased tolerance to DNA damage can be another explanation for increased resistance to cisplatin. Cells can achieve damage tolerance by bypassing DNA lesions during replication or transcription.

Translesion synthesis through cisplatin-DNA adducts became interesting because of its correlation to drug sensitivity by which cisplatin-resistant cells exhibited more translesion synthesis than drug-sensitive cells (Hicks et al., 2010). The process also conferred the mutagenic properties of cisplatin because of the nature of the replication bypass that was carried out by error-prone DNA synthesis (Bassett et al., 2003, 2004). The mutagenicity of cisplatin was closely related to the evolution of resistance of cell lines to the drug. In particular, the cisplatin-resistant human ovarian carcinoma cell lines showed a 3-5 fold increase in the replicative bypass ability to proceed past a DNA adduct compared to their respective cisplatin-sensitive cells (Hoffmann et al., 1995; Mamenta et al., 1994).

Strategies to Overcome Cisplatin Resistance and Prospectives

Cisplatin entered clinical trials in 1971 and within a relatively short time became the most widely used anticancer medicine in the world. However, its application is somewhat limited due to its severe toxicity and rapid development of drug resistance. Development of cisplatin resistance by tumors is a major clinical limitation. This is often linked to resistance to other chemotherapy drugs (doxorubicin, taxanes) from crosstalk of mechanisms involving import of these molecules across the cell membrane. Experimental strategies under investigation aim to overcome cisplatin resistance. Manipulations of transport mechanisms can alter cell sensitivity to cisplatin. A proteasome inhibitor, bortezomib, has been found to enhance platinum accumulation and overcome resistance through interfering with ubiquitination-mediated downregulation of CTR1 (Holzer et al., 2004). Novel approaches include the development of ribozymes or oligonucleotides designed to cleave specific mRNAs, and consequently decrease the levels of functional proteins in cancerous cells. In addition, liposome encapsulation of the drug as well as the introduction of miRNAs would be optimistic methods to avoid the detoxification of cisplatin in resistant tumors.

At present, the enhanced sensitivity to cisplatin and gemcitabine has been reported in a triple-negative breast cancer cell lines (Hastak et al., 2010; Koshy et al., 2010), and in BRCA1-deficient murine mammary epithelial cells (Alli et al., 2011). Sunitinib, a multi-targeted receptor tyrosine kinase inhibitor, significantly potentiated the cytotoxic effect of cisplatin in vitro and in vivo (Suddek, 2011). The results indicated that sunitinib ameliorates cisplatin-induced nephrotoxicity and potentiates its anticancer activity. This type of combination therapy could improve chemotherapeutic efficacy and have beneficial implications for patients during treatment with cisplatin. Further mechanistic studies of such synergistic interactions are promising in the future. Recently, a number of preclinical and clinical studies have revealed that breast cancer patients with BRCA dysfunction gain more benefit from cisplatin treatments, particularly for patients with a BRCA1 mutation (Byrski et al., 2009; Font et al., 2010; Quinn et al., 2007; Silver et al., 2010; Taron et al., 2004). It revealed that the response to cisplatin treatment occurred in a dose-dependent manner in human breast cancer cells (Tassone et al., 2003; Wong et al., 2011). The increased cisplatin sensitivity in the BRCA1-mutated breast cancers might be related to an impaired BRCA1 function normally responsible for repairing DNA adducts produced by cisplatin, and ultimately results in cell death (Alli et al., 2011; Price & Monteiro, 2010; Tassone et al., 2009). This was consistent with previous studies, showing that cisplatin-based chemotherapy achieved an increased response rate for triple-negative breast cancer (Silver et al., 2010; Sirohi et al., 2008). This evidence has emphasized the potential of using the BRCA1 dysfunction as an important determinant of chemotherapy responses in breast cancer (Mullan et al., 2006).

In conclusion, the emerging highlighted therapeutic strategies appear to be targeting the relevance of new proteins in the signal transduction and DNA damage response pathways, particularly those related to the DNA repair pathways (Amir et al., 2010; Helleday et al., 2008; Zhu et al., 2009) that have responded to cisplatin, chemically-modified cisplatin or combined platinum-based regimens (Ashworth, 2008). It is optimistic to believe that this trend of molecularly targeted therapy can pave the way to more individualized and effective therapies in the near future.

ACKNOWLEDGEMENTS

The author would like to thank Prince of Songkla University for financial support (PHA530188S, PHA540650S), and Dr. Brian Hodgson for the proof reading and assistance with the English.

REFERENCES

Aebi, S., Kurdi-Haidar, B., Gordon, R., Cenni, B., Zheng, H., Fink, D., et al. (1996). Loss of DNA mismatch repair in acquired resistance to cisplatin. *Cancer Res.* 56(13): 3087-3090.

Alli, E., Sharma, V. B., Hartman, A. R., Lin, P. S., McPherson, L. & Ford, J. M. (2011). Enhanced sensitivity to cisplatin and gemcitabine in Brca1-deficient murine mammary epithelial cells. *BMC Pharmacol.* 11: 7.

Amir, E., Seruga, B., Serrano, R. & Ocana A. (2010). Targeting DNA repair in breast cancer: A clinical and translational update. *Cancer Treat Rev.* 36(7): 557-565.

Andrews, P. A., Jones, J. A., Varki, N. M. & Howell, S. B. (1990). Rapid emergence of acquired cis-diamminedichloroplatinum(II) resistance in an in vivo model of human ovarian carcinoma. *Cancer Comm.* 2(2): 93-100.

Andrews, P.A., Murphy, M.P. & Howell, S.B. (1987). Metallothionein-mediated cisplatin resistance in human ovarian carcinoma cells. *Cancer Chemother Pharmacol.* 19(2): 149-154.

Araujo, S.J., Tirode, F., Coin, F., Pospiech, H., Syvaoja, J.E., Stucki, M., et al. (2000). Nucleotide excision repair of DNA with recombinant human proteins: definition of the minimal set of factors, active forms of TFIIH, and modulation by CAK. *Genes Dev.* 14(3): 349–359.

Ashworth, A. (2008). A synthetic lethal therapeutic approach: poly(ADP) ribose polymerase inhibitors for the treatment of cancers deficient in DNA double-strand break repair. *J Clin Oncol.* 26(22): 3785-3790.

Atipairin, A., Canyuk, B. & Ratanaphan, A. (2010). Cisplatin affects the conformation of apo-form, not holo-form, of BRCA1 RING finger domain and confers thermal stability. *Chem Biodivers.* 7(8): 1949-1967.

Atipairin, A., Canyuk, B. & Ratanaphan, A. (2011a). The RING heterodimer BRCA1-BARD1 is a ubiquitin ligase inactivated by the platinum-based anticancer drugs. *Breast Cancer Res Treat.* 126(1): 203-209.

Atipairin, A., Canyuk, B. & Ratanaphan, A. (2011b). Substitution of aspartic acid with glutamic acid at position 67 of BRCA1 RING domain retains ubiquitin ligase activity and zinc(II)-binding with a reduced transition temperature. *J Biol Inorg Chem.* 16(2): 217-226.

Ban, N., Takahashi, Y., Takayama, T., Kura, T., Katahira, T., Sakamaki, S., et al. (1996). Transfection of glutathione S-transferase (GST)-π antisense complementary DNA increases the sensitivity of a colon cancer cellline to adriamycin, cisplatin, melphalan, and etoposide. *Cancer Res.* 56(15): 3577-3582.

Bassett, E., King, N.M., Bryant, M.F., Hector, S., Pendyala, L., Chaney, S.G., et al. (2004). The role of DNA polymerase eta in translesion synthesis past platinum-DNA adducts in human fibroblasts. *Cancer Res.* 64(18): 6469-6475.

Bassett, E., Vaisman, A., Havener, J.M., Masutani, C., Hanaoka, F. & Chaney, S.G. (2003). Efficiency of extension of mismatched primer termini across from cisplatin and oxaliplatin adducts by human DNA polymerases beta and eta in vitro. *Biochemistry.* 42(48): 14197-14206.

Basu, A. & Cline, J.S. (1995). Oncogenic transformation alters cisplatin-induced apoptosis in rat embryo fibroblasts. *Int J Cancer.* 63(4): 597-603.

Bedford, P., Fichtinger-Schepman, A.M., Shellard, S.A., Walker, M.C., Masters, J.R.W. & Hill, B.T. (1988). Differential repair of pt-DNA adducts in human bladder and testicular tumor continuous cell lines. *Cancer Res.* 48(11): 3019-3024.

Bellon, S.F., Coleman, J.H. & Lippard, S.J. (1991). DNA unwinding produced by site-specific intrastrand cross-links of the antitumor drug cis-diamminedichloroplatinum(II). *Biochemistry.* 30(32): 8026-8035.

Berek, J.S. & Hacker, N.F. (1990). Ovary and fallopain tubes, In: Cancer treatment, (ed.) Haskell, C.M., Saunders, W.B., Philadelphia, pp. 295-325.

Berners-Price, S.J., Frenkiel, T.A., Frey, U., Ranford, J.D. & Sadler, P.J. (1992). Hydrolysis products of cisplatin: pKa determinations via [^{1}H,^{15}N] NMR spectroscopy. *J Chem Soc., Chem Commun.* 789-791.

Bernges, F. & Holler, E. (1991). The reaction of platinum(II) complexes with DNA. Kinetics of intrastrand crosslink formation in vitro. *Nucleic Acids Res.* 19(7): 1483-1489.

Bohr, V.A., Phillips, D.H. & Hanawalt, P.C. (1987). Heterogenous DNA damage and repair in the mammalian genome. *Cancer Res.* 47: 6426-6436.

Bose, R.N., Yang, W.W. & Evanics, F. (2005). Structural perturbation of a C4 zinc-finger module by *cis*-diamminedichloroplatinum(II): insights into the inhibition of transcription processes by the antitumor drug. *Inorg Chim Acta.* 358(10): 2844-2854.

Boulikas, T. (2009). Clinical overview on Lipoplatin: a successful liposomal formulation of cisplatin. *Expert Opin Invest Drugs.* 18(8): 1197-1218.

Byrski, T., Huzarski, T., Dent, R., Gronwald, J., Zuziak, D., Cybulski, C., et al. (2009). Response to neoadjuvant therapy with cisplatin in BRCA1-positive breast cancer patients. *Breast Cancer Res Treat.* 115(2): 359-363.

Casini, A., Gabbiani, C., Michelucci, E., Pieraccini, G., Moneti, G., Dyson, P.J., et al. (2009). Exploring metallodrug-protein interactions by mass spectrometry: comparisons between platinum coordination complexes and an organometallic ruthenium compound. *J Biol Inorg Chem.* 14(5): 761-770.

Casini, A., Guerri, A., Gabbiani, C. & Messori, L. (2008). Biophysical characterisation of adducts formed between anticancer metallodrugs and selected proteins: New insights from X-ray diffraction and mass spectrometry studies. *J Inorg Biochem.* 102(5-6): 995-1006.

Casini, A., Mastrobuoni, G., Temperini, C., Gabbiani, C., Francese, S., Moneti, G., et al. (2007). ESI mass spectrometry and X-ray diffraction studies of adducts between anticancer platinum drugs and hen egg white lysozyme. *Chem Commun.* 14(2): 156-158.

Chen, D., Ohta, N., Ukai, M., Masuda, M. & Yotsuyanagi T. (1994). Binding and aggregation of human γ-globulin by *cis*-diamminedichloroplatinum (II) through disulfide bond. *Biol Pharm Bull.* 17(12): 1561-1566.

Cohen, G.L., Ledner, J.A., Bauer, W.R., Ushay, H.M., Caravana, C. & Lippard, S.J. (1980). Sequence dependent binding of cis-dichlorodiammineplatinum(II) to DNA. *J Am Chem Soc.* 102(7): 2487-2488.

Coley, R.F. & Martin, D.S. (1973). Kinetics and equilibria for the acid hydrolysis of dichloro(ethylenediammine)platinum(II). *Inorg Chim Acta.* 7: 573-577.

Corda, Y., Job, C., Anin, M-F., Leng, M. & Job, D. (1991). Transcription by eukaryotic and prokaryotic RNA polymerases of DNA modified at a d(GG) or a d(AG) site by the antitumor drug *cis*-diamminedichloroplatinum(II). *Biochemistry.* 30(1): 222-230.

Corda, Y., Job, C., Anin, M.F., Leng, M. & Job, D. (1993). Spectrum of DNA- platinum adduct recognition by prokaryotic and eukaryotic DNA dependent RNA polymerase. *Biochemistry.* 32(33): 8582-8588.

Corda, Y., Anin, M.F., Leng, M. & Job, D. (1992). RNA polymerases react differently at d(ApG) and d(GpG) adducts in DNA modified by cis-diamminedichloroplatinum(II). *Biochemistry.* 31(7): 1904-1908.

Cox, M.C., Barnham, K.J., Frenkiel, T.A., Hoeschele, J.D., Mason, A.B., He, Q-Y., et al. (1999). Identification of platination sites on human serum transferrin using ^{13}C and ^{15}N NMR spectroscopy. *J Biol Inorg Chem.* 4(5): 621-631.

Crider, S.E., Holbrook, R.J. & Franz, K.J. (2010). Coordination of platinum therapeutic agents to met-rich motifs of human copper transport protein 1. *Metallomics.* 2(1): 74-83.

Cubo, L., Thomas, D.S., Zhang, J., Quiroga, A.G., Navarro-Ranninger, C. & Berners-Price, S.J. (2009). [^{1}H,^{15}N] NMR studies of the aquation of *cis*-diamine platinum(II) complexes. *Inorg Chim Acta.* 362(3): 1022-1026.

Cullinane, C., Mazur, S.J., Essigmann, J.M., Phillips, D.R. & Bohr, V.A. (1999). Inhibition of RNA polymerase II transcription in human cell extracts by cisplatin DNA damage. *Biochemistry.* 38(19): 6204-6212.

Custodio, J.B.A., Cardoso, C.M.P., Santos, M.S., Almeida, L.M., Vicente, J.A.F. & Fernandes, M.A.F. (2009). Cisplatin impairs rat liver mitochondrial functions by inducing changes on membrane ion permeability: Prevention by thiol group protecting agents. *Toxicology.* 259(1-2): 18-24.

de Paula, Q.A., Mangrum, J.B. & Farrell, N.P. (2009). Zinc finger proteins as templates for metal ion exchange: Substitution effects on the C-finger of HIV nucleocapsid NCp7 using M(chelate) species (M=Pt, Pd, Au). *J Inorg Biochem.* 103(10): 1347-1354.

Dhar, R. & Basu, A. (2008). Costitutive activation of p70 S6 kinase is associated with intrinsic resistance to cisplatin. *Int J Oncol.* 32(5): 1133-1137.

Dijt, F.J., Fichtinger-Schepman, A.M., Berends, F. & Reedijk, J. (1988). Formation and repair of cisplatin-induced adducts to DNA in cultured normal and repair-deficient human fibroblasts. *Cancer Res.* 48(21): 6058-6062.

Donahue, B.A., Augot, M., Bellon, S.F., Treiber, D.K., Toney, J.H., Lippard, S.J., et al. (1990). Characterization of a DNA damage-recognition protein from mammalian cells that binds specifically to intrastrand d(GpG) and d(ApG) DNA adducts of the anticancer drug cisplatin. *Biochemistry*. 29(24): 5872-5880.

Drummond, J.T., Anthoney, A., Brown, R. & Modrich, P. (1996). Cisplatin and adriamycin resistance are associated with MutLα and mismatch repair deficiency in an ovarian tumor cell line. *J Biol Chem*. 271(33): 19645–19648.

Du, W., Li, Z., Wang, B. & Zhang, Y. (1999). A study on the interaction between cisplatin and urease. *Thermochim Acta*. 333(2): 109-114.

Eastman, A. (1983). Characterization of the adducts produced in DNA by cis-diamminedichloroplatinum(II) and cis-dichloro(ethylenediammine) platinum(II). *Biochemistry*. 22(16): 3927-3933.

Eastman, A. (1986). Reevaluation of interaction of cis-dichloro (ethylenediamine) platinum (II) with DNA. *Biochemistry*. 25(13): 3912-3915.

Eastman, A. (1987). The formation, isolation, and characterization of DNA adducts produced by anticancer platinum complexes. *Pharmacol Ther*. 34(2): 155-166.

Esteller, M. (2007). Cancer epigenomics: DNA methylomes and histone-modification maps. *Nat Rev Genet*. 8(4): 286-298.

Fan, S., Smith, M.L., Rivet, D.J., Duba, D., Zhan, Q., Kohn, K.W. et al. (1995). Disruption of p53 function sensitizes breast cancer MCF-7 cells to cisplatin and pentoxifylline. *Cancer Res*. 55: 1649-1654.

Farmer, H., McCabe, N., Lord, C.J., Tutt, A.N., Johnson, D.A., Richardson, T.B., et al. (2005). Targeting the DNA repair defect in BRCA mutant cells as a therapeutic strategy. *Nature*. 434(7035): 917-921.

Fedier, A., Steiner, R.A., Schwarz, V.A., Lenherr, L., Haller, U. & Fink, D. (2003). The effect of loss of Brca1 on the sensitivity to anticancer agents in p53-deficient cells. *Int J Oncol*. 22(5): 1169-1173.

Fichtinger-Schepman, A.M.J., Lohman, P.H.M. & Reedijk, J. (1982). Detection and quantification of adducts formed upon interaction of diamminedichloroplatinum(II) with DNA, by anion-exchange chromatography after enzymatic degradation. *Nucleic Acids Res*. 10(17): 5345-5356.

Fichtinger-Schepman, A.M.J., van der Veer, J.L., den Hartog, J.H.J., Lohman, P.H.M. & Reedijk, J. (1985). Adducts of the antitumor drug cis-diamminedichloroplatinum(II) with DNA: formation, identification, and quantitation. *Biochemistry*. 24(3): 707-713.

Fichtinger-Schepman, A.M.J., van Oosterom, A.T., Lohman, P.H.M. & Berends, F. (1987a). Interindividual human variation in cisplatinum sensitivity, predictable in an in vitro assay. *Mutat Res*. 190(1): 59-62.

Fichtinger-Schepman, A.M.J., van Oosterom, A.T., Lohman, P.H.M. & Berends, F. (1987b). cis-Diamminedichloroplatinum(II)-induced DNA adducts in peripheral leukocytes from seven cancer patients: quantitative immunochemical detection of the adduct induction and removal after a single dose of cis-diamminedichloroplatinum(II). *Cancer Res*. 47(11): 3000-3004.

Fink, D., Nebel, S., Aebi, S., Nehme, A. & Howell, S.B. (1997). Loss of DNA mismatch repair due to knockout of MSH2 or PMS2 results in resistance to cisplatin and carboplatin. *Intl J Oncol*. 11(3): 539-542.

Fink, D., Nebel, S., Aebi, S., Zheng, H., Cenni, B., Nehme, A. et al. (1996). The role of DNA mismatch repair in platinum drug resistance. *Cancer Res*. 56(21): 4881-4886.

Fink, D., Nebel, S., Norris, P.S., Baergen, R.N., Wilczynski, S.P., Costa, M.J., et al. (1998). Enrichment for DNA mismatch repair-deficient cells during treatment with cisplatin. *Int J Cancer*. 77(5): 741-746.

Folbergrova, J., Lisa, V., Drobnik, J. & Mares, V. (1987). Cyclic AMP levels of C6 glioma cells treated with cis-dichlorodiammineplatinum (cis-DDP). *Neoplasma*. 34(1): 3-13.

Fong, P. C., Boss, D. S., Yap, T. A., Tutt, A., Wu, P., Mergui-Roelvink, M., et al. (2009). Inhibition of poly(ADP-ribose) polymerase in tumors from BRCA mutation carriers. *N Engl J Med*. 361(2): 123-134.

Font, A., Taron, M., Gago, J.L., Costa, C., Sánchez, J.J., Carrato, C., et al. (2010). BRCA1 mRNA expression and outcome to neoadjuvant cisplatin-based chemotherapy in bladder cancer. *Ann Oncol*. doi:10.1093/annonc/mdq333.

Gately, D.P. & Howell, S.B. (1993). Cellular accumulation of the anticancer agent cisplatin: A review. *Br J Cancer*. 67(6): 1171-1176.

Godwin, A.K., Meister, A., O'Dwyer, P.J., Huang, C.S., Hamilton, T.C. & Anderson, M.E. (1992). High resistance to cisplatin in human ovarian cancer cell lines is associated with marked increase of glutathione synthesis. *Proc Natl Acad Sci. USA*. 89(7): 3070-3074.

Hall, M.D., Okabe, M., Shen, D.W., Liang, X.J. & Gottesman, M.M. (2008). The role of cellular accumulation in determining sensitivity to platinum-based chemotherapy. *Annu Rev Pharmacol Toxicol*. 48: 495–535.

Hartman, A-R. & Ford, J.M. (2003). BRCA1 and p53: compensatory roles in DNA repair. *J Mol Med*. 81(11): 700-707.

Hastak, K., Alli, E. & Ford, J.M. (2010). Synergistic chemosensitivity of triple-negative breast cancer cell lines to poly(ADP-Ribose) polymerase inhibition, gemcitabine, and cisplatin. *Cancer Res*. 70(20): 7970-7980.

Helleday, T., Petermann, E., Lundin, C., Hodgson, B. & Sharma, R.A. (2008). DNA repair pathways as targets for cancer therapy. *Nat Rev Cancer*. 8(3): 193-204.

Hemminki, K. & Thilly, W.G. (1988). Binding of cisplatin to specific sequences of human DNA in vitro. *Mutat Res*. 202(1): 133-138.

Herman, J. G. & Baylin, S. B. (2003). Gene silencing in cancer in association with promoter hypermethylation. *N Engl J Med*. 349(21): 2042-2054.

Hicks, J.K., Chute, C.L., Paulsen, M.T., Ragland, R.L., Howlett, N.G., Gueranger, Q., et al. (2010). Differential roles for DNA polymerases eta, zeta, and REV1 in lesion bypass of intrastrand versus interstrand DNA cross-links. *Mol Cell Biol*. 30(5): 1217-1230.

Hofr, C. & Brabec, V. (2001). Thermal and thermodynamic properties of duplex DNA containing site-specific interstrand cross-link of antitumor cisplatin or its clinically ineffective trans isomer. *J Biol Chem*. 276(13): 9655-9661.

Hofr, C., Farrell, N. & Brabec, V. (2001). Thermodynamic properties of duplex DNA containing a site-specific d(GpG) intrastrand crosslink formed by an antitumor dinuclear platinum complex. *Nucleic Acids Res*. 29(10): 2034-2040.

Hoffmann, J.S., Pillaire, M.J., Garcia-Estefania, D., Lapalu, S. & Villani, G. (1996). In vitro bypass replication of the cisplatin-d(GpG) lesion by calf thymus DNA polymerase beta and human immunodeficiency virus type I reverse transcriptase is highly mutagenic. *J Biol Chem*. 271(26): 15386-15392.

Hoffmann, J.S., Pillaire, M.J., Maga, G., Podust, V., Hubscher, U. & Villani G. (1995). DNA polymerase beta bypasses in vitro a single d(GpG)-cisplatin adduct placed on codon 13 of the HRAS gene. *Proc Natl Acad Sci. USA*. 92(12): 5356-5360.

Holler, E. (1993). Mechanism of action of tumor-inhibiting metal complexes. In: Metal complexes in cancer chemotherapy, Keppler, B.K. (edn.) VCH, Weinhein, pp. 37-71.

Holzer, A.K. & Howell, S.B. (2006). The internalization and degradation of human copper transporter 1 following cisplatin exposure. *Cancer Res.* 66(22): 10944–10952.

Holzer, A.K., Katano, K., Klomp, L.W. & Howell, S.B. (2004a). Cisplatin rapidly downregulates its own influx transporter hCTR1 in cultured human ovarian carcinoma cells. *Clin Cancer Res.* 10(19): 6744–6749.

Holzer, A.K., Manorek, G.H. & Howell, S.B. (2006a). Contribution of the major copper influx transporter CTR1 to the cellular accumulation of cisplatin, carboplatin, and oxaliplatin. *Mol Pharmacol.* 70(4): 1390–1394.

Holzer, A.K., Samimi, G., Katano, K., Naerdemann, W., Lin, X., Safaei, R, et al. (2004b). The copper influx transporter human copper transport protein 1 regulates the uptake of cisplatin in human ovarian carcinoma cells. *Mol Pharmacol.* 66(4): 817–823.

Howell, S.B., Safaei, R., Larson, C.A. & Sailor, M.J. (2010). Copper transporters and the cellular pharmacology of the platinum-containing cancer drugs. *Mol Pharmacol.* 77(6): 887-894.

Holzer, A.K., Varki, N.M., Le, Q.T., Gibson, M.A., Naredi, P. & Howell, S.B. (2006b). Expression of the human copper influx transporter 1 in normal and malignant human tissues. *J Histochem Cytochem.* 54(9): 1041–1049.

Holliday, R. (1987). The inheritance of epigenetic defects. *Science.* 238(4824): 163-170.

Hostetter, A.A., Chapman, E.G. & DeRose, V.J. (2009). Rapid cross-linking of an RNA internal loop by the anticancer drug cisplatin. *J Am Chem Soc.* 131(26): 9250-9257.

Hromas, R.A., North, J.A. & Burns, C.P. (1987). Decreased cisplatin uptake by resistant L1210 leukemia cells. *Cancer Lett.* 36(2): 197-201.

Ishida, S., Lee, J., Thiele, D.J. & Herskowitz, I. (2002). Uptake of the anticancer drug cisplatin mediated by the copper transporter Ctr1 in yeast and mammals. *Proc Natl Acad. Sci. USA.*. 99(22): 14298–14302.

Ishidaa, R., Takaokaa, Y., Yamamotoa, S., Miyazakia, T., Otakab, M., Watanabeb, S., et al. (2008). Cisplatin differently affects amino terminal and carboxyl terminal domains of HSP90. *FEBS Lett.* 582(28): 3879-3883.

Ishikawa, T. & Ali-Osman, F. (1993). Glutathione-associated cis-diamminedichloroplatinum(II) metabolism and ATP-dependent efflux from leukemia cells. Molecular characterization of glutathione-platinum complex and its biological significance. *J Biol Chem.* 268(27): 20116-20125.

Ivanov, A.I., Christodoulou, J., Parkinson, J.A., Barnham, K.J., Tucker, A., Woodrow, J., et al. (1998). Cisplatin binding sites on human albumin. *J Biol Chem.* 273(24): 14721-14730.

Jakupec, M.A., Galanski, M. & Keppler, B.K. (2003). Tumour-inhibiting platinum complexes--state of the art and future perspectives. *Rev Physiol Biochem Pharmacol.* 146(1): 1-54.

Jandial, D.D., Farshchi-Heydari, S., Larson, C.A., Elliott, G.I., Wrasidlo, W.J. & Howell, S.B. (2009). Enhanced delivery of cisplatin to intraperitoneal ovarian carcinomas mediated by the effects of bortezomib on the human copper transporter 1. *Clin Cancer Res.* 15(2): 553–560.

Johnson, R.D., Liu, N. & Jasin, M. 1999. Mammalian XRCC2 promotes the repair of DNA double-strand breaks by homologous recombination. *Nature.* 401(6751): 397-399.

Jordan, P. & Carmo-Fonseca, M. (1998). Cisplatin inhibits synthesis of ribosomal RNA *in vivo*. *Nucleic Acids Res.* 26(12): 2831-2836.

Jung, Y. & Lippard, S.J. (2003). Multiple states of stalled T7 RNA polymerase at DNA lesions generated by platinum anticancer agents. *J Biol Chem.* 278(52): 52084-52092.

Jung, Y. & Lippard, S.J. (2006). RNA polymerase II blockage by cisplatin-damaged DNA. Stability and polyubiquitylation of stalled polymerase. *J Biol Chem.* 281(3): 1361-1370.

Kartalou, M. & Essigmann, J.M. (2001). Recognition of cisplatin adducts by cellular proteins. *Mutat Res.* 478(1-2): 1-21.

Kashani-Sabet, M., Lu, Y., Leong, L., Haedicke, K. & Scanlon, K.J. (1990). Differential oncogene amplification in tumor cells from a patient treated with cisplatin and 5-fluorouracil. *Eur J Cancer.* 26(3): 383-390.

Kawai, K., Kamatani, N., Georges, E. & Ling, V. (1990). Identification of a membrane glycoprotein overexpressed in murine lymphoma sublines resistant to cis-diamminedichloroplatinum(II). *J Biol Chem.* 265(22): 13137-13142.

Kelley, S.L., Basu, A., Teicher, B.A., Hacker, M.P., Hamer, D.H. & Lazo, J.S. (1988). Overexpression of metallothionein confers resistance to anticancer drugs. *Science.* 241(4874): 1813-1815.

Kelley, M.R. & Fishel, M.L. (2008). DNA repair proteins as molecular targets for cancer therapeutics. *Anticancer Agents Med Chem.* 8(4): 417-425.

Kelman, A.D. & Buchbinder, M. (1978). Platinum-DNA crosslinking: platinum antitumor drug interactions with native lambda bacteriophage DNA studied using a restriction endonuclease. *Biochemie.* 60: 893-899.

Kennedy, R.D., Quinn, J.E., Mullan, P.B., Johnston, P.G. & Harkin, D.P. (2004). The role of BRCA1 in the cellular response to chemotherapy. *J Natl Cancer Inst.* 96(22): 1659-1668.

Kharbanda, S., Ren, R., Pandey, P., Shafman, T.D., Feller, S.M., Weichselbaum, R.R. et al. (1995). Activation of the c-Abl tyrosine kinase in the stress response to DNA-damaging agents. *Nature.* 376(6543): 785-788.

Köberle, B., Payne, J., Grimaldi, K.A., Hartley, J.A. & Masters, J.R. (1996). DNA repair in cisplatin-sensitive and resistant human cell lines measured in specific genes by quantitative polymerase chain reaction. *Biochem Pharmacol.* 52(11): 1729-1734.

Konstantakou, E.G., Voutsinas, G.E., Karkoulis, P.K., Aravantinos, G., Margaritis, L.H. & Stravopodis, D.J. (2009). Human bladder cancer cells undergo cisplatin-induced apoptosis that is associated with p53-dependent and p53-independent responses. *Int J Oncol.* 35(2): 401-416.

Koshy, N., Quispe, D., Shi, R., Mansour, R. & Burton, G.V. (2010). Cisplatin-gemcitabine therapy in metastatic breast cancer: Improved outcome in triple negative breast cancer patients compared to non-triple negative patients. *Breast.* 19(3): 246-248.

Kraker, A.J. & Moore, C.W. (1988). Accumulaton of cis-diamminedichloroplatinum(II) and platinum analogues by platinum resistant murine leukemia cells in vitro. *Cancer Res.* 48(1): 9-13.

Kroemer, G., Zamzami, N. & Susin, S.A. (1997). Mitochondrial control of apoptosis. *Immunol Today.* 18(1): 44-51.

Kuo, Y.M., Zhou, B., Cosco, D. & Gitschier, J. (2001). The copper transporter CTR1 provides an essential function in mammalian embryonic development. *Proc Natl Acad Sci. USA.,* 98(12): 6836–6841.

Lafarge, S., Sylvain, V., Ferrara, M. & Bignon, Y.J. (2001). Inhibition of BRCA1 leads to increased chemoresistance to microtubule-interfering agents, an effect that involves the JNK pathway. *Oncogene*. 20(45): 6597-6606.

Larson, C.A., Blair, B.G., Safaei, R. & Howell, S.B. (2009). The role of the mammalian copper transporter 1 in the cellular accumulation of platinum-based drugs. *Mol Pharmacol.* 75(2): 324–330.

Lemaire, M.A., Schwartz, A., Rahmouni, A.R. & Leng, M. (1991). Interstrand cross-links are preferentially formed at the d(GC) sites in the reaction between cis-diamminedichloroplatinum(II) and DNA. *Proc Natl Acad. Sci. USA*. 88(5): 1982-1985.

Li, L., Wang, H., Yang, E.S., Arteaga, C.L. & Xia, F. (2008). Erlotinib attenuates homologous recombinational repair of chromosomal breaks in human breast cancer cells. *Cancer Res.* 68(22): 9141-9146.

Lin, X., Okuda, T., Holzer, A. & Howell, S.B. (2002). The copper transporter CTR1 regulates cisplatin uptake in *Saccharomyces cerevisiae*. *Mol Pharmacol.* 62(5): 1154–1159.

Loehrer, P.J. & Einhorn, L.H. (1984). Drug five years later. Cisplatin, *Annals of Internal Medicine,* 100, pp. 704–713.

Lujambio, A., Ropero, S., Ballestar, E., Fraga, M.F., Cerrato, C., Setien, F., et al. (2007). Genetic unmasking of an epigenetically silenced microRNA in human cancer cells. *Cancer Res.* 67(4): 1424-1429.

Lyakhovich, A. & Shekhar, M. P. V. (2004). Supramolecular complex formation between Rad6 and proteins of the p53 pathway during DNA damage-induced response. *Mol Cell Biol.* 23(7): 2463-2475.

Mamenta, E.L., Poma, E.E., Kaufmann, W.K., Delmastro, D.A., Grady, H.L. & Chaney, S.G. (1994). Enhanced replicative bypass of platinum-DNA adducts in cisplatin-resistant human ovarian carcinoma cell lines. *Cancer Res.* 54(13): 3500-3505.

Mann, S.C., Andrews, P.A. & Howell, S.B. (1988). Comparison of lipid content, surface membrane fluidity, and temperature dependence of cis-diamminedichloroplatinum(II) accumulation in sensitive and resistant human ovarian carcinoma cells. *Anticancer Res.* 8(6): 1211-1215.

Mann, S.C., Andrews, P.A. & Howell, S.B. (1990). Short-term cis-diamminedichloro-platinum(II) accumulation in sensitive and resistant human ovarian carcinoma cells. *Cancer Chemother Pharmacol.* 25(4): 236-240.

Mann, S.C., Andrews, P.A. & Howell, S.B. (1991). Modulation of cis-diamminedichloro-platinum(II) accumulation and sensitivity by forskolin and 3-isobutyl-I-methylxanthine in sensitive and resistant human ovarian carcinoma cells. *Int J Cancer.* 48(6): 866-872.

Mansouri, A., Ridgway, L.D., Korapati, A.L., Zhang, Q., Tian, L., Wang, Y., et al. (2003). Sustained activation of JNK/p38 MAPK pathways in response to cisplatin leads to Fas ligand induction and cell death in ovarian carcinoma cells. *J Biol Chem.* 278(21): 19245-19256.

Mullan, P.B., Gorski, J.J. & Harkin, D.P. (2006). BRCA1 - a good predictive marker of drug sensitivity in breast cancer treatment? *Biochim Biophys Acta.* 1766(2): 205-216.

Musah, R.A. (2004). The HIV-1 nucleocapsid zinc finger protein as a target of antiretroviral therapy. *Curr Top Med Chem.* 4(15): 1605-1622.

Neault, J.F., Benkirane, A., Malonga, H. & Tajmir-Riahi, H.A. (2001). Interaction of cisplatin drug with Na,K-ATPase: drug binding mode and protein secondary structure. *J Inorg Biochem.* 86(2-3): 603-609.

Neault, J.F. & Tajmir-Riahi, H.A. (1998). Interaction of cisplatin with human serum albumin. Drug binding mode and protein secondary structure. *Biochim Biophys Acta.* 1384(1): 153-159.

Nehme, A., Baskaran, R., Aebi, S., Fink, D., Nebel, S., Cenni, B. et al. (1997). Differential induction of c-Jun NH_2-terminal kinase and c-Abl kinase in DNA mismatch repair-proficient and –deficient cells exposed to cisplatin. *Cancer Res.* 57(15): 3253-3257.

Noda, S., Yoshimura, S., Sawada, M., Naganawa, T., Iwama, T., Nakashima, S., et al. (2001). Role of ceramide during cisplatin-induced apoptosis in C6 glioma cells. *J Neurooncol.* 52(1): 11-21.

Ober, M. & Lippard, S.J. (2008). A 1,2-d(GpG) cisplatin intrastrand cross-link influences the rotational and translational setting of DNA in nucleosomes. *J Am Chem Soc.* 130(9): 2851-2861.

O'Byrne, K.J., Barr, M.P. & Gray, S.G. (2011). The role of epigenetics in resistance to cisplatin chemotherapy in lung cancer. *Cancer.* 3: 1426-1453.

Oldenburg, J., Begg, A.C., van Vugt, M.J.H., Ruevekamp, M., Schornagel, J.H., Pinedo, H.M. & G. Los, G. (1994). Characterization of resistance mechanisms to cis-diamminedichloroplatinum(II) in three sublines of the CC531 colon adenocarcinoma cell line in vitro. *Cancer Res.* 54(2): 487-493.

Pabla, N., Murphy, R.F., Liu, K. & Dong, Z. (2009). The copper transporter Ctr1 contributes to cisplatin uptake by renal tubular cells during cisplatin nephrotoxicity. *Am J Physiol Renal Physiol.* 296(3): F505–F511.

Parker, R.J., Eastman, A., Bostick-Bruton, F. & Reed, E. (1991). Acquired cisplatin resistance in human ovarian cancer cells is associated with enhanced repair of cisplatin-DNA lesions and reduced drug accumulation. *J Clin Invest.* 87(3): 772-777.

Parker, R.J., Poirier, M.C., Bostick-Bruton, F., Vionnet, J., Bohr, V.A. & Reed, E. (1990). The use of peripheral blood leukocytes as a surrogate marker for cisplatin drug resistance studies of adduct levels and ERCC1. *Basic Life Sci.* 53: 251-261.

Peklak-Scott, C., Smitherman, P.K., Townsend, A.J. & Morrow, C.S. (2008). Role of glutathione S-transferase P1-1 in the cellular detoxification of cisplatin. *Mol Cancer Ther.* 7(10): 3247-3255.

Pillaire, M.J., Margot, A., Villani, G., Sarasin, A., Defais, M. & Gentil, A. (1994). Mutagenesis in monkey cells of a vector containing a single d(GpG *cis*-diamminedichloroplatinum(II) adduct placed on codon 13 of the human *H-ras* protooncogene. *Nucleic Acids Res.* 22(13): 2519-2524.

Pinto, A.L. & Lippard, S.J. (1985). Binding of the antitumor drug cis-diamminedichloroplatinum(II)(cisplatin) to DNA. *Biochim Biophys Acta..* 780(3): 167-180.

Pogribny, I.P., Filkowski, J.N., Tryndyak, V.P., Golubov, A., Shpyleva, S.I. & Kovalchuk, O. (2010). Alterations of microRNAs and their targets are associated with acquired resistance of MCF-7 breast cancer cells to cisplatin. *Int J Cancer.* 127: 1785-1794.

Powell, S.N. & Bindra, R.S. (2009). Targeting the DNA damage response for cancer therapy. *DNA Repair.* 8(9): 1153-1165.

Pratt, W.R., Ruddon, R.W., Ensminger, W.D & Maybaum, J. (1994). The anticancer drugs 2nd, Oxford University press, New York, USA.

Price, M. & Monteiro, A.N.A. (2010). Fine tuning chemotherapy to match BRCA1 status. *Biochem Pharmacol.* 80(5): 647-653.

Qiu, Y.Y., Mirkin, B.L. & Dwivedi, R.S. (2005). Inhibition of DNA methyltransferase reverses cisplatin induced drug resistance in murine neuroblastoma cells. *Cancer Detect Prev.* 29: 456-463.

Quinn, J.E., Carser, J.E., James, C.R., Kennedy, R.D. & Harkin, D.P. (2009). BRCA1 and implications for response to chemotherapy in ovarian cancer. *Gynecol Oncol.* 113(1): 134-142.

Quinn, J.E., James, C,R., Stewart, G.E., Mulligan, J.M., White, P., Chang, G.K., et al. (2007). BRCA1 mRNA expression levels predict for overall survival in ovarian cancer after chemotherapy. *Clin Cancer Res.* 13(24): 7413-7420.

Quinn, J.E., Kennedy, R.E., Mullan, P.B., Gilmore, P.M., Carty, M., Johnston, P.G., et al. (2003). BRCA1 functions as a differential modulator of chemotherapy-induced apoptosis. *Cancer Res.* 63(19): 6221-6228.

Ratanaphan, A., Canyuk, B., Wasiksiri, S. & Mahasawat, P. (2005). In vitro platination of human breast cancer suppressor gene1 (BRCA1) by the anticancer drug carboplatin, *Biochim Biophys Acta.* 1725(2): 145-151.

Ratanaphan, A., Wasiksiri, S., Canyuk, B. & Prasertsan P. (2009). Cisplatin-damaged BRCA1 exhibits altered thermostability and transcriptional transctivation. *Cancer Biol Ther.* 8(10): 890-898.

Reed, E. Ozols, R.F., Tarone, R., Yuspa, S.H. & Poirier, M.C. (1987). Platinum-DNA adducts in leukocyte DNA correlate with disease response in ovarian cancer patients receiving platinum-based chemotherapy. *Proc Natl Acad Sci. USA.* 84(14): 5024-5028.

Reed, J.C. (2002). Apoptosis-based therapies. *Nat Rev-Drug Discov.* 1(2): 111-121.

Reeves, R. (1984). Transcriptionally active chromatin. *Biochim Biophys Acta.* 782(4): 343-393.

Rosenberg, B., VanCamp, L. & Krisgas, T. (1965). Inhibition of cell devision in *Escherichia coli* by electrolysis products from a platinum electrod. *Nature.* 205(4972): 698- 699.

Rosenberg, B., Renshaw, E., VanCamp, L., Hartwick, J. & Drobnik. J. (1967). Platinum induced filamentous growth in *Escherichia coli. J Bacteriol.* 93(2): 716-721.

Rosenberg, B., VanCamp, L., Trosko, J.E. & Mansour, V.H. (1969). Platinum compounds: a new class of potent antitumor agents. *Nature.* 222(191): 385-386.

Rosenberg, J. M. & Sato, P. H. (1988). Messenger RNA loses the ability to direct in vitro peptide synthesis following incubation with cisplatin. *Mol Pharmacol.* 33(6): 611-616.

Rosenberg, J.M. & Sato, P.H. (1993). Cisplatin inhibits in vitro translation by preventing the formation of complete initiation complex. *Mol Pharmacol.* 43(3): 491-497.

Royer - Pokora, B., Gordon, I. K. & Haseltine, W. A. (1981). Use of exonuclease III to determine the site of stable lesions in defined sequences of DNA: the cytobutane pyrimidine dimmer and cis- and trans- dichlorodiammineplatinum(II) examples. *Nucleic Acids Res.* 9(18): 4595-4609.

Safaei, R. (2006). Role of copper transporters in the uptake and efflux of platinum containing drugs. *Cancer Lett.* 234(1): 34–39.

Safaei, R., Katano, K., Samimi, G., Naerdemann, W., Stevenson, J. L., Rochdi, M., et al. (2004). Cross-resistance to cisplatin in cells with acquired resistance to copper. *Cancer Chemother Pharmacol.* 53(3): 239–246.

Safaei, R., Otani, S., Larson, B. J., Rasmussen, M. L. & Howell, S.B. (2008). Transport of cisplatin by the copper efflux transporter ATP7B. *Mol Pharmacol.* 73(2): 461-468.

Saga, Y., Hashimoto, H., Yachiku, S., Iwata, T. & Tokumitsu, M. (2004). Reversal of acquired cisplatin resistance by modulation of metallothionein in transplanted murine tumors. *Int J Urol.* 11(6): 407-415.

Saito, Y., Liang, G., Egger, G., Friedman, J.M., Chuang, J.C., Coetzee, G.A., et al. (2006). Specific activation of micro RNA-127 with downregulation of the proto-oncogene BCL6 by chromatin-modifying drugs in human cancer cells. *Cancer Cell.* 9(6): 435-443.

Sato, K., Hayami, R., Wu, W., Nishikawa, T., Nishikawa, H., Okuda, Y., et al. (2004). Nucleophosmin/B23 is a candidate substrate for the BRCA1-BARD1 ubiquitin ligase. *J Biol Chem.* 279(30): 30919-30922.

Sato, P.H., Rosenberg, J.M. & Sato, R.I. (1996). Differences in the inhibition of translation by cisplatin, transplatin, and certain related compounds. *Biochem Pharmacol.* 52(12): 1895-1902.

Scanlon, K.J., Kashani-Sabet, M., Miyachi, H., Sowers, L.C. & Rossi, J.J. (1989). Molecular basis of cisplatin resistance in human carcinomas: model systems and patients. *Anticancer Res.* 9(5): 1310-1312.

Selvakumaran, M., Pisarcik, D.A., Bao, R., Yeung, A.T. & Hamilton, T.C. (2003). Enhanced cisplatin cytotoxicity by disturbing the nucleotide excision repair pathway in ovarian cancer cell lines. *Cancer Res.* 63(6): 1311-1316.

Sherman, S.E. & Lippard, S.J. (1987). Structural aspects of platinum anticancer drug interactions with DNA. *Chem Rev.* 87(5): 1153-1181.

Silver, D.P., Richardson, A.L., Eklund, A.C., Wang, Z.C., Szallasi, Z., Li, O., et al. (2010). Efficacy of neoadjuvant cisplatin in triple-negative breast cancer. *J Clin Oncol.* 28(7): 1145-1153.

Sirohi, B., Arnedos, M., Popat, S., Ashley, S., Nerurkar, A., Walsh, G., et al. (2008). Platinum-based chemotherapy in triple-negative breast cancer. *Ann. Oncol.* 19(11): 1847-1852.

Sklar, M. (1988). Increased resistance to cis-diamminedichloroplatinum(II) in NIH 3T3 cells transformed by ras oncogenes. *Cancer Res.* 48(4): 793-797.

Suddek, G.M. (2011). Sunitinib improves chemotherapeutic efficacy and ameliorates cisplatin-induced nephrotoxicity in experimental animals. *Cancer Chemother Pharmacol.* 67(5): 1035-1044.

Sun, X., Tsang, C-N. & Sun, H. (2009). Identification and characterization of metallodrug binding proteins by (metallo)proteomics. *Metallomics.* 1(1): 25-31.

Swisher, E.M., Sakai, W., Karlan, B.Y., Wurz, K., Urban, N. & Taniguchi, T. (2008). Secondary BRCA1 mutations in BRCA1-mutated ovarian carcinomas with platinum resistance. *Cancer Res.* 68(8): 2581-2586.

Taron, M., Rosell, R., Felip, E., Mendez, P., Souglakos, J., Ronco, M.S., et al. (2004). BRCA1 mRNA expression as an indicator of chemoresistance in lung cancer. *Hum Mol Genet.* 13(20): 2443-2449.

Tassone, P., Martino, M.T.D., Ventura, M., Pietragalla, A., Cucinotto, I., Calimeri, T., et al. (2009). Loss of BRCA1 function increases the antitumor activity of cisplatin against human breast cancer xenografts in vivo. *Cancer Biol Ther.* 8(7): 648-653.

Tassone, P., Tagliaferri, P., Perricelli, A., Blotta, S., Quaresima, B., Martelli, M.L., et al. (2003). BRCA1 expression modulates chemosensitivity of BRCA1-defective HCC1937 human breast cancer cells. *Br J Cancer.* 88(8): 1285-1291.

Teicher, B.A., Holden, S.A., Kelley, M.J., Shea, T.C., Cucchi, C.A., Rosowsky, A., et al. (1987). III. Characterization of a human squamous carcinoma cell line resistant to cis-diamminedichloroplatinum(II). *Cancer Res.* 47(2): 388-393.

Timerbaev, A.R., Hartinger, C.G., Aleksenko, S.S. & Keppler, B.K. (2006). Interactions of antitumor metallodrugs with serum proteins: advances in characterization using modern analytical methodology. *Chem Rev.* 106(6): 2224-2248.

Tornaletti, S., Patrick, S.M., Turchi, J.J. & Hanawalt, P.C. (2003). Behavior of T7 RNA polymerase and mammalian RNA polymerase II at site-specific cisplatin adducts in the template DNA. *J Biol Chem.* 278(37): 35791-35797.

Treiber, D.K., Zhai, X., Jantzen, H.M. & Essigmann, J.M. (1994). Cisplatin-DNA adducts are molecular decoys for the ribosomal RNA transcription factor hUBF (human upstream binding factor). *Proc Natl Acad. Sci. USA.* 91(12): 5672-5676.

Tullius, T.D. & Lippard, S.J. (1981). Cis-Diamminedichloroplatinum(II) binds in a unique manner to oligo(dG)oligo(dC) sequences in DNA-A new assay using exonuclease III. *J Am Chem Soc.* 103(15): 4620-4622.

Vichi, P., Coin, F., Renaud, J-P., Vermeulen, W., Hoeijmakers, J.H.J., Moras, D. et al. (1997). Cisplatin- and UV-damaged DNA lure the basal transcription factor TFIID/TBP. *EMBO J.* 16(24): 7444-7456.

Wang, D. & Lippard, S.J. (2005). Cellular processing of platinum anticancer drugs. *Nat Rev Drug Discov.* 4(4): 307-320.

Wang, W. & Figg, W.D. (2008). Secondary BRCA1 and BRCA2 alterations and acquired chemoresistance. *Cancer Biol Ther.* 7(7): 1004-1005.

Waud, W.R. (1987). Differential uptake of cis-diamminedichloroplatinum(II) by sensitive and resistant murine L1210 leukemia cells. *Cancer Res.* 47: 6549-6555.

Wilkins, R. J. & Hart, R. W. (1974). Preferential DNA repair in human cells. *Nature.* 247(5435): 35-36.

Wong, S.W., Tiong, K.H. & Kong, W.Y. (2011). Rapamycin synergizes cisplatin sensitivity in basal-like breast cancer cells through up-regulation of p73. *Breast Cancer Res Treat.* 128(2): 301-313.

Wu, B., Droege, P. & Davey, C.A. (2008). Site selectivity of platinum anticancer therapeutics. *Nat Chem Biol.* 4(2): 110-112.

Wu, Z., Liu, Q., Liang, X., Yang, X., Wang, N., Wang, X., et al. (2009). Reactivity of platinum-based antitumor drugs towards a Met- and His-rich 20 mer peptide corresponding to the N-terminal domain of human copper transporter 1. *J Biol Inorg Chem.* 14(8): 1313-1323.

Young, R.C., Fuks, Z. & Hoskins, W.J. (1989). Cancer of the ovary, In: Cancer principles and practice of oncology, (ed.) Devita, Jr., V.T., et al., Lippincott, J.B., Philadelphia, pp. 1162-1196.

Zamble, D.B. & Lippard, S.J. (1995). Cisplatin and DNA repair in cancer therapy. *Trends Biochem Sci.* 20(10): 435-439.

Zamble, D.B., Mu, D., Reardon, J.T., Sancar, A. & Lippard, S.J. (1996). Repair of cisplatin-DNA adducts by the mammalian excision nuclease. *Biochemistry*. 35: 1004-1013.

Zhao, T., King, F.L. (2009). Direct determination of the primary binding site of cisplatin on cytochrome c by mass spectrometry. *J Am Soc Mass Spectrom*. 20(6): 1141-1147.

Zhen, W., Link, Jr.C.J., O'Connor, P.M., Reed, E., Parker, R., Howell, S.B., et al. (1992). Increased gene-specific repair of cisplatin interstrand cross-links in cisplatin-resistant human ovarian cancer cell lines. *Mol Cell Biol.* 12(9): 3689-3698.

Zhu, Y., Hub, J., Hu, Y. & Liu, W. (2009). Targeting DNA repair pathways: a novel approach to reduce cancer therapeutic resistance. *Cancer Treat Rev.* 35(7): 590-596.

Zwelling, L.A. & Kohn, K.W. (1982). Platinum complexes. In: Chabner BA, edn. Pharmacologic principle of cancer treatment. Philadelphia: WB Saunders: USA.

In: Cisplatin: Pharmacology, Clinical Uses and Adverse Effects ISBN: 978-1-61942-359-6
Editors: Toshiko Kojima and Yoko Morita

Chapter II

DRUG DELIVERY SYSTEM WITH CISPLATIN ENCAPSULATED IN LIPOSOME TARGETING E-SELECTIN

M. Hirai,[1] K. Igarashi[1] and M. Seno[2]

[1]RandD Division, Katayama Chemical Industries Co.,LTD, Minoh, Osaka, Japan
[2]Department of Medical and Bioengineering Science,
Graduate School of Natural Science and Technology,
Okayama University, Okayama, Japan

ABSTRACT

Although administration of anti-cancer drugs in high doses results in serious side effects due to their strong toxicity, many kinds of chemical compounds and recombinant proteins are used against various types of cancer. It would be more beneficial for cancer patients if they could take an effective dose without unexpected and unwanted side effects. Cisplatin (CDDP) is one example. It is one of the most effective anti-cancer agents. It requires an appropriate drug delivery system (DDS). Encapsulation of drug molecules into liposomes is one typical DDS strategy, but it is still necessary to improve the combination of drug and lipids to obtain the best efficiency of incorporation. Our first approach was to establish a highly-efficient method to prepare liposomes incorporating CDDP. We exploited cis-diamminedinitratoplatinum (CDDP3), which is highly soluble in water and labile in the presence of chloride ions converting into CDDP, to prepare liposomes containing CDDP at high concentration, because the insolubility of CDDP in water considerably inhibits incorporation. As expected, the loading efficiency of CDDP into liposomes was dramatically improved with CDDP3 in chloride-ion-free conditions, compared with CDDP used by itself.

Furthermore, the liposomes were conferred with the ability to target a specific locus of tumor *in vivo*, being conjugated with Sialyl Lewis X (SLX) on the surface. The SLX liposome (SLX-Lip) is considered to mimic leucocyte accumulating in the inflammatory region of arthritis and tumors with high affinity to E-selectin expressed on the vascular endothelial cells. CDDP encapsulated into SLX-Lip (CDDP-SLX-Lip) was then evaluated *in vivo* as a sophisticated active targeting DDS.

The acute toxicity of CDDP was markedly reduced by the use of liposome. Intravenous administration of CDDP-SLX-Lip at doses of 18 and 25 mg CDDP/kg weight to normal mice showed a survival rate of 75 % even at 14 days after injection, while CDDP at the same doses showed survival rates of 25 and 0 %. Decrease of body weight was 20 to 25 % for 3 days after administration of these liposomes, but recovered in a couple of days within the loss of 10 %. Histologically, no abnormality was observed in the kidney, spleen or liver of normal mice after administration of CDDP-SLX-Lip at a dose of 25 mg CDDP/kg weight.

The anti-tumor effect of CDDP-SLX-Lip or CDDP-Lip administered via tail veins was evaluated in tumor-bearing mice. The amount of CDDP accumulated in tumors at 48 h after injection was 6 times more when CDDP-SLX-Lip was administered than with CDDP-Lip. The anti-tumor effect at the dose of 25 mg/kg weight in lung carcinoma-bearing mice was shown to be significant when CDDP was actively directed to tumors suppressing the growth.

Thus, CDDP at high doses was demonstrated to be incorporated into liposome and specifically directed to tumors *in vivo*, showing a practical anti-tumor effect. It may be worth doing further evaluation for a clinical study.

Abbreviations

CDDP, *cis*-diamminedichloroplatinum(II) or Cisplatin; CDDP3, *cis*-diamminedinitratoplatinum(II); SLX, Sialyl Lewis X; Cy5.5-SLX-Lip, liposomes modified with SLX containing Cy5.5; Cy5.5-Lip, liposomes containing Cy5.5; HUVEC, Human umbilical vein endothelial cell; EAT, Ehrlich ascites tumor; HE, hematoxylin and eosin;TUNEL, terminal deoxynucleotidyl transferase mediated dUTP nick end labeling;LEL, *lycopersion esculentum* lectin; CDDP-SLX-Lip, liposomes modified with SLX containing CDDP; CDDP-Lip, liposomes containing CDDP; NMR, nuclear magnetic resonance spectroscopy; FAAS, flameless atomic absorption spectrophotometry; RES, reticular endothelial systems; TAPS, N-trismethyl-3-aminopropanesulfonic acid buffer; CBS, hydrogencarbonate saline buffer; PBS, phosphate buffered saine; HEPES, 2-[4-(2-hydroxyethyl)-1-piperazineethanesulfonicacid;Tris, tris(hydroxymethyl)aminomethane; BS_3, bis(sulfosuccinimidyl)suberate;DTSSP, 3,3-dithiobis(sulfosuccinimidylpropionate); HSA, human serum albumin; FBS, fetal bovine serum; MRI, magnetic resonance imaging; VEGF, vascular endothelial cell growth factor; EPR, enhanced permeability and retention effect.

1. Introduction

Cisplatin (cis-diamminedichloroplatinum, CDDP) is one of the most widely used chemotherapeutic agents in the clinical treatment of a variety of tumors, such as lung, ovarian, cervical and gastric carcinomas [1]. However, administration of escalating doses of CDDP is limited because of severe side effects such as nephrotoxicity, hematopoietic injury and deafness [2-5]. In spite of the efforts to decrease these deleterious side effects by screening various CDDP derivatives and by developing improved forms of dosage or methods of medication, there have been few successful results [6-9].Some medicines encapsulated into liposomes are successfully designed to target carcinomas as drug delivery system (DDS), which has already clinically been available [10, 11]. However, an efficient DDS for CDDP has not yet to be developed [12-14]. Among the several liposomal formulations of CDDP, the latest is SPI-077, in which CDDP is encapsulated with pegylation as stealth liposomes [13]. Although preclinical studies showed that SPI-077 exhibited improved stability, prolonged circulation time, increased antitumor effect and reduced side effects when compared with the free drug [13, 14], little antitumor activity of SPI-077 was observed in Phase I/II studies [15-17]. The major problem of conventional liposomal formulations of CDDP, including SPI-077, was the extremely low drug to lipid weight ratio due to water insolubility and low lipophilicity of CDDP, which failed toadequately deliver of the drug to tumors [12, 18]. In contrast, cis-diamminedinitratoplatinum (II) (CDDP3), one of the various CDDP derivatives, is highly water soluble and is easily converted to CDDP in the presence of chloride ions [19]. Recently, we applied this character of CDDP3 to establish an efficient procedure of CDDP encapsulation into liposomes at a high concentration [20].

The DDS with liposome, so-called passive delivery, depends on the particle size and the electric charge of the surface for the distribution and the delivery of medicines to the targets [21-23]. The conjugation of various ligands such as antibody, transferrin, folic acid, monosaccharide, etc. on the surface of liposomes is considered to confer the liposomes to the active targeting potential [23,24]. While few trials have proved successful so far, the cationic liposomes conjugated with 3,5-dipentadecyloxybenzamidine hydrochloride (TRX-20) encapsulating CDDP have been shown to suppress tumor growth and liver metastasis targeting chondroitin sulfate proteoglycans on the malignant cell surface [25].

Recently, the specific affinity of lectin for sugar chain was exploited for active targeting with liposome [26, 27]. A large number of studies have shown that the animal lectins possess specific affinity for sugar chains. Based on the primary structure, lectin molecules, including (1) C-type lectin, (2) Galectin, (3) I-type lectin, (4) P-type lectin, and (5) Pentraxin, are classified into fourteen types [28-30]. The specific interaction of E-selectin, which is classified into the C-type lectin, and Sialyl Lewis X (SLX) has been best characterized in inflammation. In inflammation, and even in tumors, the vascular endothelial cells are usually activated by inflammatory cytokines, such as TNF‒α, IL-1β, IL-6 and IL-8, which induce E-selectin expression on the surface. SLX is a sugar chain present on the surface of leucocytes which crawls on the vascular endothelial cells in the inflammatory regions due to their affinity for E-selectin. This phenomenon is called “rolling”. Rolling through the gaps of the vascular endothelium made by inflammation, leucocytes invade tissues. This explains the specific accumulation of leucocytes in inflammatory region [31, 32].

We came to the idea that the liposomes can be accumulated specifically and efficiently in inflammation and tumor regions, mimicking leucocytes when the surface is modified with SLX [33]. Liposomes incorporating fluorescent Cy5.5 were shown to accumulate in the inflammatory and tumor regions and to penetrate into the surrounding tissues *in vivo* when conjugated with SLX [33].

When conjugated with anti-E-selectin antibody in place of SLX, the liposomes failed in targeting E-selectin *in vivo* while it was successful *in vitro* [34-37]. The reason was considered to be that the liposomes conjugated with antibodies were rapidly depleted *in vivo* because of the phagocytosis by macrophages after being entrapped by the reticular endothelial systems (RES) in the liver and spleen or bound to opsonin proteins in blood [23, 24, 34]. Sufficient retention in the blood was considered to be required to target to target E-selectin expressing endothelial cells. However, a recent *in vivo* imaging method to target tumor cells allowed successful results with liposomes conjugated with anti-E-selectin antibody on the surface, implying even short retention was enough for quick imaging by a highly sensitive camera detecting near-infrared fluorescent dye [38].

In this review, we described a new protocol of encapsulation of CDDP into anionic liposomes for the specific delivery of CDDP to tumor regions. The conjugation of SLX helped specific and efficient accumulation of CDDP in tumor *in vivo* targeting E-selectin [33,39]. The rolling movement of the liposomes with SLX on the tumor vascular endothelial cells was captured simultaneously. These liposomes were also observed to enter the gaps of the vascular walls, where permeability is augmented by tumor angiogenesis [31, 40, 41].

2. Design of Liposomes Targeting Endothelial Cells

2.1. Preparation of SLX-Lip

The liposomes were prepared using the improved cholate dialysis method [42, 43] as shown schematically in Figure 1. Dipalmitoylphosphatidylcholine (16.8 mg), cholesterol (10.1 mg), dicetylphosphate (1.8 mg), ganglioside GM3 (14.6 mg), dipalmitoylphosphatidylethanolamine (2.3 mg), and sodium cholate (46.9 mg) were mixed. The mixture was dissolved with 3 ml of chloroform/methanol (1:1, v/v) solution. The solvent was evaporated by a rotary evaporator at 30 °C and the lipid film was formed after drying under vacuum. This lipid film was dissolved in 3 ml of tris-(hydroxymethyl) methylaminopropanesulfonic acid buffer (TAPS, pH 8.4), and the micelle suspension was obtained after sonicating.

Three milliliters of human serum albumin (HSA) with Cy5.5 solution was mixed with the micelle suspension described above, and this was ultrafiltrated with TAPS (pH 8.4) by PM10 membrane to remove residual HSA with Cy5.5, then 10 ml of liposome solution was obtained. In addition, the solution was ultrafiltrated with sodium hydrogencarbonate buffer (CBS, pH 8.5) by XM300 membrane (Amicon) to exchange buffer. Ten milligrams of bis(sulfosuccinimidyl)suberate (BS_3, Pierce), a crosslinking reagent, was added to 10 ml of liposome solution, and stirred at 20–25 °C for 2 h, then further stirred overnight at 4 °C. BS_3 was combined to the liposome surface. Then, 40 mg of tris(hydroxymethyl)aminomethane (Tris) was added, and stirred at 20–25 °C for 2 h, then further stirred overnight at 4 °C to bind Tris to BS_3. This was ultrafiltrated with TAPS (pH 8.4) by XM300 membrane to remove residual Tris. To bind HSA to the liposome surface, the coupling method was used [42, 43]. To oxidize the liposome surface, 10.8 mg of sodium periodate was added to 10 ml of liposome solution and stirred at 4 °C overnight. To remove residual sodium periodate, it was ultrafiltrated with phosphate buffered saline (PBS, pH 8.0) by XM300 membrane. Twenty milligram of HSA was added to it and stirred at 20–25 °C for 2 h. Then 3.13 mg of sodium cyanoborohydrate was added, and stirred at 20–25 °C for 2 h and further overnight at 4 °C. To remove residual sodium cyanoborohydrate, the solution was ultrafiltered with CBS (pH 8.5) by XM300 membrane. Sugar chains were combined on the liposome surface through 3,3-dithiobis(sulfosuccinimidylpropionate) (DTSSP, Pierce). DTSSP was used as a cross-linking reagent. Ten milligrams of DTSSP was added to 10 ml of liposome solution and stirred at 20–25 °C for 2 h, and further overnight at 4 °C. To remove residual DTSSP, the solution was ultrafiltrated with CBS (pH 8.5) by XM300 membrane. The amination of the reducing group terminal of sugar chain was done by the glycosyl amination reaction. Two milligrams of SLX (Calbiochem) was dissolved in 0.5 ml of distilled water. 0.25 g of NH_4HCO_3 was added and stirred at 37 °C for 3 days. Aminated SLX was added to reach a final concentration of 100 µg/ ml and stirred at 25 °C for 2 h. Then, Tris was added to reach a final concentration of 132 mg/ml, and stirred overnight at 4 °C for repeated hydrophilization of the liposome surface. To remove residual SLX and Tris, the solution was ultrafiltrated with n-(2-hydroxyethyl)piperazine-n'-(2-ethanesulfonic acid) (HEPES, pH 7.2) byXM300 membrane. The preparation of liposome without sugar chains was similar to the Cy5.5-SLX- Lip case except for the process for binding sugar chains.

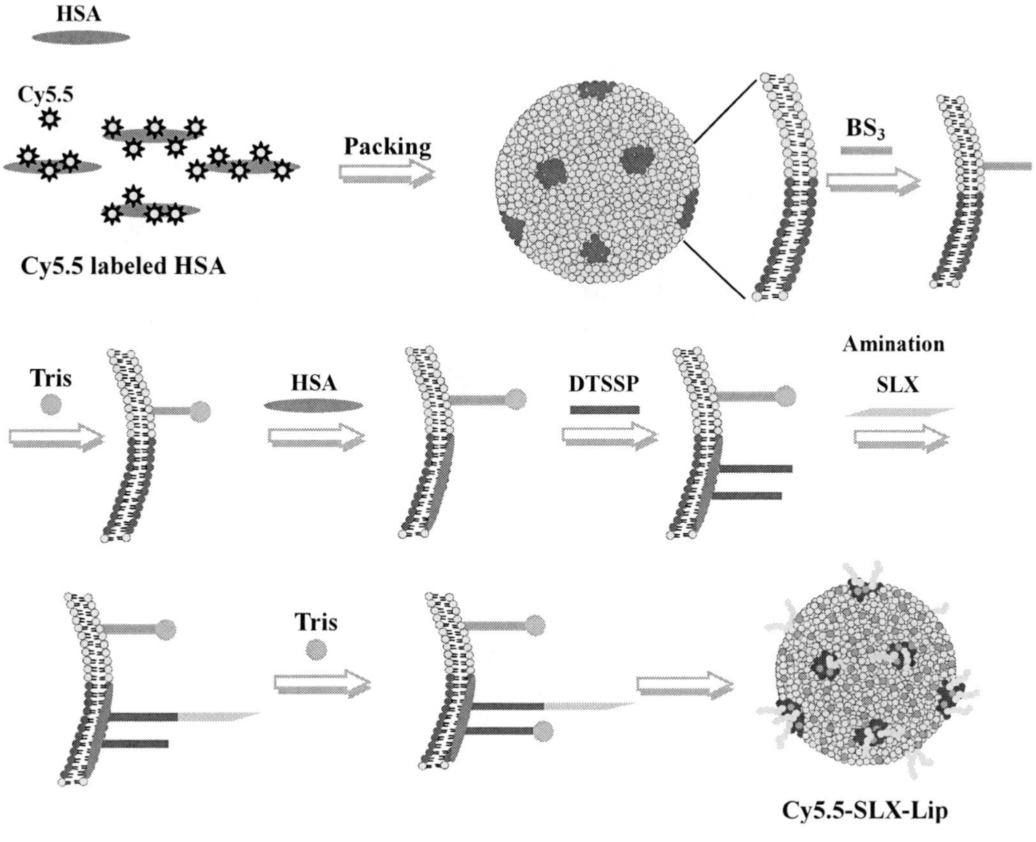

Figure 1. Preparation scheme of liposome with sugar chain. HSA, BS_3, Tris, DTSSP, and SLX denote the following: HSA, human serum albumin; BS_3, bis(sulfosuccinimidyl) suberate; Tris, Tris(hydroxymethyl)aminomethane; DTSSP, 3,3-dithiobis(sulfosuccinimidylpropionate); SLX, Sialyl Lewis X.

2.2. Properties of SLX-Lip

The contents of lipid and protein in Cy5.5-SLX-Lip was 3.7 and 1.2 mg/mL, respectively. For Cy5.5-Lip, 3.8 mg/mL lipid and 1 mg/mL protein content were obtained. The distribution of particle sizes of both Cy5.5-SLX-Lip and Cy5.5-Lip was almost uniform and the mean particle size was approximately 100 nm. The electric charge of the membrane surface of the liposome was negative, showing a zeta-potential of −40 mV for both types of liposome. Even after storage for 6 months at 4 °C, the particle size distribution was almost the same as that just after the preparation, so that the liposomes should be stable. Electron microscopic observation revealed almost all Cy5.5-SLX-Lip spheres with a diameter of approximately 100 nm (data not shown). This particle size is consistent with those measured by laser scattering (Zetasizer Nano ZS, Malvern).

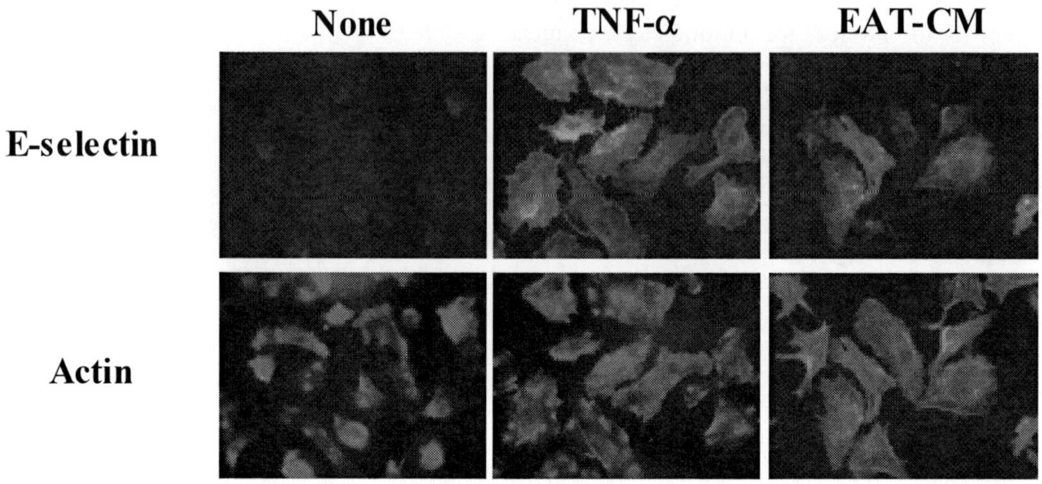

Figure 2. Evaluation of E-selectin expressed on HUVEC. Cells were cultured in medium for HUVEC supplemented 10 % FBS (None), with 10 ng/mL of TNF-α (TNF-α)or with EAT conditioned medium (EAT-CM) for 4 h. To detect E-selectin, anti-E-selectin antibody was used followed by FITC labeled anti-mouse IgG polyclonal antibody (E-selectin). Actin filaments were stained with rhodamine labeled phalloidin (Actin). Total magnification was 400×.

2.3. Tumor Cells Induce E-selectin on Endothelial Cells *In Vitro*

Since the liposomes were designed to target E-selectin, it is important to assess the expression of E-selectin on vascular endothelial cells in the tumors.

Anti-E-selectin monoclonal antibody was prepared from the ascites fluid of female Balb/c mice (8 weeks), which received CL-3 hybridoma (ATCC). Human umbilical vein endothelial cells (HUVEC) were seeded at 1×10^5 per well in 12-well chamber slide and incubated in 500 μL of medium at 37 °C for 24 h. Ehrlich Ascites Tumor (EAT) cells were cultured until 100 % confluent. Five hundred μL of the supernatant culture medium of EAT or the complete medium of EAT was added to 500 μL of the culture medium of HUVEC. As a control of inflammatory response to induce E-selectin, TNF-α was separately added at 10 ng/mL and HUVEC were cultured at 37 °C for 4 h under an atmosphere of 5 % CO_2. After 4 h, HUVEC were then fixed with 3.7 % formaldehyde in PBS by incubation at room temperature for 15 min and washed twice with PBS and 0.1 % TritoX-100 in PBS. PBS containing 0.1 % of BSA was added to each well and the incubation was continued at room temperature for 20 min. The fixed cells were then incubated with anti-E-selectin monoclonal mouse antibody at 10 μg/mL at room temperature for 1 h, washed twice with PBS, stained with 5 μg/mL FITC labeled anti-mouse polyclonal antibody at room temperature for 1 h and washed twice with PBS. For staining the cytoskeleton, rhodamine phalloidin was added at 5 U/mL to HUVEC cultures and incubated at room temperature for 20 min and washed twice with PBS and water. The fluorescence of FITC and rhodamine was observed with a fluorescent microscope (Model CKX41, Olympus, Tokyo, Japan). As shown in Figure 2, TNF-α stimulated E-selectin expression on HUVEC. Although tumors may not always produce TNF-α, it is conceivable that tumors should secrete some cytokines, which can directly or indirectly induce E-selectin expression on surrounding endothelial cells through paracrine mechanism. In fact, the conditioned medium of EAT cells induced E-selectin expression on HUVEC *in vitro* while the control medium did not.

A.

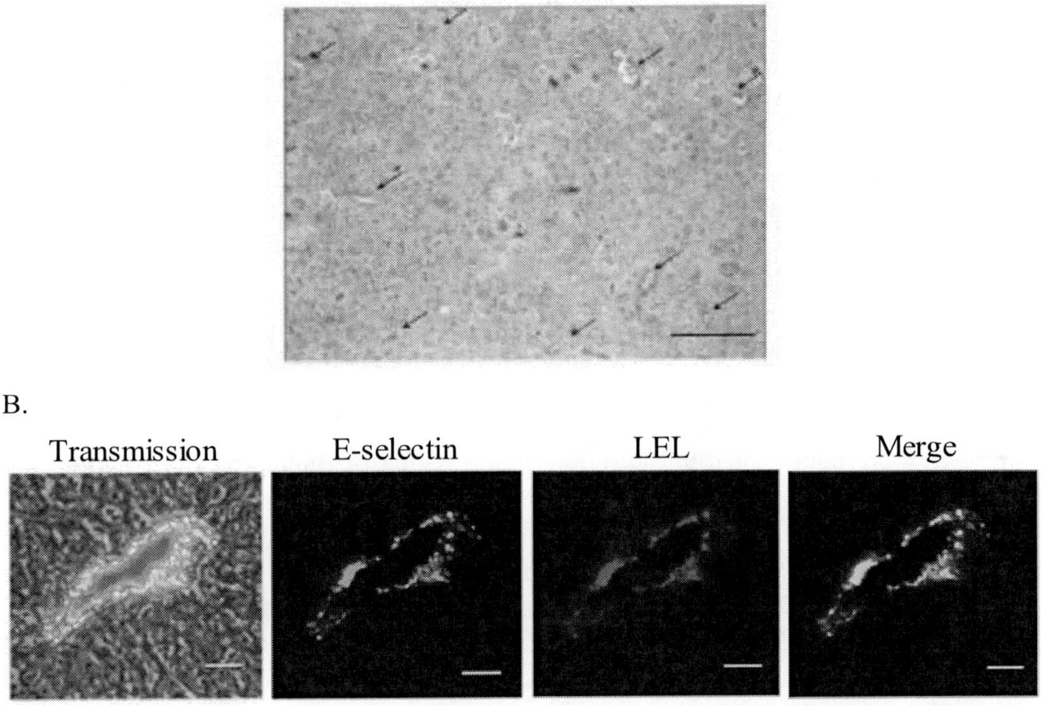

Figure 3. The expression of E-selectin in vascular vessels of solid EAT. (A) HE staining of the section. Arrows indicated locations of vascular vessels. Scale bar: 100 μm. (B) Vascular vessel stained for E-selectin and for LEL. After being deparaffinized, the section was incubated with anti-E-selectin antibody (10 μg/mL) for 1 h at 37 °C, then incubated with FITC labeled goat anti-mouse IgG and LEL conjugated with Texas red for 1 h at room temperature. Merge, colocalization of E-selectin and vascular endothelial cells are shown in yellow. Scale bar showed 20 μm.

2.4. Vascular Endothelial Cells in Tumors Express E-selectin *In Vivo*

EAT cells (5×10^6 cells/mouse) were transplanted subcutaneously in the back of female BALB/C nude mice. After 10 days, tumors were excised and fixed in 10 % neutral formalin solution (Wako) for 24 h. After fixation, the tissues were dehydrated, cleared, infiltrated and embedded with paraffin. Then 4-μm thick sections were cut out for hematoxylin and eosin (HE) staining and for immunohistochemistry. For immunological staining, sections were deparaffinized and blocked with 10 % goat serum containing 3 % TritonX-100 at room temperature for 1 h, sections were then incubated with anti-E-selectin antibody (10 μg/mL) for 1 h at 37 °C and rinsed three times in PBS for 5 min each. Then the sections were further incubated with FITC labeled anti-mouse IgG goat antibody (Santa Cruz) and lycopersicon esculentum lectin (LEL) conjugated with Texas red (Vector Labs) for 1 h at room temperature followed by washing three times with PBS for 5 min. The sections were mounted with glycerol–PBS (9:1) and observed under an IX81 microscope (Olympus) equipped with a light fluorescence device (Olympus). The thin section prepared from the solid EAT tissue was subjected to assessment for the expression of E-selectin on vascular endothelial walls in the tumor. As shown in Figure 3, E-selectin and blood vessels in the section were stained with anti-E-selectin antibody and LEL, which has specific affinity to fucose on the vascular endothelial cells. Since the sites of E-selectin expression agreed well with the vascular walls, the vascular endothelial cells were judged to express E-selectin in the tumor tissue. These results as well as those in HUVEC suggest that the angiogenic vascular endothelial cells in EAT can be stimulated by cytokines or factors that are secreted from EAT cells to induce E-selectin expression.

2.5. Liposomes Conjugated with SLX Accumulate in Tumors *In Vivo*

EAT cells (5×10^6cells/mouse) were transplanted to the right femoral region of ddY mice (male, 7 weeks of age), and the mice were used for experiments 7–10 days later. For the observation by scanning fluorescent microscope IV-100 (Olympus), EAT cells (2×10^6 cells/mouse) were transplanted to the right femoral region of Balb/c mice (female, 8weeks old).

To anesthetize, 200 μL of Nembutal solution (Dainippon Pharmaceutical) diluted 10 times with saline was administered into the peritoneal cavity. Then, 200 μL of Cy5.5-SLX-Lip or Cy5.5-Lip was administered from the tail vein. Using eXplore Optix (ART), a fluorescent signal of Cy5.5 was monitored in the tumor region (right femoral region) of the same mouse before injection and at 0, 24, 48 and 96 h after injection (excitation: 680 nm, emission: 700 nm).

To stain leucocytes and vascular endothelial cells, 150 μL of 0.5 % acridine orange (AO) was administered from the tail vein of the mouse right before the observation. A hundred μL of Cy5.5-SLX-Lip or Cy5.5-Lip was administered from the tail vein. Scanned by IV-100, the fluorescence was monitored under the following conditions. Cy5.5 and AO were excited by a HeNe-R laser at 633 nm and an argon laser at 488 nm, respectively, and emission from Cy5.5 was captured in the range 660–730 nm and that from AO in the range 505–525 nm just the same as for green fluorescent protein (GFP) . The blood vessels and the surrounding tissues of the tumor region (right femoral region) were observed at 48 h after injection.

The tumor region of the same mouse (right femoral region) was observedat 0, 24, 48, 72, and 96 h after administration by eXplore Optix, (excitation at 680 nm, emission at 700 nm). As shown in Figure 4a, Cy5.5-SLX-Lip accumulated significantly in the tumor region and the accumulation increased gradually until 48 h. On the other hand, the accumulation of Cy5.5-

Lip was lower than that of Cy5.5-SLX-Lip and constant until 72 h later. In addition, the accumulation of liposome with other sugar chain to the tumor region was as low as Cy5.5-Lip, indicating that Cy5.5-SLX-Lip accumulated specifically in the tumor region (data not shown). To examine the distribution of fluorescence in the body, the whole body was scanned at 72 h after injection. As shown in Figure 4b, strong fluorescence signals were detected in the liver, bladder and tumor region. These signals were analyzed by the lifetime of fluorescence. In the tumor region, only Cy5.5 bound to HSA (lifetime, 1.8 ns) was detected. However, in the liver and bladder, it was confirmed that both free-Cy5.5 (lifetime, 1.5 ns) and Cy5.5 bound to HSA existed (lifetime, 1.8 ns).

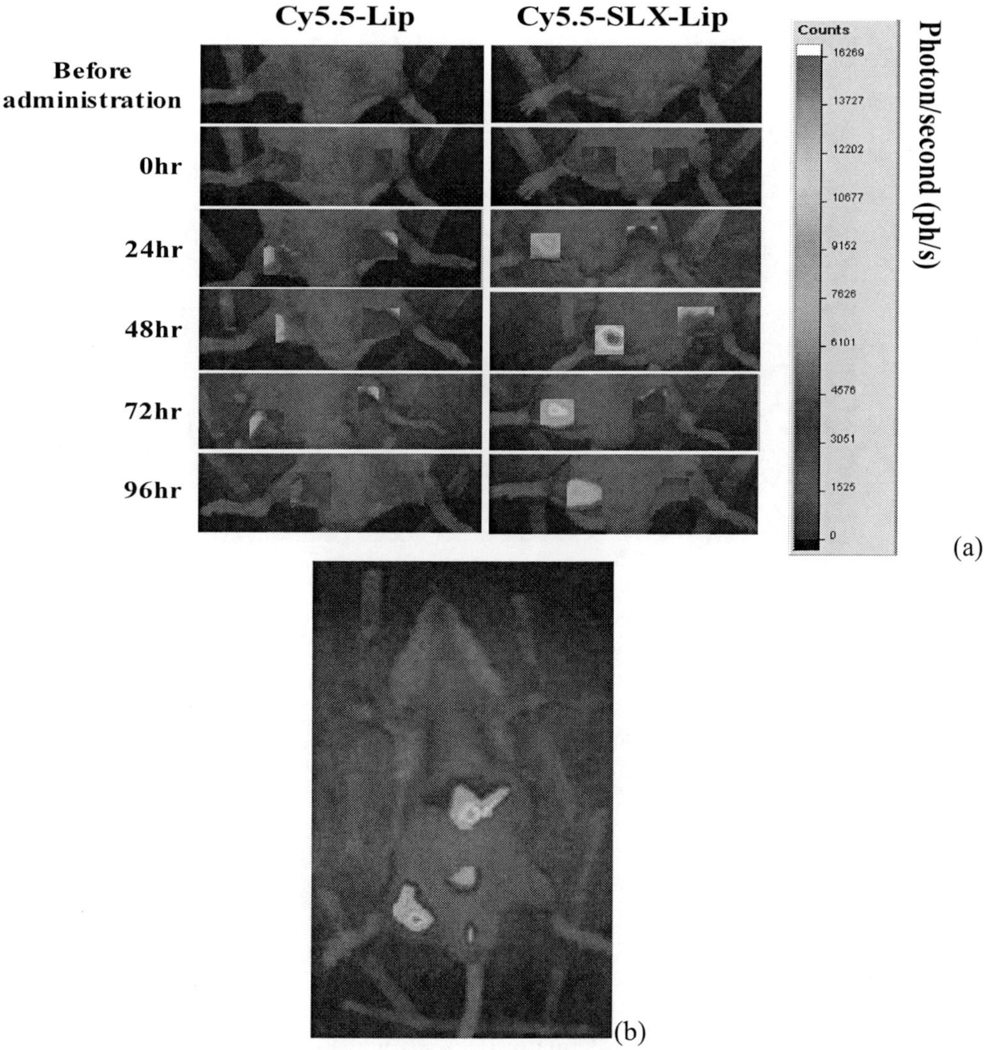

Figure 4 (a).Accumulation of Cy5.5-SLX-Lip to the tumor region in a tumor-bearing mouse. Cy5.5-SLX-Lip or Cy5.5-Lip was administered from the tail vein (200 μL/mouse), and the tumor region (right femoral region) of the same mouse was observed using eXplore Optix (Ex: 680 nm, Em: 700 nm). Before and 0, 24, 48, 72, and 96 h after injection. Data were normalized.(b) Distribution of fluorescence in the mouse body. Cy5.5-SLX-Lip was administrated from the tail vein (200 μL/mouse) and whole body was scanned by eXplore Optix (Ex: 680 nm, Em: 700 nm) at 72 h after injection.

To confirm whether this accumulation in the tumor region had occurred in the blood vessels or the surrounding tissues, the tumor region was observed by IV-100 after injection of Cy5.5-SLX-Lip or Cy5.5-Lip. As shown in Figure 5, fluorescence signals shifted from the blood vessels to the surrounding tissues at 48 h after injection, and it was also detected even in the cells of the tissues. In addition, the rolling of leucocytes was observed on the blood vessel endothelium of the tumor region by movie, indicating that Cy5.5-SLX-Lip was recognized by E-selectin expressed with tumor growth, and as a result, it was accumulated in the tumor region. Cy5.5-Lip was accumulated in the surrounding tissues of blood vessels, but the amount of accumulation was less than Cy5.5-SLX-Lip. It was thought that Cy5.5-Lip was passively shifted to the tissues from the gaps of the blood vessel endothelium around the tumor.

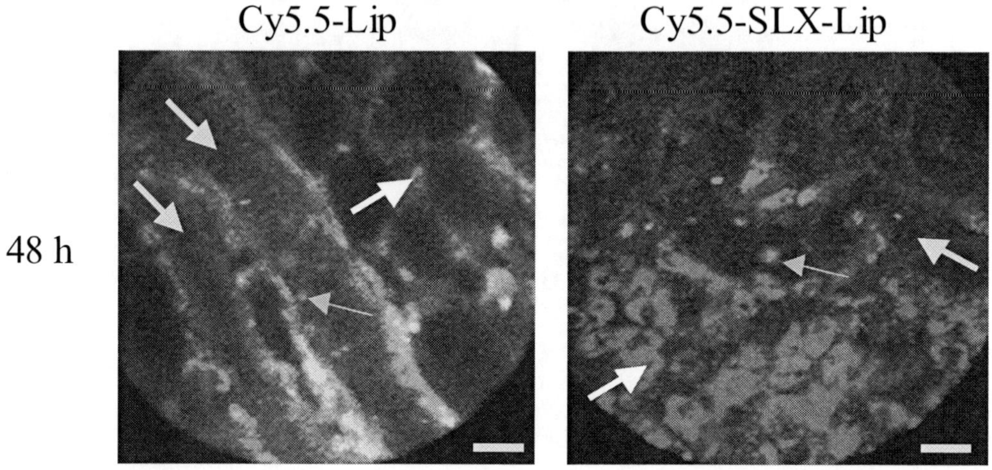

Figure 5. Shift of fluorescence from blood vessels to the surrounding tissues in tumor region. Cy5.5-SLX-Lip or Cy5.5-Lip was administrated from the tail vein (100 μL/mouse), and the blood vessels and the surrounding tissues of the tumor region (right femoral region) were observed by IV-100 (Olympus) at 48 h after injection. To dye leucocytes and vascular endothelial cells, 150 μL of AO was administered from the tail vein right before the observation. Cy5.5 is shown with red (Ex: 633 nm, Em: 693 nm) and acridine orange (AO) is shown with green (Ex: 488 nm, Em: 526 nm). Bar: 20 μm. Yellow arrow: blood vessel. White arrow: tumor tissue (tumor cell). Blue arrow: Leukocyte.

3. Drug Delivery with SLX-Lip Containing CDDP

3.1. CDDP3, a Cool Derivative of CDDP

CDDP was purchased from Sigma. CDDP3 was synthesized by the method of Dhara [19]. Briefly, potassium tetrachloroplatinate (II) (4.15 g, 10 mmol) was dissolved in distilled water. Potassium iodide (6.64 g, 40 mmol) was then added and stirred on ice for 5 min under a nitrogen atmosphere and light shielding. Ammonia aqueous solution (28 %, 1.35 mL) was added to this reaction solution, and stirred on ice for 3 h. The yellow crystals formed were washed with distilled water and ethanol, and dried at 40 °C for 10 h under decompression. At this stage, 4.49 g of cis-diamminediiodeplatinum (II) (CDDP2) was obtained. CDDP2 (2.41

g, 5 mmol) was suspended in distilled water. Silver nitrate (1.68 g, 9.9 mmol) was then added and stirred on ice for 24 h under light shielding. The reaction solution was passed through a paper filter to remove any silver iodide. The filtrate was then concentrated using a rotating evaporator and white crystals were obtained. These crystals were washed with iced distilled water and ethanol, and then dried at 40 °C for 10 h under decompression. The final yield of CDDP3 was 1.0 g.

CDDP has a structure coordinating chloride ions at the cis location (Figure 6A) while CDDP3 has nitrate ions in place of chloride (Figure 6B) with solubility in water about 10 times higher than that of CDDP. The absorption spectra showed that CDDP3 gradually converted to CDDP during incubation in 150 mM NaCl for 24 h (Figure 6C).

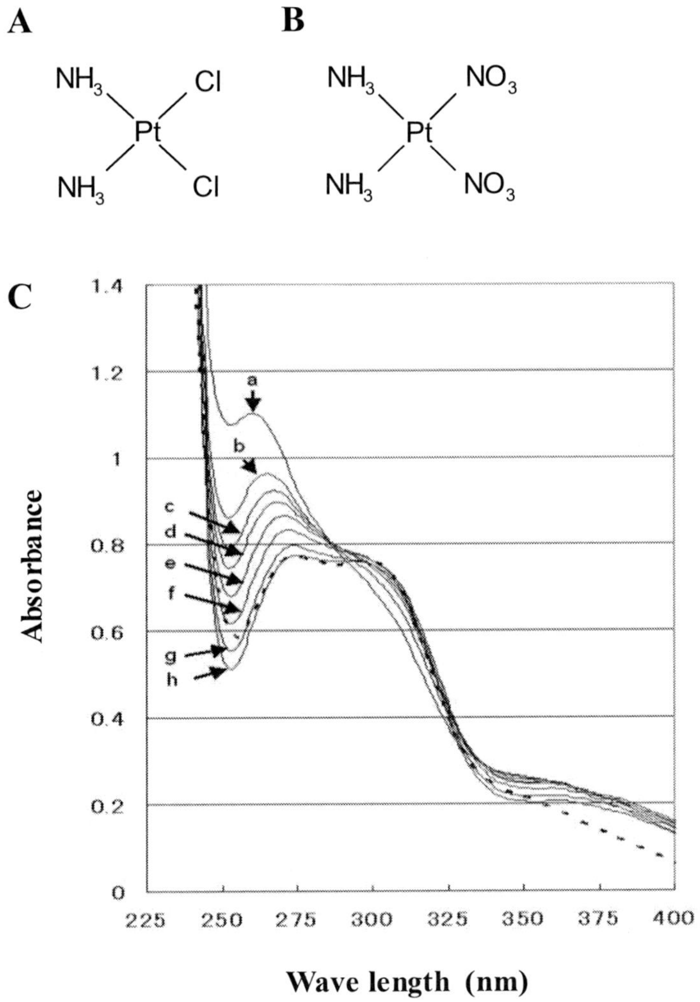

Figure 6. Conversion from cis-diamminedinitratoplatinum (II) (CDDP3) to CDDP.Chemical structures of CDDP (A) and CDDP3 (B). (C) Time-dependent shifts in absorption spectrum of 13.7 mM CDDP3 placed in 150 mM NaCl solution for a, 0; b, 5; c, 10; d, 15; e, 30; f, 60; g, 120; h, 180 min. The dotted line shows the absorption spectrum of 6.6 mM CDDP solution at 24 h after dissolving in 150 mM NaCl solution.

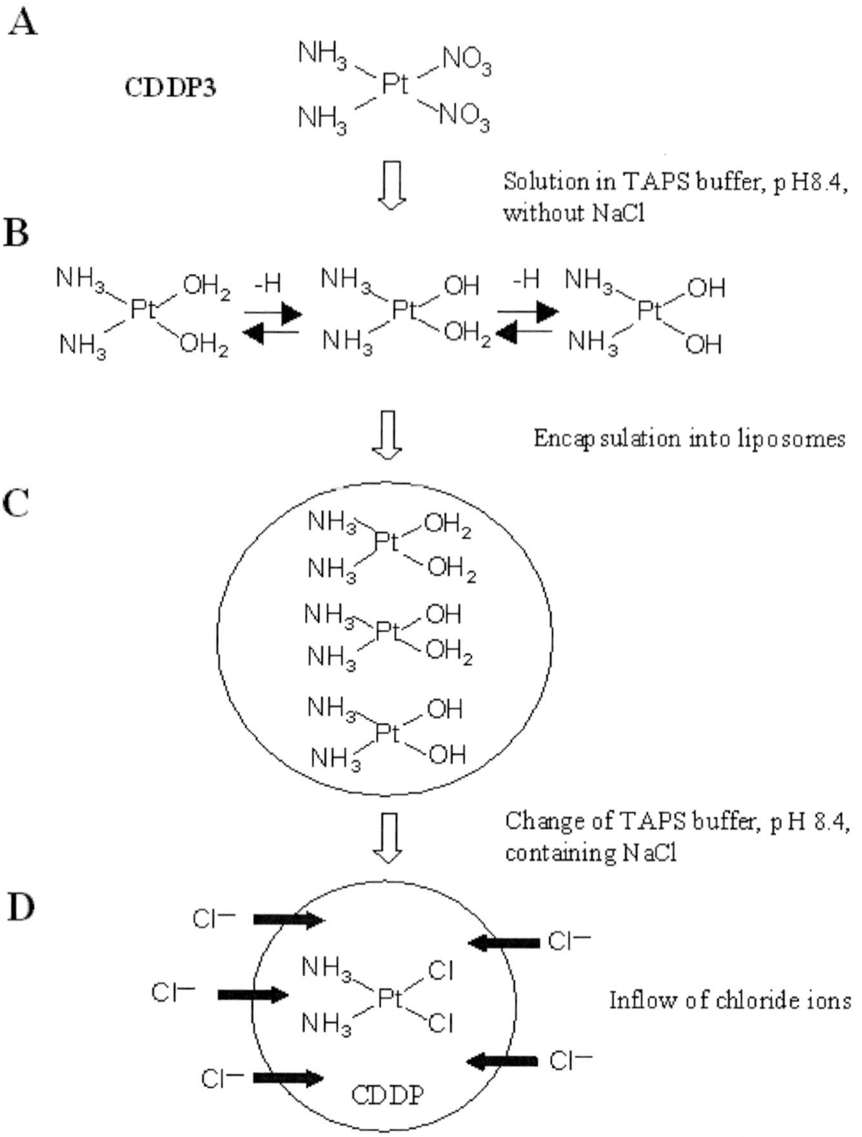

Figure 7. Scheme of CDDP encapsulation into liposomes using CDDP3. (A) CDDP3 in TAPS, pH 8.4, without NaCl. (B) CDDP3 is in a reversible equilibrium state where H_2O molecules are coordinated due to high solubility of CDDP3 in water. (C) CDDP3 are incorporated in liposomes at this stage, they will show various molecular forms in the liposomes. (D) Change to buffer TAPS (pH 8.4) containing 150 mM NaCl makes a flow of chloride ions into the liposomes and then CDDP is generated by forming coordinate bonds preferentially with chloride ions.

3.2. A Unique Encapsulation Method of CDDP into Liposomes

Since CDDP3 is soluble in water and stable under chloride-ion-free conditions, a high amount of encapsulation of CDDP3 into liposomes should be efficient as depicted in Figure 7 while the insolubility in water impairs encapsulation of CDDP into liposomes. CDDP3 was encapsulated into liposomes conjugated with SLX and was converted to CDDP in the presence of chloride ions. This conversion was monitored as the chemicalshift (δ) by ^{195}Pt NMR, which was referenced to sodium hexachloroplatinate (δ =0 ppm). After incubation of CDDP3-encapsulated liposomes with chloride ion for 96 h, the chemical shift (δ) indicated only −2160 ppm, which is identical to the chemical shift (δ) of CDDP (Figure 8). No chemical shift of CDDP3 (δ =−1620 ppm) was detected, implying that CDDP3 in SLX liposomes should be efficiently converted to CDDP in the presence of chloride ions. The chemical shifts of −1620 ppm and −2160 ppm are consistent with those of CDDP3 and CDDP, respectively, as previously described by Rosenberg [44].

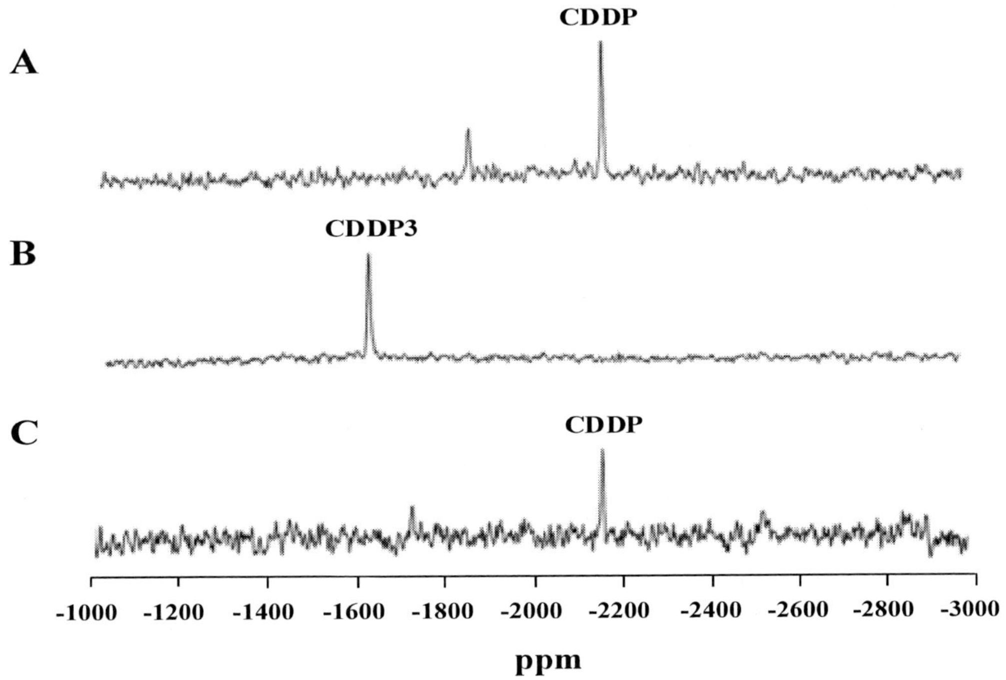

Figure 8. Conversion of CDDP3 in the liposomes with SLX to CDDP detected by ^{195}Pt NMR. (A) 6.6 mM of CDDP in deuterium oxide; (B) 137 mM of CDDP3 in deuterium oxide; (C) CDDP3 encapsulated liposomes with SLX were treated with 150 mM NaCl for 96 h.

3.3. Preparation of CDDP Encapsulated Liposomes

The liposomes were prepared by the same method as described in "2-1 preparation of Cy5.5-encapsulated liposomes" except CDDP3 was employed instead of Cy5.5 bound HSA. One gram of CDDP3 was completely dissolved in 70 mL of 10 mM TAPS (pH 8.4), without NaCl and the pH was readjusted to 8.4 with 1M NaOH. The CDDP3 solution was then added to the micelle suspension described in 2-1. To subsequently remove cholic acid and free CDDP3, the micelle solution was ultrafiltrated with 10mM TAPS (pH 8.4) using an ultrafiltration cell holder (Amicon model 8200, Millipore) fitted with an ultrafiltration disc membrane (molecular cut off 10,000) (Amicon PM10, Millipore). One hundred mL of the liposome encapsulated CDDP3 was obtained. To convert CDDP3 in the liposomes into CDDP, the buffer was exchanged to 10mM TAPS, pH 8.4, containing 150 mM NaCl by ultrafiltration through an ultrafiltration disc membrane (molecular cut off: 300,000) (Amicon XM300, Millipore). Hydrophilization treatment and SLX conjugation on the surface of liposomes were carried out as described previously [33].

3.4. Properties of CDDP Liposomes Prepared from CDDP3

Encapsulation of CDDP in liposomes under various conditions is summarized in Table 1. When encapsulation was started with 10 mg of CDDP3 and 4.5 mg of lipid, the resultant quantity of CDDP incorporated into SLX-Lip was 211 μg CDDP/3.5 mg lipid/mL and the loading efficiency was 6×10^{-2}.

Table 1. Physicochemical characteristics of CDDP liposomes with CDDP or CDDP3(n=3)

	Method of encapsulation			
	I[a]	II[b]		
CDDP (mg)[c]	1.4	0	0	0
CDDP3 (mg)[c]	0	10	10	10
Lipid (mg)[c]	4.5	4.5	9	9
Lipid concentration (mg/mL)[d]	3.5±0.4	3.5±0.3	7.8±0.5	16.5±0.8
Particle size (nm)[e]	158±6.5	150±5.7	152±5.5	160±6.2
ζ potential (mV)	-57±5.3	-55±2.8	-50±3.8	-54±5.2
CDDP concentration (μg/mL)[f]	0.7±0.2	211±8	402±0.5	821±0.3
CDDP encapsulation efficiency (%)[g]	0.05	2.11	4.02	8.21
CDDP loading efficiency[h]	2×10^{-3}	6×10^{-2}	5×10^{-2}	5×10^{-2}

[a] Direct encapsulation of CDDP into liposomes.

[b] Encapsulation of CDDP3 into liposomes followed by conversion into CDDP in TAPS buffer containing NaCl.

[c] Initial amount used to prepare 1 mL of CDDP liposome.

[d] Total cholesterol in CDDP liposome solution was measured using a Determiner TC555 kit.

[e] Measured by photon correlation spectroscopy with a Nano-ZS (Malvern). Polydispersity index was between 0.1 and 0.5 in each case.

[f] The amount of platinum was measured and the amount of CDDP was calculated as defined follwing formula.

CDDP concentration = A×300/195.

Where A is the concentration of platinum, 300 is the molecular weight of CDDP, and 195 is the molecular weight of platinum.

[g] Encapsulation efficiency were defined by the following formula.

Encapsulation efficiency (%) = amount of CDDP in liposomes/initial amount of CDDP×100

[h] Loading efficiency was defined by following formula.

Loading efficiency = CDDP concentration (mg/mL)/lipid concentration (mg/mL).

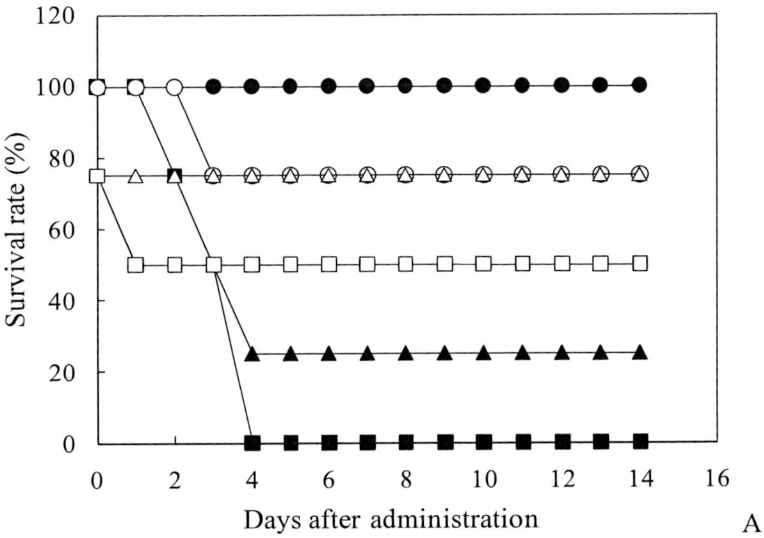

A.

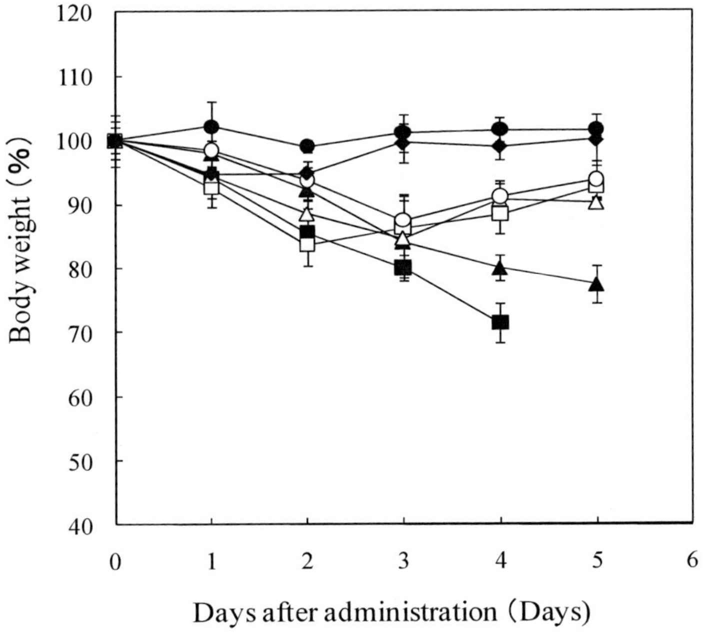

B.

Figure 9. Survival rate and body weight change of normal mice that received CDDP-SLX-Lip. (A) Survival rate (%); (B) body weight (%). Keys: ▲, CDDP solution (18 mg CDDP/kg body weight); ■, CDDP solution (25 mg CDDP/kg body weight); ○, CDDP-SLX-Lip (18 mg CDDP/kg body weight); △,CDDP-SLX-Lip (25mg CDDP/kg body weight); □, CDDP-SLX-Lip (50mg CDDP/kg body weight); ♦, empty liposomes; ●, saline solution. Each sample was injected into normal mice (female, 8 weeks) via tail veins. Results are expressed as the mean (n = 4); bars, ±SE. *P < 0.005; **not significant (P > 0.05).

It is important to note that the quantity of CDDP in SLX-Lip increased from 211 μg to 821 μg depending on the amount of lipid.However, it was difficult to make the encapsulation efficiency higher than 10 %.Since we found the loading efficiency was almost constant during the course of the experiment, we took the loading efficiency as a parameter specific to the encapsulation method. On the other hand, the quantity of CDDP in SLX-Lip was 0.7 μg CDDP/3.5 mg lipid/mL and the loading efficiency was 2×10^{-3} when CDDP was directly encapsulated into liposomes. Actually 1.4 mg was the maximum amount of CDDP for encapsulation while 10 mg was available for CDDP3 in a similar condition. Thus, CDDP3 dramatically improved CDDP encapsulation by almost 300 times in quantity and 42 times in encapsulation efficiency when compared with direct encapsulation of CDDP into liposomes at the initial lipid amount of 4.5 mg. The CDDP loading efficiency appeared to be improved 30 times. The CDDP loading efficiency was improved by almost 4 times when compared with that of 1.4×10^{-2} for SPI-077 [15, 16]. We successfully concentrated CDDP-SLX-Lip and CDDP-Lip up to 4.2 mg CDDP/70 mg lipid/mL, which was 20 times more than the concentration of CDDP in SPI-077. Dynamic laser scattering of the CDDP-SLX-Lip prepared from CDDP3 showed a mean diameter of about 160 nm (Table 1). The ζpotential of the liposomes was negative irrespective of the method of encapsulation (Table 1). Even after 6 months of storage at 4 °C, the leakage of CDDP from liposomes was only about 6 % of the total amount of CDDP incorporated into liposomes just after preparation.

3.5. CDDP-SLX-Lip Shows no Toxic Effect in Normal Mice

The acute toxicity of CDDP-SLX-Lip was evaluated in normal mice by injection via tail veins. The mice were observed for 14 days after injection. The survival rate was 75 % when mice received CDDP-SLX-Lip at doses of 18 or 25 mg CDDP/kg body weight. In contrast, the survival rates were 25 % and 0 % when mice received CDDP at doses of 18 and 25 mg CDDP/kg body weight, respectively (Figure 9A). The mice did not die when they received empty liposomes with SLX. From these results encapsulation of CDDP in liposomes was found remarkably effective to protect mice from toxicity. This effect of encapsulation was not only recognized in the survival rate but also in the loss of body weight. When CDDP was administered at doses of 18 mg CDDP/kg body weight and 25 mg CDDP/kg body weight, the loss of body weight was 20 % over 5 days and 25 % over 4 days, respectively. The mice which received CDDP-SLX-Lip at the dose of 18, 25 and 50 mg CDDP/kg body weight showed a loss of body weight of about 15 % during 3 days and recovered to less than 10 % loss of body weight over 5 days (Figure 9B). Liposomes without CDDP had no significant effect on the body weight. These results support the possibility that CDDP-SLX-Lip can significantly reduce the toxicity of CDDP *in vivo*.

The effect of CDDP-SLX-Lip and CDDP on normal tissues of mice was histologically evaluated (Figure 10). Kidney, spleen and liver were excised from the mice which received a dose of 25 mg CDDP/kg body weight. Since the mice died at day 3 from the injection of CDDP, the tissues were prepared at day 3 after injection. Tissues were stained with HE and by terminal deoxynucleotidyl transferase mediated dUTP nick end labeling (TUNEL) method to assess for apoptosis.

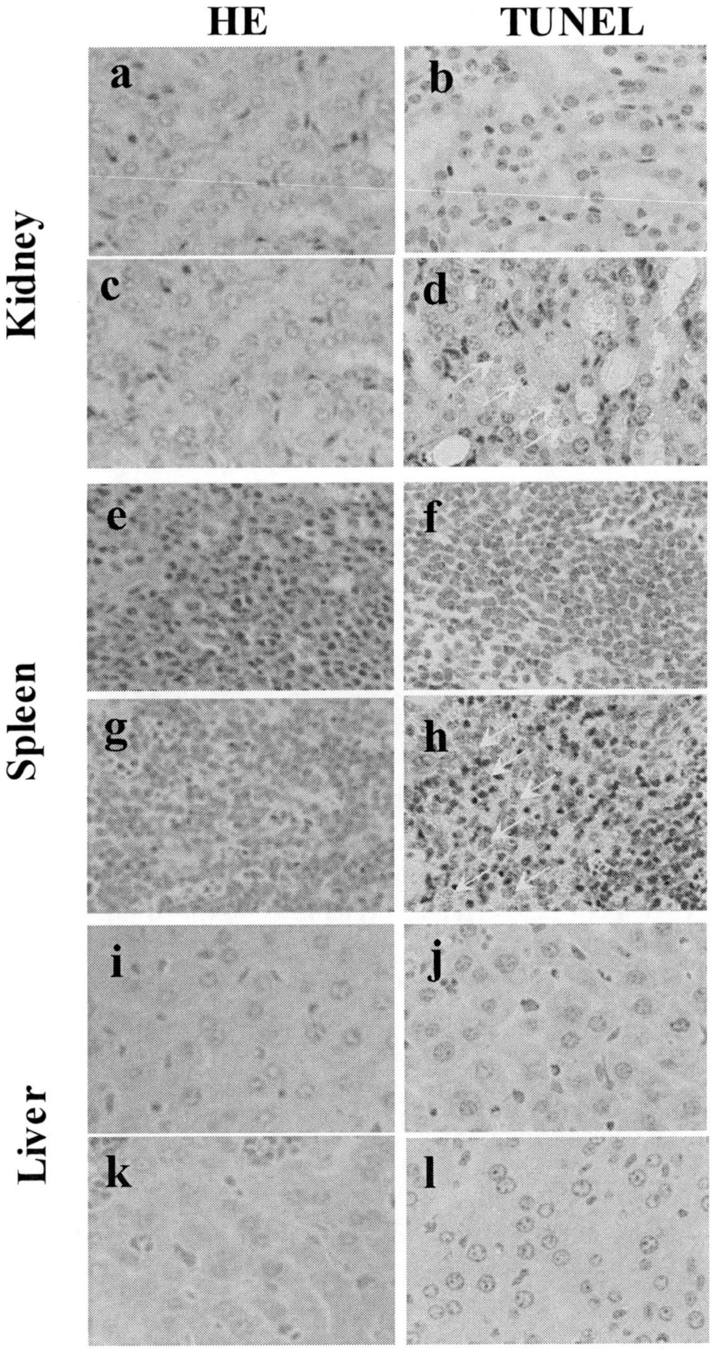

Figure 10. Histochemical analysis of organs, which received CDDP-SLX-Lip or CDDP. CDDP-SLX-Lip (a, b, e, f, i, j) or CDDP (c, d, g, h, k, l) was injected into each normal mouse (Balb/c, female, 8-week-old) via tail veins at the dose of 25mg CDDP/kg body weight. At 3 days after administration, kidney (a, b, c, d), spleen (e, f, g, h) and liver (i, j, k, l) were excised and fixed. HE staining (a, c, e, g, i and k) and TUNEL immunohistochemical staining (b, d, f, h, j and l) of the slices were observed. Yellow arrows indicate TUNEL positive cells. Objective lens was 60×.

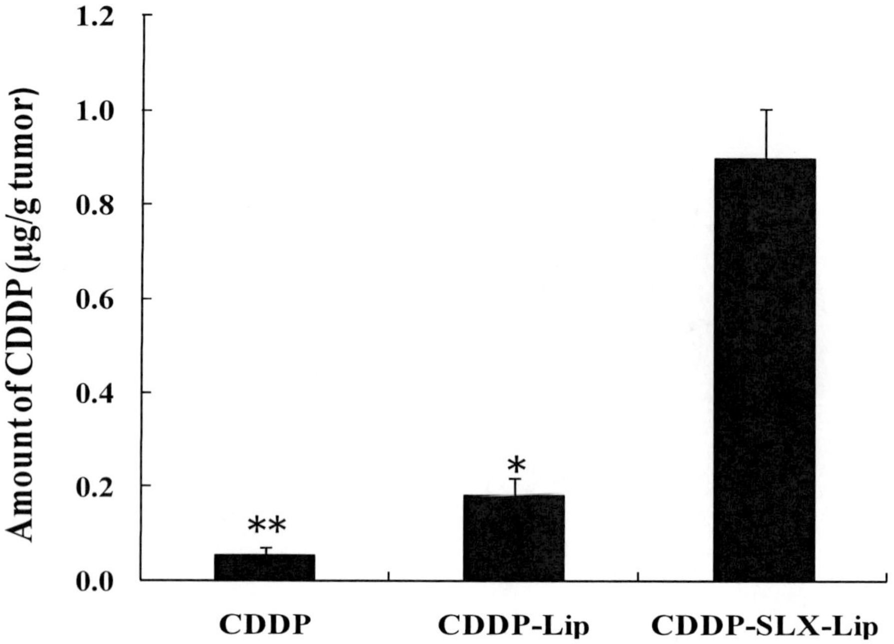

Figure 11. Accumulation of CDDP in the tumor *in vivo*. At day 10 after transplantation of EAT cells, CDDP-SLX-Lip, CDDP-Lip or CDDP (2 mg/kg body weight as CDDP) were administered from tail veins of mice. At 48 h after injection the tumor tissues were excised and the amount of platinum was measured by FAAS. Results are expressed as the mean ±SD (n = 3). *P < 0.01 compared with CDDP-Lip. **P < 0.005 compared with CDDP.

Abnormal changes were not found in the kidney in mice which received both CDDP-SLX-Lip and CDDP (Figure 10a, c) but TUNEL positive tubular epithelial cells were sporadically detected after CDDP treatment (Figure 10d). CDDP-SLX-Lip treatment also did not produce any abnormal changes in the spleen (Figure 10e, f). However, CDDP treatment of mice induced atrophy of the follicles with necrosis and a decrease in cell number in the white pulp (Figure 10g). In follicles, phagocytosed dead lymphocytes were observed. TUNEL positive cells were also found in the white pulp (Figure 10h). In the liver, no abnormal cells and TUNEL positive cells were found after the administration of either CDDP-SLX-Lip (Figure 10i, j) or CDDP (Figure 10k, l). Even when CDDP was injected at 25 mg CDDP/kg bodyweight, significant toxicity in the kidney was not obvious by HEstaining (Figure 10c) and the TUNEL assay showed only a small numberof positive cells in the kidney (Figure 10d). In this part of the study,the period between administration of CDDP and removal of tissueswas 3 days, which was probably too short for CDDP to exhibit anysignificant nephrotoxicity. To observe more dramatic nephrotoxiceffects of CDDP would probably require longer periods of administrationat lower doses of CDDP.

3.6. CDDP-SLX-Lip Increases Accumulation of CDDP Efficiently in Tumors

To prepare EAT bearing mice, 5×10^6 cells were subcutaneously injected into the right femoral region of 6-week-old female BALB/c mice. Ten days after injection, CDDP-SLX-Lip, CDDP-Lip and CDDP were injected into the tail veins at a dose of 2 mg CDDP/kg body weight. At 48 h after administration, the tumors were excised and soaked in 1mL of 70 % HNO_3 per 0.1 g of each tumor tissue followed by incubation in a water-bath at 60 °C for 1 h. After being cooled to room temperature, supernatant was diluted 4-fold with distilled water. To determine the recovery of platinum, blank tumor tissues samples were spiked with 125 ng CDDP for 1 h, followed by digestion with nitric acid and dilution with distilled water. The amount of platinum in the tumor tissues was measured by flameless atomic absorption spectrophotometer (FAAS) (AA-6700, Shimadzu) and the amounts of CDDP were calculated. The recovery of platinum after incubation of tumor tissues with CDDP was in the range from 82 to 95 %, which was statistically analyzed using the standard Student's t-test. As shown in"2-5",the maximum level of accumulation of liposomes with SLX in the tumor achieved at 48 h after injection when evaluated by *in vivo*imaging using Cy5.5-encapsulated liposomes with SLX [33]. On the basis of these data, the accumulation of CDDP-SLX-Lip in tumors was evaluated at 48 h after injection. The accumulation of CDDP from CDDP-SLX-Lip in the tumors was 6 times higher than that by CDDP-Lip, implying the targeting potential of CDDP-SLX-Lip *in vivo*(Figure 11).

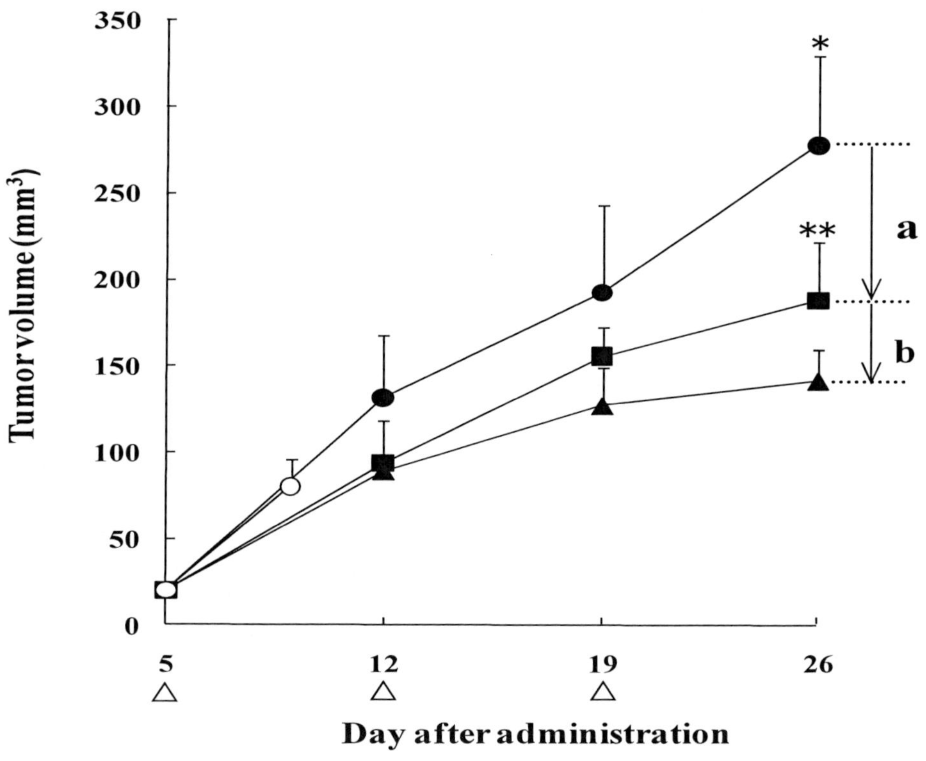

Figure 12. Comparison of tumor growth suppression with CDDP-SLX-Lip, CDDP-Lip and CDDP in A549-bearing mice. Keys: ▲, CDDP-SLX-Lip (25 mg CDDP/kg body weight); ■, CDDP-Lip (25 mg CDDP/kg body weight); ○, CDDP solution (25 mg CDDP/kg body weight); ●, saline. Each sample was injected via tail veins of A549-bearing mice on days 5, 12 and 19 after tumor cell transplantation. At each day of 5, 12, 19 and 26 after transplantation, each tumor volume (mm^3) was measured. Each open triangle at the horizontal axis shows the time of administration. Results are expressed as the mean ± SD (n = 4). *P < 0.01 compared with saline. **P < 0.05 compared with CDDP-Lip. Vertical arrows indicate the effects of EPR (a) and active targeting (b).

3.7. CDDP-SLX-Lip Enhances Antitumor Activity *In Vivo*

The antitumor effect of CDDP-SLX-Lip and CDDP-Lip was evaluated in a mouse xenograft model of human lung carcinoma A549 cells because CDDP is widely used for the treatment of lung cancers. To prepare tumor-bearing mice, 1×10^7 cells were subcutaneously injected into the right femoral region of 6-week-old female BALB/c mice at 5, 12 and 19 days after injection, CDDP-SLX-Lip, CDDP-Lip and CDDP were independently injected into the tail veins at a dose of 25 mg CDDP/kg body weight ($n = 4$). Saline solution was injected into the control group ($n=4$). At 5, 12, 19 and 26 days after injection, the length and width of the tumors were measured using digital calipers (Model CD-20C, Mitsutoyo, Japan), and tumor volume was calculated by the following formula: volume (mm^3) = length $\times$ width$^2\times$ 0.5.

The statistical analysis was carried out using the standard Student's t-test. When CDDP was administrated at 25 mg/kg body weight, all the mice died at day 4 after injection. The volume of the tumors that were exposed to either CDDP-Lip or CDDP-SLX-Lip was significantly smaller than that of the non-treated tumors. A difference in tumor volumes between the two different CDDP-containing liposomes could not be detected until 12 days after injection. CDDP-SLX-Lip suppressed the growth of tumors much more effectively than CDDP-Lip 19–26 days after injection. Suppression of tumor growth by CDDP-Lip as indicated with the arrow "a" in Figure 12 could be attributed to an enhanced permeability and retention effect (EPR). Further suppression induced by CDDP-SLX-Lip as indicated with the arrow "b" in Figure 12 might be accounted for by the effect of active targeting through the binding of SLX to the tumor vascular endothelial cells.

4. Discussion

First of all, we focused on the establishment of the drug carrier for the pin point targeting delivery. Vascular endothelial cells in a solid tumor of EAT should conceivably be stimulated to express E-selectin *in vivo* as well as *in vitro* (Figure 2 and 3), resulting in the tumor specific accumulation of liposomes with SLX [33] or with anti-E-selectin antibody [38]. In our previous study, when liposomes were conjugated with SLX, the fluorescence in tumors achieved a maximum at 48 h after injection and then gradually decreased by 96 h after injection [33]. In contrast, photon counts of fluorescence from Cy5.5-labeled liposomes in the tumors increased during 72 h and were maintained at a high level up to 96 h after injection when the liposomes were conjugated with anti-E-selectin antibody [38]. The high affinity of liposomes to E-selectin might account for the difference in retention time of fluorescence between the SLX and anti-E-selectin antibody. Considering the fact that pin-point active targeting *in vivo* has been extremely difficult so far [23, 24, 34], the modification of the liposome surface with a negative charge that was used in this study should also be important. We introduced a negative charge on the surface of liposomes since this modification allowed liposomes that had been conjugated with SLX and antibody to have a long half-life in blood, resulting in efficient and active targeting of tumors *in vivo* [26,42,43,45]. Simultaneously, a hydrophilic surface was established on the liposomes. The repulsive force between the liposomes and the wall of the blood vessels should enhance the retention in the vascular system. All of these modifications might assist the liposomes for *in vivo* imaging of tumor by targeting E-selectin and escaping from RES, opsonin proteins in blood plasma and uptake by phagocytic macrophages. However, *in vivo* imaging from the abdominal side of the animal showed high fluorescence in the liver 72 h after administration (data not shown). As a result, efficient and specific accumulation of liposome-conjugated SLX or antibodies could be observed in the final target region with the exception of the liver [33, 38]. Here we successfully demonstrated visualization of tumors, in which tumor-associated vascular endothelial cells were expressing E-selectin presumably as a consequence of angiogenic factors that were secreted from the tumor, with liposomes conjugated to SLX or anti-E-selectin antibody. Recently, nanoparticles conjugated with SLX which were designed for MRI imaging have been reported to image regions of inflammation in the brain for a short time [46]. In this context, E-selectin targeting should also be useful for visualization of inflammatory regions *in vivo*. While it is important to distinguish these two different states of tissues, E-selectin targeting should be significantly useful for diagnosis and treatment, since inflammation is a well-known risk factor for tumor development and correlates with increased invasiveness and prognosis in a variety of cancers [47]. In the previous reports, the maximum accumulation of liposomes conjugated with SLX in tumors was achieved 48 h after administration. Although the background was still higher, presumably due to the majority of liposomes circulating in blood, the accumulation of the liposomes started right after administration and the tumor region could be visualized even 1 h after administration.

One of the most important points to establish the drug delivery system is how efficiently you can encapsulate the drug into the carriers. Here, we describe a unique, simple and novel method to encapsulate CDDP intoliposomes at significantly high concentrations [20]. This procedure was applied to the above liposomes conjugated withSLX selectively targeting tumors without deleterious and toxic side effects even if a high dose of CDDP was administered. CDDP3 was exploited here to encapsulate CDDPinto liposomes to achieve high concentrations that are practically useful for the administration of CDDP. Since CDDP3 is an extremely hydrophilic CDDP derivative that readily converts to CDDP inthe presence of chloride ions (Figure 6C), the entire process of encapsulation could be performed in an aqueous phase. Namely, CDDP3 was first dissolved at a saturated concentration ina buffer without chloride ions and encapsulated into liposomes (Figure 7).CDDP3 in the liposomes was then converted into CDDP by replacing the buffer containing 150 mM NaCl. As a result, theCDDP encapsulation efficiency and the CDDP loading efficiencywere dramatically improved when compared with the conventionalmethod of encapsulating CDDP as itself. The CDDP loading efficiencyin CDDP-SLX-Lip was improved by almost 4 times evenwhen compared with the antecedent CDDP liposome called SPI-077 [15, 16]. The higher efficiency of CDDPencapsulation achieved in this study could beaccounted for by the good solubility of CDDP3 in water. As described above, the surface of the liposomes wasdesigned to have negative charge to avoid being trapped by blood proteins such as opsonin,as well as to enhance the retention in blood. On the other hand, CDDP3 in aqueoussolution has positive charge, so that electrostatic attractive force should get CDDP3 close enough to lipids to efficiently be encapsulated into liposomes.

The mean diameter of the CDDP-SLX-Lip particle in the presentstudy was about 160 nm (Table 1). Due to the SLX moiety, CDDP-SLX-Lip should bind to the E-selectin expressed on the tumor vascularendothelial cells. The gaps in the range between 100 and 300 nm are considered to be formed between the endothelial cells of the capillary bed, through whichCDDP-SLX-Lip should penetrate into the tumor [48-52].

Simultaneously, CDDP-SLX-Lip was evaluated *in vivo*for acute toxicity and antitumoractivity with targeting potential. The acute toxicity of CDDP wasremarkably reduced by the encapsulation of CDDPin SLX liposomes. Our conclusion is that CDDP-SLX-Lip is relatively safe as a therapeutic agent when comparedto CDDP with an excellent survival rate as shown in Figure 9. Itis noteworthy that CDDP-SLX-Lip loading of 25 mg CDDP/kg bodyweight showed significant antitumor activity *in vivo* (Figure 12). Whilean EPR effect should allow the accumulation of CDDP-Lip in tumors[53], active targeting by CDDP-SLX-Lipexhibited an additive effect. In this context, CDDP-SLX-Lip wasmore effective than CDDP-Lip at 19 and 26 days after administration(Figure 12). The accentuated antitumor activity appearing in thelate stages may be related to leakage of CDDP from CDDP-SLX-Lipinto the tumor. Furthermore, the expression of E-selectin ontumor vascular endothelial cells may be upregulated by tumor-derived vascular endothelial cell growth factor (VEGF) [54], which could account for the enhanced antitumor activity ofCDDP-SLX-Lip versus CDDP-Lip. CDDP-SLX-Lip might therefore bemore effective than unconjugated CDDP on a wide range of tumorsbecause a number of tumors are sensitive to VEGF-induced angiogenesis[55].

Recently, the number of E-selectin-positive vessels was foundto be higher in invasive microcapillary breast carcinoma than ininvasive ductal carcinoma which was correlated with histologicalgrade [56].Furthermore, TNF-α expression, which isknown to induce E-selectin in vascular endothelial cells [57], showed a significant positive correlation with therate of proliferation, histological grade, lymph node metastasis andmicrovessel density [58]. Targeting E-selectin shouldbe a feasible and practical therapeutic strategy for breast carcinomawith poor prognosis. Further detailed studies such as distribution,clearance, toxicity, application for various tumor cells and doseswith CDDP-SLX-Lip are underway.

Conclusions

1. We successfully established a novel efficient technology to encapsulate CDDP in liposomes at high concentrations.
2. E-selectin on the vascular endothelial cells in tumor tissues is considered a good candidate for a selective target to deliver CDDP in liposomes with SLX.
3. The increased loading efficiency of CDDP together with the ability of targeting E-selectin is expected to enhance the pharmaceutical availability of CDDP and to improveits therapeutic index.
4. CDDP-SLX-Lip should provide a way of developing novel antitumor therapy with CDDP, decreasing the side effects without sparing the antitumor activity.

Acknowledgements

We thank Prof. T. Ema (Okayama University) for his kind support and help in analysis of CDDP structure by NMR, and Prof. L. Fu (Tianjin Medical School) and Prof. M.Chikuma (Osaka University of Pharmaceutical Sciences) for helpful discussions.

REFERENCES

[1] Comis, R.L., 1994. Cisplatin: the future. *Semin. Oncol.* 21, 109–113.

[2] Cvitkovic, E., Spaulding, J., Bethune, V., Martin, J., Whitmore, W.F., 1977. Improvement of cis-dichlorodiammineplatinum therapeutic index in an animal model. *Cancer.* 39, 1357–1361.

[3] Hayes, D.M., Cvitkovic, E., Golbey, R.B., Scheiner, E., Helson, L., Krakoff, I.H., 1977.High dose cis-platinum diammine dichloride: amelioration of renal toxicity by mannitol diuresis. *Cancer.* 39, 1372–1381.

[4] Von Hoff, D.D., Schilsky, R., Reichert, C.M., Reddick, R.L., Rozencweig, M., Young, R.C., Muggia, F.M., 1979. Toxic effects of cis-dichlorodiammineplatinum (II) in man. *Cancer Treat. Rep.* 63, 1527–1531.

[5] Goldstein, R.S., Noordewier, B., Bond, J.T., Hook, J.B., Mayor, G.H., 1981. Cis-dichlorodiammineplatinum nephrotoxicity: time course and dose response of renal functional impairment. *Toxicol. Appl. Pharmacol.* 60, 163–175.

[6] Borch, R.F., Markman, M., 1989. Biochemical modulation of cisplatin toxicity. *Pharmacol.Ther.* 41, 371–380.

[7] Ogilvie, G.K., Fettman, M.J., Jameson, V.J., Walters, L.M., Lafferty, M.H., Cooper, M.F., Powers, B.E., Ciekot, P.A., Atwater, S.W., Withrow, S.J., 1992. Evaluation of a one-hour saline diuresis protocol for administration of cisplatin to dogs. *Am. J. Vet. Res.* 53, 1666–1669.

[8] Legha, S.S., Hodges, C., Ring, S., 1992. Efficacy of ondansetron against nausea and vomiting caused by dacarbazine containing chemotherapy. *Cancer.* 70, 2018–2020.

[9] Navari, R.M., Kaplan, H.G., Gralla, R.J., Grunberg, S.M., Palmer, R., Fitts, D., 1994. Efficacy and safety of granisetron, a selective 5-hydroxytryptamine-3 receptor antagonist, in the prevention of nausea and vomiting induced by high-dose cisplatin. *Clin. Oncol.* 12, 2204–2210.

[10] Gabison, A., Shmeeda,H., Barenholz,Y., 2003. Pharmacokinetics ofpegylated liposomal Doxorubicin: review of animal and humanstudies. *Clin. Pharmacokinet.* 42, 419–436.

[11] Unezaki, S., Maruyama, K., Ishida, O., Takahashi, T., Iwatsuru, M., 1993. Enhanced tumor targeting of Doxorubicin by gangliosideGM1-bearing long-circulating liposomes. *J. Drug Target.* 1,287–292.

[12] Bandak, S., Goren, D., Horowitz, A., Tzemach, D., Gabizon, A., 1999. Pharmacological studies of cisplatin encapsulated in long-circulating liposomes in mouse tumor models. *Anticancer Drugs.* 10, 911–920.

[13] Newman, M.S., Colbern, G.T., Working, P.K., Engbers, C., Amantea, M.A., 1999. Comparative pharmacokinetics, tissue distribution, and therapeutic effectiveness of cisplatin encapsulated in long-circulating, pegylated liposomes (SPI-077) in tumor-bearing mice. *Cancer Chemother. Pharmacol.* 43, 1–7.

[14] Vaage, J., Donovan, D., Wipff, E., Abra, R., Colbern, G., Uster, P., Working, P., 1999. Therapy of a xenografted human colonic carcinoma using cisplatin or doxorubicin encapsulated in long-circulating pegylated stealth liposomes. *Int. J. Cancer.* 80, 134–137.

[15] Harrington, K.J., Lewanski, C.R., Northcote, A.D., Whittaker, J., Wellbank, H., Vile, R.G., Peters, A.M., Stewart, J.S., 2001. Phase I–II study of pegylated liposomal

cisplatin (SPI-077) in patients with inoperable head and neck cancer. *Ann. Oncol.* 12, 493–496.

[16] Kim, E.S., Lu, C., Khuri, F.R., Tonda, M., Glisson, B.S., Liu, D., Jung, M., Hong, W.K., Herbst, R.S., 2001. A phase II study of STEALTH cisplatin (SPI-077) in patients with advanced non-small cell lung cancer. *Lung Cancer*. 34, 427–432.

[17] Veal, G.J., Griffin, M.J., Price, E., Parry, A., Dick, G.S., Little, M.A., Yule, S.M., Morland, B.,Estlin, E.J., Hale, J.P., Pearson, A.D., Welbank, H., Boddy, A.V., 2001. A phase I study in paediatric patients to evaluate the safety and pharmacokinetics of SPI-77, a liposome encapsulated formulation of cisplatin. *Br. J. Cancer*. 84, 1029–1035.

[18] Meerum Terwogt, J.M., Groenewegen, G., Pluim, D., Maliepaard, M., Tibben, M.M., Huisman, A., ten Bokkel Huinink, W.W., Schot, M.,Welbank, H., Voest, E.E., Beijnen, J.H., Schellens, J.M., 2002. Phase I and pharmacokinetic study of SPI-77, a liposomal encapsulated dosage form of cisplatin. *Cancer Chemother. Pharmacol*. 49, 201–210.

[19] Dhara, S., 1970. A rapid method for the synthesis of cis-[Pt(NH3)Cl2]. *Indian J. Chem.* 7, 193–194.

[20] Hirai, M., Minematsu, H., Hiramatsu, Y., Kitagawa, H., Otani,T., Iwashita,S., Kudoh, T., Chen, L., Li, Y., Okada, M., salmon, D.S., Igarashi, K., Chikuma, M., Seno, M., 2010. Novel and simple loading procedure of cisplatin into liposomes and targeting tumor endothelial cells. *Int. J. Pharm*. 391, 274-283.

[21] Maruyama, K., Yuda, T., Okamoto, A., Kojima, S., Suginaka, A., Iwatsuru, M., 1992. Prolonged circulation time *in vivo* of large unilamellarliposomes composed of distearoyl phosphatidylcholine and cholesterolcontaining amphipathic poly (ethylene glycol). *Biochim. Biophys.Acta*. 1128, 44–49.

[22] Gabizon, A., Papahadjopoulos, D., 1988. Liposome formulation withprolonged circulation time in blood and enhanced uptake by tumors.*Proc. Natl. Acad. Sci. USA*. 85, 6949–6953.

[23] Vyas, S.P., Singh, A., Sihorkar, V., 2001. Ligand-receptor-mediated drugdelivery: an emerging paradigm in cellular drug targeting. *Crit. Rev.Ther. Drug Carrier Syst.* 18, 1–76.

[24] Willis, M., Forssen, E., 1998. Ligand-targeted liposomes. *Adv. Drug Deliv.Rev*. 29, 249–271.

[25] Lee, C.M., Tanaka, T., Murai, T., Kondo, M., Kimura, J., Su, W., Kitagawa, T., Ito, T., Matsuda, H., Miyasaka, M., 2002. Novel chondroitin sulfate-binding cationic liposomes loaded with cisplatin efficiently suppress the local growth and liver metastasis of tumor cells *in vivo*. *Cancer Res*. 62, 4282–4288.

[26] Yamazaki, N., Kojima, S., Yokoyama, H., 2005. Biomedical nanotechnology for active drug delivery systems by applying sugar-chain molecular functions. *Curr. Appl. Phys*. 5, 112–117.

[27] Yamazaki, N., 2006. Active targeting DDS. *Farumashia*. 42 (2), 125–129.

[28] Ehrhardt, C., Kneuer, C., Bakowsky, U., 2004. Selectins-an emerging target for drug delivery. *Adv. Drug Deliv. Rev*. 56, 527–549.

[29] Dodd, R.B., Drickamer, K., 2001. Lectin-like proteins in model organisms: implications for evolution of carbohydrate-binding activity. *Glycobiology*. 11, 71R–79R.

[30] Kilpatrick, D.C., 2002. Animal lectins: a historical introduction and overview. *Biochim. Biophys. Acta*. 1572, 187–197.

[31] Bevilacqua, M.P., Stengelin, S.,Gimbrone Jr, M.P., Seed B., 1989. Endothelial leukocyte adhesion molecule 1: an inducible receptor for neutrophils related to complement regulatory proteins and lectins. *Science*. 243, 1160–1165.

[32] Vestweber, D., Blanks, J.E., 1999. Mechanisms that regulate the function of the selectins and their ligands. *Physiol. Rev*. 79, 181–213.

[33] Hirai, M., Minematsu, H., Kondo, N., Oie, K., Igarashi, K., Yamazaki, N., 2007. Accumulation of liposome with Sialyl Lewis X to inflammation and tumor region: application to *in vivo*bio-imaging. *Biochem. Biophys. Res. Commun*. 353, 553–558.

[34] Spragg, D.D., Alford, D.R., Greferath, R., Larsen, C.E., Lee, K.D., Gurtner, G.C., Cybulsky, M.I., Tosi, P.F., Nicolau, C., 1997. Immunotargeting of liposomes to activated vascular endothelial cells; A strategy for site-selective delivery in the cardiovascular systems. *Proc. Natl. Acad. Sci. USA* 94, 8795–8800.

[35] Stahn, R., Grittner, C., Zeisig, R., Karsten, U., Felix, S.B., Wenzel, K., 2001. Sialyl Lewis (X)–liposomes as vehicles for site-directed, E-selectin mediated drug transfer into activated endothelial cells. *Cell Mol. Life Sci*. 58, 141–147.

[36] Tan, P.H., Manunta, M., Ardjomand, N., Xue, S.A., Larkin, D.F., Haskard, D.O., Taylor, K.M., George, A.J., 2003. Antibody targeted gene transfer to endothelium. *J. Gene Med*. 5, 311–323.

[37] Zeising, R., Stahn, R., Wenzel, K., Behrens, D., Fichtner, I., 2004. Effect of Sialyl LewisX-glycoliposomes on the inhibition of E-selectin-mediated tumor cell adhesion *in vitro*. *Biochim. Biophys. Acta*. 1660, 31–40.

[38] Hirai, M., Hiramatsu, Y., Iwashita, S., Otani,T., Chen, L., Li, Y., Okada, M., Oie, K., Igarashi, K., Wakita, H., Seno, M., 2010. E-selectin targeting to visualize tumors *in vivo*. *Contrast Media Mol.Imaging*.5, 70-77.

[39] Hirai, M., Oie, K., Igarashi, K., 2007. *In vivo* imaging reagent with liposome with sugar chain. *Med. Sci. Digest*. 33, 826–828.

[40] Mayer, B., Spatz, H., Funke, I., Johnson, J.P., Schildberg, F.W., 1998. *De novo* expression of the cell adhesion molecule E-selectin on gastric cancer endothelium. *Langenbeck's Arch.Surg*. 383, 81–86.

[41] Liu, F.T., Rabinovich, G.A., 2005. Galectins as modulators of tumor progression. *Nat. Rev. Cancer*. 5, 29–41.

[42] Yamazaki, N., 1989. Analysis of the carbohydrate-binding specificity of lectin-conjugated lipid vesicles which interact with polysaccharide fragments. *J. Membr. Sci*. 41, 249–267.

[43] Yamazaki, N., Kodama, M., Gabius, H.J., 1994. Neoglycoprotein–liposome and lectin–liposome conjugates as tools for carbohydrate recognition research. *Methods Enzymol*. 242, 56–65.

[44] Rosenberg, B., 1978. Platinum complex–DNA interactions and anticancer activity. *Biochimie* 60, 859–867.

[45] Hashida, N., Ohguro, N., Yamazaki, N., Arakawa, Y., Oiki, E., Mashimo, H., Kurikawa, N., Tano, Y., 2008. High-efficacy site-directed drug delivery system using Sialyl–Lewis X conjugate liposome. *Exp. Eye Res*. 86, 138–149.

[46] Van Kasteren, S.I., Campbell, S.J., Serres, S., Anthony, D.C., 2009. Glyconanoparticles allow pre-symptomatic *in vivo* imaging of brain disease. *Proc. Natl. Acad. Sci. USA*106, 18–23.

[47] Coussens, L.M., Web, Z., 2002. Inflammation and cancer. *Nature* 420, 860–867.

[48] Drummond, D.C., Meyer, O., Hong, K., Kirpotin, D.B., Papahadjopoulos, D., 1999. Optimizing liposomes of chemotherapeutic agents to solid tumors. *Pharmacol. Rev.*51, 691–743.

[49] Gabizon, A.A., 1992. Selective tumor localization and improved therapeutic index of anthracyclines encapsulated in long-circulating liposomes. *Cancer Res.* 52, 891–896.

[50] Huang, S.K., Mayhew, E., Gilani, S., Lasic, D.D., Martin, F.J., Papahadjopoulos, D., 1992. Pharmacokinetics and therapeutics of sterically stabilized liposomes in mice bearing C-26 colon carcinoma. *Cancer Res.* 52, 6774–6781.

[51] Huang, S.K., Martin, F.J., Jay, G., Vogel, J., Papahadjopoulos, D., Friend, D.S., 1993. Extravasation and transcytosis of liposomes in Kaposi's sarcoma-like dermal lesions of transgenic mice bearing the HIV tat gene. *Am. J. Pathol.* 143, 10–14.

[52] Wu, N.Z., Da, D., Rudoll, T.L., Needham, D., Whorton, A.R., Dewhirst, M.W., 1993. Increased microvascular permeability contributes to preferential accumulation of stealth liposomes in tumor tissue. *Cancer Res.* 53, 3765–3770.

[53] Matsumura, Y., Maeda, H., 1986. A new concept for macromolecular therapeutics in cancer chemotherapy: mechanism of tumoritropic accumulation of proteins and the antitumor agent smancs. *Cancer Res.* 46, 6387–6392.

[54] Aoki, M., Kanamori, M., Yudoh, K., Ohmori, K., Yasuda, T., Kimura, T., 2001. Effects of vascular endothelial growth factor and E-selectin on angiogenesis in the murine metastatic RCT sarcoma. *Tumour Biol.* 22, 239–246.

[55] Szekanecz, Z., Halloran, M.M., Haskell, C.J., Shah, M.R., Polverini, P.J., Koch, A.E., 1999. Mediators of angiogenesis: the role of cellular adhesion molecules. *Trends Glycosci. Glycotechnol.* 11, 73–93.

[56] Wei, J., Cui, L., Liu, F., Fan, Y., Lang, R., Gu, F., Guo, X., Tang, P., Fu, L., 2010. E-selectin and Sialyl Lewis X expression is associated with lymph node metastasis of invasive micropapillary carcinoma of the breast. *Int. J. Surg. Pathol.* 18, 193-200.

[57] Murakami, T., Mataki, C., Nagao, C., Umetani, M., Wada, Y., Ishii, M., Tsutsumi, S., Kohro, T., Saiura, A., Aburatani, H., Hamakubo, T., Kodama, T., 2000. The gene expression profile of human umbilical vein endothelial cells stimulated by tumor necrosis factor alpha using DNA microarray analysis. *J. Atheroscler. Thromb.* 7, 39–44.

[58] Cui, L.F., Guo, X.J., Wei, J., Liu, F.F., Fan, Y., Lang, R.G., Gu, F., Zhang, X.M., Fu, L., 2008. Overexpression of TNF-α and TNFRII in invasive microcapillary carcinoma of the breast: clinicopathological correlations. *Histopathology*. 53, 381–388.

In: Cisplatin: Pharmacology, Clinical Uses and Adverse Effects ISBN: 978-1-61942-359-6
Editors: Toshiko Kojima and Yoko Morita

Chapter III

CISPLATIN, PHARMACOLOGY AND CLINICAL APPLICATIONS

Suthinee Ithimakin
Division of medical oncology, Department of Medicine, Faculty of Medicine Siriraj Hospital, Mahidol University, Bangkok, Thailand

ABSTRACT

Cisplatin, cis-diamminedichloroplatium, was firstly discovered of its antitumor activity during a study on the effects of electric current on bacterial growth in 1965 (1) and was later developed to be the cornerstone of modern chemotherapy in early 1970s. Cisplatin plays an important role as one of the most widely used and the most effective chemotherapy for various epithelial cancers. Cisplatin-based chemotherapy is responsible for high cure rate of germ cell tumor, high response and remission rate of ovarian cancer. It is capable of stabilizing various cancers, including non-small cell lung cancer, small cell lung cancer as well as other cancers: head and neck, bladder, stomach, anal and cervix. Cisplatin, when use concurrently with radiotherapy, is a potent radiation sensitizer, therefore, it has been widely used to improve local control in head and neck, lung, cervix, esophagus and anal cancer. The clinical use of cisplatin, however, has been impeded by several adverse effects, such as renal toxicity, electrolyte imbalance, severe nausea with vomiting, neuropathy and ototoxicity. All these unfavorable effects can be minimized by applying some strategies as will be mentioned later. This review article covers cisplatin application on various aspects: pharmacology, current evidence-based clinical use, side effects and prevention.

PHARMACOLOGY

Mechanism of Action

Cisplatin covalently binds to DNA to form intra-and inter-strand DNA crosslinks which lead to DNA breakage during replication and alteration of the DNA template. This inhibits DNA transcription, other nuclear functions with arrest cancer cell proliferation and tumor growth. Other proposed mechanisms of cisplatin are activation of signal transduction leading to apoptosis and modulation of some cytoplasmic proteins. Cisplatin also has synergistic effects to radiation and other chemotherapeutic agents. Cisplatin is able to inhibit repair of radiation-induced injury. (2) The synergistic effect to other chemotherapy is probably due to enhancement of cisplatin binding ability, changing mode of DNA damage and disruption of repairing process.

Dosage

Cisplatin, when given as a single agent or in combination with other cytotoxic agent, is usually administered as a single intravenous dose of 50-100 mg/m^2 in 250 ml of normal saline as 1- to 4-hour infusion every 3-4 weeks, either single dose or divided dose over 5 days. One hour infusion is the most common practice. Cisplatin should be diluted in physiologic saline because of its instability with possibly more toxic if dilute in the solution without chloride ions. Other dosing regimens may be used in selected conditions, such as weekly cisplatin infusion concurrently with radiotherapy for cervical cancer treatment. It is important that the patient is well-hydrated with at least with 2 liters of intravenous fluid for high urine flow maintenance. Dose reduction with extensive precaution strategies or consideration of alternative agent is indicated if the 24-hour creatinine clearance is less than 60 ml/min.

Pharmacokinetics

Oral bioavailability is poor. Following intravenous infusion, there is rapid distribution to tissue with more than 90 percent of plasma protein bound. Half-life of unbound cisplatin after short infusion is about 20-30 minutes but the terminal half-life is 60 minutes because of tissue retention. Of the portion eliminated, renal excretion is 90 percent, most during the first few hours to a day, while 10 percent was excreted in bile. Approximately one-fourth of drug is excreted via urine in the first 24 hours. Hemodialysis is partially effective with 8% efficacy to remove cisplatin from circulation. (3) After intraperitoneal administration, the concentration of cisplatin in peritoneal-lining tissue was 2.5-8 folds greater than achieve by intravenous cisplatin. (4) Intraperitoneal administration, with potential increase exposure to intraperitoneal tumor, is associated with increase efficacy in advanced ovarian cancer. Small amount of cisplatin can be detected in cerebrospinal fluid after intravenous administration of cisplatin, but whether this level reach the therapeutic efficacy remains unclear. (5, 6)

Drug Interactions

Because of potential synergistic effects of renal toxicity and ototoxicity, diuretic or other nephrotoxic or ototoxic drug should be avoided when the patient is scheduled to receive cisplatin. Along with cisplatin administration, the use of other chemotherapy with mainly excreted by kidney, such as etoposide, methotrexate, bleomycin and ifosfamide, must be done cautiously. Cisplatin may reduce the creatinine clearance, thereby increase toxicity of these drugs. Cisplatin should be administered after paclitaxel when they are used in combination, to avoid delayed paclitaxel excretion.

CLINICAL APPLICATIONS

Significant activity of cisplatin has been established in various cancers, either combined with other chemotherapeutic agents or concurrently used with radiotherapy. This article reviews current use of cisplatin in common cancers in which cisplatin plays a major role for treatment.

Germ Cell Tumors

Germ cell tumor of testis is the most common cancer in young men. Although ninety-five percent of germ cell tumor occurs in testis, occasionally extragonadal germ cell tumor occurs. Considerable therapeutic improvement, especially from cisplatin-based chemotherapy, provides extremely high response rate and leads to improvement of cure rate as well as survival. Staging and prognosis of testicular cancer depend on the type of cancer (seminoma or non-seminoma), nodal or distant metastasis and level of Beta-Human Chorionic Hormone (β-HCG) or Alfa-fetoprotein (AFP) or lactate dehydrogenase (LDH).

Primary treatment of stage IA, IB pure seminoma is one of the followings; surveillance, radiotherapy or single dose carboplatin. Although mainstay therapy of stage IIA or IIB seminoma is radiotherapy, cisplatin-based chemotherapy (4 cycles of cisplatin and etoposide [EP] or 3 cycles of cisplatin, etoposide and bleomycin [BEP]) is an alternative treatment to radiotherapy, especially in stage IIB seminoma. For treatment of non-seminoma, surveillance or nerve-sparing retroperitoneal node dissection (RPNLD) is optional for stage IA, whereas either RPNLD or chemotherapy (2 cycles of BEP) is standard treatment for stage IB. The treatment of non-seminoma with regional lymph node metastasis, with the size of lymph node less than 5 cm (stage IIA, IIB), is either RPNLD or chemotherapy (4 cycles of EP or 3 cycles of BEP). Cisplatin-based chemotherapy (both EP and BEP regimen) is the cornerstone of treatment in germ cell tumor, both seminoma and non-seminoma, with huge lymph node (> 5 cm) or distant metastasis. Risk stratification is the important marker to determine suitable amount and regimen of chemotherapy. Currently, standard regimen of good risk non-seminoma are both 4 cycles of EP or 3 cycles of BEP with the cure rate of more than 90 percent. (7) For the worse prognostic patients, cure rate are 70 and less than 50 percent of patients have durable complete response with 4 cycles of BEP in intermediate and poor-risk non-seminoma, respectively. (7-9)

Cisplatin is also a backbone of the second-line chemotherapy for germ cell tumor. The conventional second-line chemotherapy for favorable patients (complete response from first-line treatment, testicular primary site, low-volume of disease and serum marker after orchiectomy) includes cisplatin and ifosfamide with either vinblastine or paclitaxel. (10) High-dose regimen, including high-dose chemotherapy with autologous stem cell transplantation is an option for patients with unfavorable features. (11)

Small Cell Lung Cancer (SCLC)

Small cell lung cancer accounts for 20 percent of total lung cancer patients. Nearly all of these cancer cases are attributed to cigarette smoking. The aim of treatment in limited stage is to achieve a cure by combination treatment of chemotherapy and radiotherapy. In patients with extensive disease, the main treatment is palliative chemotherapy and/or palliative radiation to achieve clinical response which might lead to lessen symptoms and prolong survival.

Chemotherapy, especially platinum-based regimen, is the essential component of the treatment in both limited and extensive-stage SCLC. Cisplatin plus etoposide (EP) is the most common first-line combination regimen. The EP has been shown its superiority in terms of efficacy and toxicity to the older anthracycline/alkylator-based regimen. (12) Concurrent EP with radiotherapy has been accepted for standard treatment for limited-stage SCLC. (13, 14) With the efficacy of EP plus concurrent chemotherapy, response rate of 70-90% is expected in limited-stage SCLC. Compared with extensive-stage patients, response rate can be achieved in 60-70 percent from combination chemotherapy. (15) Unfortunately, despite dramatic response from chemotherapy, recurrence often occurs in short period in most cases. Therefore, median survival period of limited- and extensive-stage SCLC patients are only 14-20 and 9-11 months, respectively.

Four to six cycles of combination chemotherapy is standard for extensive stage SCLC. Maintenance or consolidation chemotherapy beyond 6 cycles produced minor prolongation of progression-free period, but does not influence to survival with increase cumulative toxicity. (16)

Other combinations have been evaluated for extensive SCLC to enhance the efficacy of standard EP regimen. Irinotecan plus cisplatin, in a study from Japan, was shown to have superiority to the EP in terms of median survival (12.8 vs 9.4 months, p=0.002). (17) Subsequently, however, two large phase III trials from the United State failed to demonstrate significant difference among these two regimens. (18, 19)

Addition of ifosfamide (or cyclophosphamide plus anthracycline) to EP regimen has been evaluated in 2 trials. The combination provided significant improvement in response rate, progression-free and overall survival. (20, 21) However, the beneficial effects are not uniformly observed in other trials with increase hematotoxicity compared to standard EP regimen. (22) Similarly, addition of paclitaxel to EP initially showed promising results in phase II trial, but subsequent larger phase III study demonstrated no beneficial effect with higher toxicity compared to EP regimen. (23)

Non-small Cell Lung Cancer (NSCLC)

Surgery, radiation and chemotherapy are main modalities used for NSCLC treatment. Chemotherapy usually is used as single modality for adjuvant treatment in resectable cases or palliative intent for metastatic disease or concurrently used with radiotherapy in locally-advanced cases. Platinum-based chemotherapy is the major backbone for majority of doublet chemotherapy for NSCLC. Dosage and schedules depend on status of disease and combination modality.

Cisplatin and carboplatin both are major component of chemotherapy for NSCLC with different toxicity profiles. Cisplatin associates with higher rate of nausea or vomiting, nephrotoxicity and neurotoxicity, while carboplatin's main side effect is myelosuppression. Many studies have investigated the equivalence of these two agents in terms of survival benefit. (24, 25) Given that carboplatin has relatively lower toxicity, carboplatin may become the most popular chemotherapy for NSCLC if it is proved non-inferiority to the established cisplatin.

Benefit of cisplatin-doublet chemotherapy has been established from the International Adjuvant Lung Cancer Trial (IALT). (26) Significant survival benefit at 5-year was found in patients who received cisplatin-based adjuvant chemotherapy. However, benefit of chemotherapy at 7.5 years decreased overtime because of more death was found in chemotherapy group. Later, two large randomized control studies demonstrated the efficacy of adjuvant cisplatin plus vinorelbine in stage IB-III NSCLC patients. (27, 28) Both studies showed the superiority of adjuvant chemotherapy to observation in terms of overall survival. From subset analysis, the benefits of adjuvant chemotherapy were significant in stage II and III, but not in stage I. Another meta-analysis (the Lung Adjuvant Cisplatin Evaluation: LACE) confirmed the benefit of postoperative cisplatin-based chemotherapy with absolute benefit in survival of 5.4%. There was no difference among those in chemotherapy regimen. The benefit was greater in stage II and III patients with good performance status. (29)

The CALGB 9633 trial assessed the benefit of adjuvant carboplatin plus paclitaxel in stage IB NSCLC. Initial report of 3-year overall survival was significantly greater in patients who received chemotherapy (79 vs 70%, $p=0.045$). However, update follow up did not show improvement of survival from carboplatin and paclitaxel. (30) To date, adjuvant chemotherapy for NSCLC has been recommended in stage II and III resectable NSCLC. Cisplatin-based chemotherapy is preferable in this adjuvant setting. Carboplatin should only be used in patients who have contraindication, eg. Renal impairment, existing neuropathy, or cannot tolerate to cisplatin.

Cisplatin plus etoposide concurrently with definitive thoracic radiation is the preferred option for locally advanced NSCLC. Patients further received 2 cycles of cisplatin with etoposide for consolidation phase. From phase II study of the Southwest Oncology Group, (31) 33 out of 50 patients completed radiation treatment. Five-year overall survival was 15 percent. A subsequent randomized phase III trial of stage III NSCLC assessed the benefit of consolidation chemotherapy after completing chemoradiotherapy. (32) Patients were treated with chemoradiotherapy concurrently with cisplatin plus etoposide, then either received 3 cycles of docetaxel as consolidation chemotherapy or observation. Median survival was 21.5 and 24.1 months in consolidation and observation arm, respectively ($p=0.94$). Moreover, patients who received consolidation chemotherapy experienced higher rate of hospitalization, infection and treatment-related toxicity.

Patients with metastatic NSCLC, who has good performance status, benefit from palliative chemotherapy in terms of symptom relieve and also increase survival. The useful agents include platinum (cisplatin or carboplatin) as a backbone, combine with one of the followings; gemcitabine, paclitaxel, docetaxel, vinorelbine, pemetrexed or etoposide. Combination platinum-based chemotherapy is superior to single agent and produces 1-year survival rate of 30-40 percent. (33, 34) Phase III randomized control trial has shown similar efficacy among these platinum-based chemotherapy for advanced NSCLC. (33)

Head and Neck Cancer

Treating patients with head and neck cancer is complicate and need multimodality approach. Options for treatment depend on the site of cancer, stage, pathology finding, as well as preference of organ sparing. Single modality of either surgery or radiotherapy accounts for 30-40 percent of stage I, II head and neck cancer patients. In contrast, combined modality is recommended for locally advanced head and neck cancer patients. Role of chemotherapy in head and neck cancer includes concurrently use with radiotherapy in locally advanced disease, as either postoperative treatment, part of definitive chemoradiation or induction chemotherapy, and as palliative chemotherapy in metastatic disease.

Concurrent chemoradiation with cisplatin every 3 weeks is better than radiation alone in treatment of head and neck cancer after curative surgery in terms of recurrence and progression-free survival. High risk head and neck cancer usually recurs at the surgical bed even after getting adequate surgery and proper radiotherapy. High risk features include positive margin and/or extracapsular involvement. Patients with one of these features should receive postoperative chemoradiation. The addition of chemotherapy with radiotherapy may be considered in patients with presence of other minor adverse factors-multiple positive nodes, vascular/lymphatic/perineural invasion, pT3 or pT4 primary or positive level 4 or 5 lymph node. Cisplatin is a potent radiosensitizer which enhance the efficacy of radiation. Two randomized control trials from RTOG (35) and EORTC (36) demonstrated significant improvement of locoregional control and disease-free survival in patients receiving cisplatin with radiotherapy compared with postoperative radiation alone. However, significantly higher toxicity in patients with chemoradiotherapy was found. The main side effects of patients receiving cisplatin concurrent with radiotherapy are increase incidence and degree of mucositis as well as side effects of cisplatin itself such as nausea, vomiting, nephrotoxicity, electrolyte imbalance and neuropathy.

Recently, more effective triplet chemotherapy regimen has been proved of its superiority to traditional cisplatin plus 5FU as induction chemotherapy for locally advanced head and neck cancer. Several randomized controlled studies compared induction cisplatin plus 5FU with or without taxane followed by the same locoregional treatment. (37-40) The results are consistent among the trials. There was superiority of triplet chemotherapy in terms of recurrence, disease-free or overall survival. However, the clear survival benefit of addition of induction chemotherapy to standard concurrent chemoradiotherapy in locally advanced head and neck cancer has not been established yet. (41)

Principle of metastatic head and neck cancer treatment are palliative chemotherapy in patients with good performance and nutritional status as well as adequate symptom control. The active agents are cisplatin, carboplatin, 5FU, taxane, methotrexed and gemcitabine. Active combination includes cisplatin or carboplatin plus 5FU and cisplatin or carboplatin plus a taxane. From randomized studies, combination chemotherapy provided significant higher response rate, but failed to clearly demonstrate survival benefit. (42-44) Historically, median survival of metastatic head and neck cancer patients with palliative chemotherapy was 6 months. (43) In addition, there was no difference in survival benefit in patients given cisplatin plus 5FU compared to who received cisplatin plus paclitaxel. (45)

Gynecological Cancer

Role of cisplatin in gynecological cancer is established for cervical, ovarian and endometrial cancer. Weekly cisplatin concurrent with external radiotherapy followed by brachytherapy is a standard treatment for extensive local cervical cancer (stage IIb and beyond). Several randomized phase III trials supported the benefit of cisplatin as a radiosensitizer for invasive cervical cancer in terms of progression-free and overall survival. (46-48) Cisplatin is a major agent for treatment of metastatic cervical cancer with response rate of approximately 20 percent. However, the duration of response usually does not last longer than 3-4 months. The objective response mostly occurs in non-radiated area and in chemotherapy-naïve patients. Because of widely use of cisplatin for primary treatment for locally advanced cervical cancer, activity of cisplatin toward recurrent disease following radiotherapy plus cisplatin remains problematic.

For endometrial cancer, cisplatin is one of the most active chemotherapy for metastatic disease. Other agents that have been demonstrated biologic activity included carboplatin, paclitaxel and doxorubicin. The overall response rate of these single agents is 25-35 percent. Combination of cisplatin and doxorubicin produced a higher objective response compared to doxorubicin alone, but no survival benefit. (49) Addition of either doxorubicin or paclitaxel to cisplatin increases response rate. (50) A report from randomized study noted that combination of cisplatin, doxorubicin and paclitaxel resulted in small but significant improvement of survival compared to cisplatin plus doxorubicin. (51) However, the triple-drug regimen associated with higher toxicity, especially neurotoxicity.

Standard treatment for advanced ovarian cancer is platinum agent (cisplatin or carboplatin) plus taxane. Although Cisplatin and carboplatin have comparable efficacy with respect to survival in overian cancer patients, carboplatin is preferable option because of its significantly less toxicity and easier administration. (52-55) Moreover, 24-hour paclitaxel infusion, instead of 3-hour infusion, is required if cisplatin is concomitantly used with paclitaxel to avoid severe neurotoxicity. (55) Intraperitoneal cisplatin administration as primary treatment for small-volume residual advanced ovarian cancer compared with systemic administration has been studied. These studies showed superiority of regional treatment in terms of progression-free and overall survival. (56-58) Despite concern of excessive local toxicity, requirement of catheter administration and the necessity to use cisplatin rather than carboplatin, available data demonstrated intraperitoneal cisplatin can be safely done for treatment of small-volume residual ovarian cancer in selected case.

Adverse Effects and Prevention

Renal Toxicity

Kidney is the principle excretion organ of cisplatin. Concentration of cisplatin in renal cortex is much higher than plasma level or other organs. Autoradiography study showed radiolabeled cisplatin had greater uptake in the segment of S3 nephron or so called "proximal straight tubule". Therefore, the proximal straight tubule is the principle area of vulnerability to cisplatin toxicity. As a result, salt wasting nephropathy is one of the most common patterns of renal adverse effect.

The clinical use of cisplatin is hindered by the nephrotoxicity, especially reduction of glomerular filtration rate (GFR) which is the main dose-limited toxicity of cisplatin. Decline GFR is in proportion to the repeated cycles of chemotherapeutic use. Progressive and partially-irreversible decrease of renal function may develop in each successive course. With the cisplatin withdrawal and adequate hydration, renal function may totally or partially recover or indefinitely impaired. In addition, cisplatin may directly induce necrosis and apoptosis of renal tubular cells. The proposed mechanisms are p53 mediated activations of caspase-2, -8 and -3 in renal cell induced apoptosis and TNF alpha synthesis via P38 MAPK phosphorylation. (59) Despite of adequate hydration prior and during cisplatin administration, some degree of renal impairment may occur. A prospective study assessed renal function in testicular cancer patients who received 5- day cisplatin of 20 $mg/m^2/day$. All patients received 15% mannitol before cisplatin infusion with 4-liter of saline infusion per 24 hours. There was 23% decrease of glomerular filtration rate at the end of induction therapy and 6-week thereafter was seen without significant difference of serum creatinine. (60)

Polyuria usually accompanies cisplatin administration in two distinct phases; first 24-48 hours and 72-96 hours. Early polyuria occurs in the first 48 hours after administration with normal renal function and spontaneously ameliorated. A second phase of polyuria, between 72-96 hours after cisplatin, usually accompanies with permanent decrease renal function and salt losing.

Hypomagnesemia is a common consequence of cisplatin use. The presence of magnesium excretion in the situation of severe hypomagnesemia suggested the tubular defect of magnesium reabsorption, or transportation of juxtamedullary nephron or collecting duct. Hypokalemia and hypocalcemia may accompany this condition.

The incidence of cisplatin-induced hyponatremia is as high as 43 percent. The mechanisms of inducing hyponatremia are controversial. The most promising mechanisms are renal salt wasting and syndrome of inappropriate antidiuretic hormone (SIADH). Cisplatin can induce tubular necrosis with associated sodium, potassium and magnesium loss. The evidence of cisplatin-induced tubular necrosis was confirmed by the autopsy report of patients who was treated with cisplatin by Gonzales-Vitale et al (61), acute tubular necrosis, mostly at distant convoluted tubule and collecting ducts, was found. Once hyponatremia occurs, it is frequently combined with other metabolic derangements. In patients with cisplatin-induced salt-wasting, inappropriately high sodium in urine is compatible with abnormal regulation of sodium reabsorption. Signs of volume depletion, such as orthostatic hypotension, may be found in these patients due to abnormally high urine output secondary to high sodium excretion and polyuria after cisplatin administration. There is no correlation between dosage, number of cisplatin cycles and occurrence of renal salt wasting described. Time to occurrence ranged from a few days to several months after starting chemotherapy. Hyponatremia from salt wasting may persist for a few days, months or become irreversible. (62) Treatment of this condition is mainly oral supplement of sodium. (63, 64)

Other reports of patients with hyponatremia after cisplatin administration are consistent with SIADH. (65-68) Clinical characteristics are different from renal salt wasting. Hyponatremia occurred more rapidly after 1-2 days, last for few days and usually reversible. The patients usually do not have sign of volume depletion or accompanying metabolic abnormalities as a result of salt wasting syndrome. Main treatment is fluid restriction, associated with furosemide and hypertonic saline in some symptomatic cases.

Prevention of Cisplatin-induced Nephrotoxicity

Up to 70% of patients receiving cisplatin in early drug development experienced renal failure. (69, 70) Aggressive hydration with normal saline is able to reduce the incidence, but renal failure still occasionally happens. There are attempts to prevent this serious complication, either using other compounds or alternating method of administration.

Although several reports have suggested that furosemide or mannitol can reduce concentration of platinum in urine and decrease nephrotoxicity (71, 72), some reports suggested they may aggravate renal toxicity. (73) A randomized study (74) compared the renal protection effect of mannitol, using hydration with or without mannitol in melanoma patients who scheduled to receive cisplatin of 100 mg/m^2. Patients receiving mannitol experienced less moderate, severe and life-threatening renal toxicity. The renal protection effect of mannitol was most convincing in the first cycle. Moreover, these patients can tolerate more dosage of cisplatin with comparable other side effects. Another randomized study (75) compared the renal protection effect of saline alone, saline plus furosemide and saline plus mannitol in patients receiving 75 mg/m^2 of cisplatin. The decrease of creatinine clearance was similar between patients receiving saline only and saline plus furosemide ($p=0.66$). Interestingly, creatinine clearance significantly reduced in patients who got saline with mannitol ($P=0.02$). Well hydration in 12-hour ahead with induction of urine flow of more than 100 ml/hour is a suggested strategy. Urine flow should be maintained at 3-4 liter in preceding day and the next 2-3 days.

Schedule of administration of cisplatin has been reported to affect renal function. Fractionation or continuous infusion of cisplatin over 3-5 days, instead of one-time bolus injection, provided comparable efficacy but probably spare renal function. (76) Adequate prevention of nausea and vomiting is another important strategy to prevent dehydration and subsequent prerenal renal failure which may aggravate deterioration of renal function by cisplatin itself.

The administration, simultaneously with cisplatin, of other nephrotoxic agents, such as aminoglycoside, non-steriodal inflammatory drugs, and contrast agents, should be avoided. These agents can potentiate the renal toxic effects. There was a report that showed greater renal toxicity in patients receiving cisplatin concomitant with aminoglycoside compared to those who received cisplatin alone. (77)

There is insufficient data for determination of serum creatinine after administration of cisplatin. However, measurement of serum creatinine at day3-5 may help diagnose transient rise of creatinine which may be responsible for cumulative renal damage and lead to progressive renal function impairment in subsequent cycles. In addition, measuring of serum Magnesium should be done and supplemented routinely in all patients receiving cisplatin-based chemotherapy. (78)

Nausea and Vomiting

Chemotherapy-induced nausea and vomiting (CINV) is among the most feared and distressing side effects of chemotherapy. The optimal control of CINV in first cycle contributed to prevent anticipatory emesis in subsequent cycle. (79) The likelihood of developing emesis depends on 2 main factors, patients' characteristics and chemotherapeutic agents. High-dose cisplatin ($\geq$ 50 mg/m^2) is considered as high-emetogenic chemotherapy (Hesketh level 4). Over 90 percent of patients receiving such dose of cisplatin without any antiemetic prophylaxis subsequently develop vomiting. Patient's characteristics that increase likelihood of CINV include female gender, younger age, history of morning sickness during pregnancy and previously experienced motion sickness. On the other hand, patients with a history of high alcohol consumption have lower risk of CINV. (80)

Without effective antiemesis, virtually all patients receiving cisplatin experience nausea and vomiting within the first 1-2 hours and usually subside at 18-24 hours after cisplatin administration. Then, second episode usually develops and reach the peak at 48-72 hours. Based on the model of cisplatin pattern of emesis, emesis occurring within first 24 hours and after 24 hours has been defined as acute and delayed emesis, respectively. Cisplatin is a prototype of chemotherapeutic agent with distressing delayed emesis property. Other chemotherapy that produces delayed emesis includes cyclophosphamide, carboplatin and anthracycline. Anticipatory emesis, another subset of CINV, represented learned response of nausea and vomiting in previous cycle of chemotherapy. Patients may develop CINV even prior to administration of current cisplatin cycle. Adequate control of emesis in first cycle can prevent anticipatory emesis in subsequent cycles.

The fundamental principle for prevention of CINV is to explore antiemetic treatment that completely prevents nausea and vomiting, using appropriate, evidence-based preventive strategies. There is variety of antiemetic agents responsible for high-emetogenic chemotherapy, 5-HT3 antagonist, corticosteroid and neurokinin-1 receptor antagonists.

Selective 5-HT3 Receptor Antagonist

The introduction of selective 5-HT3 receptor antagonist in 1990s was a cornerstone of emetic prophylaxis for patients receiving chemotherapy. It has been proved and widely used for its efficacy using for prevention of CINV over decades. To date, there are five 5-HT3 receptor antagonists that are widely accessible: ondansetron, granisetron, dolasetron, tropisetron and most recently approved of palanosetron. Dosage and schedules of 5-HT3 receptor antagonist for prevention of CINV for patients receiving cisplatin is provided in table 1. There was multiple randomized trials supported equivalent efficacy among those 4 old of 5-HT3 receptor antagonists. (81, 82) The common adverse effects of this class are mild headache, constipation and mild transient elevation of liver enzyme. Palanosetron, a new 5-HT3 receptor antagonist with prolonged half life of approximately 40 hours, was approved in 2003. A randomized controlled trial (83) compared the efficacy of single intravenous palanosetron prior to high-emetogenic chemotherapy administration to ondansetron. Palanosetron plus dexamethasone was superior to ondansetron plus dexamethasone in terms of complete response rate over 5-days and delayed period with comparable toxicity. Addition of steroid provides more effective control of CINV for high-emetogenic chemotherapy and was recommended by the National Cancer Cancer Network (NCCN) in 2007 for patients receiving highly emetogenic chemotherapy.

Corticosteroid

The most beneficial effect of corticosteroid for emesis prevention has been demonstrated when concomitant use with 5-HT3 receptor antagonists. Corticosteroid is effective for both acute and delayed emesis. However, the mechanism of steroid for emesis prophylaxis is poorly understood. The widest experience of corticosteroid for CINV prevention was found for dexamethasone use when combined with 5-HT3 receptor antagonist with the dosage of 20 mg intravenous prior to cisplatin infusion and 8 mg orally twice daily from day 2-4. The dosage of dexamethasone should be reduced approximately by half if using with aprepitant, a cytochrome p450 3A4 inhibitor (12 mg intravenous prior to cisplatin infusion, then 8 mg orally once daily from day 2-4).

Neurokinin-1 Receptor Antagonist

Neurokinin-1 receptor antagonist, aprepitant, represented the newest class of antiemetic drug for CINV prophylaxis. Aprepitant added to previously standard couple drugs of 5-HT3 receptor antagonist with corticosteroid have been approved for CINV prevention in patients receiving highly emetogenic chemotherapy. Several phase III studies was conducted to demonstrate the superiority of aprepitant when combined with previous standard couple of 5-HT3 receptor antagonist and dexamethasone and that couple alone. (84-86) Addition of aprepitant led to significant reduction of emetic rate and need for rescue medication over the 5-day period. The most common adverse effects of aprepitant include fatigue, hiccup and dyspepsia.

Antiemetic Agents with Low Therapeutic Index

There are some low therapeutic index for CINV prevention, including dopamine receptor antagonist (metoclopramide, domperidone), phenothiazine, antihistamine (dimenhydrinate) and benzodiazepine. These drugs alone are not effective for CINV in patients receiving cisplatin. Adding metoclopramide to standard treatment of ondansetron with dexamethasone provided only reduction of rescue treatment, but not improvement of overall rate of vomiting. (87) Currently, with the introduction of NK1 receptor antagonist, role of these agents to prevent CINV for cisplatin has diminished. However, these agents probably add some benefit if using as adjunct to other antiemetic drug for breakthrough treatment. Benzodiazepine has been accepted for its benefit along with behavioral therapy for anticipatory emesis.

Table 1. Recommended dose and schedule of antiemetics to prevent cisplatin-induced emesis (88)

Agents	Before injection of cisplatin	Single daily dose
Selective 5-HT3 receptor antagonist -ondansetron -Granisetron -Dolasetron -Palanosetron -Tropisetron	 Oral:24 mg or iv: 8 mg (0.15 mg/kg) Oral:2 mg or iv: 1 mg (0.01 mg/kg) Oral:100 mg or iv: 100 mg (1.8 mg/kg) Iv: 0.25 mg Oral or iv: 5 mg	
Corticosteroid	Oral: 12 mg	Oral: 8 mg daily day 2-4
Aprepitant	Oral: 125 mg	Oral: 80 mg daily day 2-3

iv: intravenous administration.

Currently, using selective 5-HT3 receptor antagonist, NK1 receptor antagonist with corticosteroid is the most effective combination in preventing cisplatin induced nausea and vomiting. Moreover, adequate hydration and closed monitoring with prompt adjunctive treatment in case of failure of fist-line prevention is still the mainstay of treatment for patients receiving cisplatin.

Neurotoxicity

Most of patients who complete full-course of cisplatin experience some degree of neurotoxicity. Peripheral neuropathy shown by sensory paresthesia or loss of proprioception/vibration is the most common pattern. Motor impairment rarely occurs and often is the dose-limiting toxicity. Cisplatin occasionally causes reversible posterior leukoencephalopathy. Patients' common manifestations are acute occipital blindness or partial loss of vision or seizure. (89)

A study from the United Kingdom assessed the incidence and prognosis of cisplatin-induced neurotoxicity in 29 metastatic germ-cell tumor patients. (90) Assessment included symptom evaluation as well as physiologic test of sural nerve conduction velocity and vibration threshold. At the end of 3 or 4 cycles of cisplatin-based chemotherapy, 11 percent of patients had paresthesia. Interestingly, the incidence dramatically rose up to 65 percent in 3 months later. Majority of patients completely resolved within 3-12 months after discontinuation of chemotherapy, but 17 percent of patients still have persistent symptoms after years. Among those who had persistent symptoms, all of them received full 4 cycles of chemotherapy. It can be implied that accumulative dosage might influence to the long-term neuropathy.

Several possible neuroprotective agents, including amifostine, vitamin E, acetylcysteine, calcium and magnesium, have been studied. The review of total 27 randomized controlled trials (1,537 patients) showed insufficient data to conclude that any of proposed neuroprotective agents can limit cisplatin-induced neurotoxicity. (91)

Ototoxicity

Ototoxicity is another adverse effect of cisplatin which usually irreversible and unpreventable. Symptoms of ototoxicity from cisplatin include tinnitus, ear pain and subjective hearing loss. Up to 36 percent of patients receiving cisplatin developed tinnitus. (92) Cisplatin induced hearing loss is usually bilateral and irreversible, especially in pediatric population. It is observed, however, that the symptoms were transient in some patients and not all patients developed audiometry abnormalities. High-frequency threshold usually is affected first. Although audimetric abnormalities seems to be the first sign of ototoxicity preceding clinical symptoms, only evidence of laboratory high-frequency defect without clinical symptoms do not designate as a surrogate to alternate dosage of cisplatin when the treatment is clearly indicated.

Degree of ototoxicity is more severe in patients receiving higher cumulative dose, higher individual dose and got bolus dosage of cisplatin. (92) Cisplatin-induced ototoxicity may occur within hours to days after drug administration. Cumulative effect of cisplatin-induced ototoxicity has been reported in pediatric patients who received cisplatin up to 400 mg/m^2 ultimately developed hearing loss after cisplatin administration for years. (93) Audiographic abnormalities were demonstrated only 5 percent at the end of therapy while the incidence significantly rose to 44 percent after more than 2 years. This finding confirmed the cumulative ototoxicity effect of cisplatin.

Intravenous amifostine was studied as a protectant agent of ototoxicity in pediatric medulloblastoma patients who scheduled to receive cisplatin with craniospinal radiotherapy. Thirteen patients (37.1%) in control and nine (14.5%) in amifostine group, respectively, developed at least grade 3 ototoxicity or requiring hearing aid at 1year after treatment (p=0.005). (94) The side effects of amifostine were mild and well-tolerated. However, protectant effect of amifostine was failed to demonstrate for germ cell cancer patients who receiving cispltin, bleomycin and etoposide. (95, 96) To date, there is no ideal oto-protectant agent in clinical used.

Hematotoxicity

Myelosuppression is generally not a significant side effect of cisplatin. Mild suppression in all lineages are reported, especially when concurrently use with other chemotherapeutic agent. Among the suppression of all blood cells lineages, cisplatin-induced anemia is the most common with the incidence of up to 40 percent of patients. (97-99) Serious adverse effects such as febrile neutropenia or severe infection are very rare with cisplatin administration alone.

Anemia in cancer patients are often multifactorial; nutritional deficiency, blood loss, anemia of malignancy, bone marrow infiltration of cancer and the effect of chemotherapeutic agent. Cisplatin is the common agent that produces significant anemia. The diagnosis of this condition needs the exclusion of other possible treatable causes. Cisplatin may directly affect and suppress synthesis of red blood cell precursors or impair the synthesis of erythropoietin because of its nephrotoxic property. The myelosuppressive effect of cisplatin is likely accumulative over the course of repeated administration of chemotherapy, resulting in increased incidence and severity of anemia in late cycle. (100) Decision for specific treatment for cisplatin-induced anemia individually bases on several factors; level of hemoglobin, symptoms of patients and preexisting comorbidities.

Main therapies of chemotherapy-induced anemia are blood transfusion and erythropoietin therapy. Blood transfusion has been used with the benefit of rapid increase hemoglobin level. Therefore, blood transfusion is an ideal option for patients who need immediate correction, for example, those are symptomatic or cardiovascular compromised. Target hemoglobin varies according to patients' conditions. Asymptomatic anemic patients usually maintain their hemoglobin of 7-9 g/dl while patients with coronary syndrome need much higher hemoglobin goal of 10 g/dl. Transfusion associated risk includes transfusion reaction, volume overload, bacterial and some viral infections. Erythropoietin treatment has become alternative treatment for cancer- or chemotherapy-related anemia with the advantage of avoidance or at least decrease transfusion. (101-103) Unlike immediate effect of transfusion, erythropoietin takes weeks to reach hemoglobin response and can be maintained with repeated administration. Erythropoietin treatment became popular treatment until evidences of potential detrimental effect of erythropoietin to cancer treatment outcome has emerged. Starting from 2007, the

FDA made a major revision regarding to erythropoietin treatment based on results on randomized controlled trials that showed decrease survival and tumor control in advanced breast, head and neck, cervical and non-small cell lung cancer. (104-108) Moreover, these adverse outcomes of erythropoietin use have been confirmed by meta-analyses. (109-111)

All in all, there is no effective prevention for myelosuppression from cisplatin. Treatment goals are relieving symptoms and improve quality of life. Blood transfusion is a mainstay treatment for cisplatin-induced anemia, especially in the patients with curative intent.

CONCLUSION

The availability of cisplatin has been a significant advance in cancer chemotherapy. Cisplatin plays major role in curative combination chemotherapy for germ cell tumor. In addition, cisplatin is an active drug for treatment of cancer of lung, head and neck, cervix and ovary. Main short-term adverse effects are nausea and vomiting, which has been alleviated with new antiemetic agents. Nephrotoxicity has become less significant problem with by adequate hydration and avoidance of simultaneous use of nephrotoxic agent. Despite important roles of cisplatin in present-day cancer management, the use of cisplatin should be surrounded by expertise to cope with unfavorable toxicity and with essential preventive measures to minimize its side effects.

REFERENCES

[1] Rosenberg B, Vancamp L, Krigas T. Inhibition of cell division in escherichia coli by electrolysis products from a platinum electrode. *Nature*. 1965 Feb 13;205:698-9.

[2] Lippard SJ. New chemistry of an old molecule: cis-[Pt(NH3)2Cl2]. *Science*. 1982 Dec 10;218(4577):1075-82.

[3] Moran RE, Straus MJ. Effects of pulse and continuous intravenous infusion of cis-diamminedichloroplatinum on L1210 leukemia in vivo. *Cancer Res.* 1981 Dec;41(12 Pt 1):4993-6.

[4] Pretorius RG, Petrilli ES, Kean CK, Ford LC, Hoeschele JD, Lagasse LD. Comparison of the iv and ip routes of administration of cisplatin in dogs. *Cancer Treat Rep.* 1981 Nov-Dec;65(11-12):1055-62.

[5] Bonnem EM, Litterst CL, Smith FP. Platinum concentrations in human glioblastoma multiforme following the use of cisplatin. *Cancer Treat Rep.* 1982 Aug;66(8):1661-3.

[6] Gormley PE, Gangji D, Wood JH, Poplack DG. Pharmacokinetic study of cerebrospinal fluid penetration of cis-diamminedichloroplatinum (II). *Cancer Chemother Pharmacol.* 1981;5(4):257-60.

[7] Jones RH, Vasey PA. Part II: testicular cancer--management of advanced disease. *Lancet Oncol.* 2003 Dec;4(12):738-47.

[8] de Wit R, Stoter G, Sleijfer DT, Neijt JP, ten Bokkel Huinink WW, de Prijck L, et al. Four cycles of BEP vs four cycles of VIP in patients with intermediate-prognosis metastatic testicular non-seminoma: a randomized study of the EORTC Genitourinary

Tract Cancer Cooperative Group. European Organization for Research and Treatment of Cancer. *Br J Cancer.* 1998 Sep;78(6):828-32.

[9] Frohlich MW, Small EJ. Stage II nonseminomatous testis cancer: the roles of primary and adjuvant chemotherapy. *Urol Clin North Am.* 1998 Aug;25(3):451-9.

[10] Loehrer PJ, Sr., Gonin R, Nichols CR, Weathers T, Einhorn LH. Vinblastine plus ifosfamide plus cisplatin as initial salvage therapy in recurrent germ cell tumor. *J Clin Oncol.* 1998 Jul;16(7):2500-4.

[11] Einhorn LH, Williams SD, Chamness A, Brames MJ, Perkins SM, Abonour R. High-dose chemotherapy and stem-cell rescue for metastatic germ-cell tumors. *N Engl J Med. 2007* Jul 26;357(4):340-8.

[12] Sundstrom S, Bremnes RM, Kaasa S, Aasebo U, Hatlevoll R, Dahle R, et al. Cisplatin and etoposide regimen is superior to cyclophosphamide, epirubicin, and vincristine regimen in small-cell lung cancer: results from a randomized phase III trial with 5 years' follow-up. *J Clin Oncol.* 2002 Dec 15;20(24):4665-72.

[13] Pignon JP, Arriagada R, Ihde DC, Johnson DH, Perry MC, Souhami RL, et al. A meta-analysis of thoracic radiotherapy for small-cell lung cancer. *N Engl J Med.* 1992 Dec 3;327(23):1618-24.

[14] Warde P, Payne D. Does thoracic irradiation improve survival and local control in limited-stage small-cell carcinoma of the lung? A meta-analysis. *J Clin Oncol.* 1992 Jun;10(6):890-5.

[15] Simon M, Argiris A, Murren JR. Progress in the therapy of small cell lung cancer. *Crit Rev Oncol Hematol.* 2004 Feb;49(2):119-33.

[16] Schiller JH, Adak S, Cella D, DeVore RF, 3rd, Johnson DH. Topotecan versus observation after cisplatin plus etoposide in extensive-stage small-cell lung cancer: E7593--a phase III trial of the Eastern Cooperative Oncology Group. *J Clin Oncol.* 2001 Apr 15;19(8):2114-22.

[17] Noda K, Nishiwaki Y, Kawahara M, Negoro S, Sugiura T, Yokoyama A, et al. Irinotecan plus cisplatin compared with etoposide plus cisplatin for extensive small-cell lung cancer. *N Engl J Med.* 2002 Jan 10;346(2):85-91.

[18] Hanna N, Bunn PA, Jr., Langer C, Einhorn L, Guthrie T, Jr., Beck T, et al. Randomized phase III trial comparing irinotecan/cisplatin with etoposide/cisplatin in patients with previously untreated extensive-stage disease small-cell lung cancer. *J Clin Oncol.* 2006 May 1;24(13):2038-43.

[19] Lara PN, Jr., Natale R, Crowley J, Lenz HJ, Redman MW, Carleton JE, et al. Phase III trial of irinotecan/cisplatin compared with etoposide/cisplatin in extensive-stage small-cell lung cancer: clinical and pharmacogenomic results from SWOG S0124. *J Clin Oncol.* 2009 May 20;27(15):2530-5.

[20] Loehrer PJ, Sr., Ansari R, Gonin R, Monaco F, Fisher W, Sandler A, et al. Cisplatin plus etoposide with and without ifosfamide in extensive small-cell lung cancer: a Hoosier Oncology Group study. *J Clin Oncol.* 1995 Oct;13(10):2594-9.

[21] Pujol JL, Daures JP, Riviere A, Quoix E, Westeel V, Quantin X, et al. Etoposide plus cisplatin with or without the combination of 4'-epidoxorubicin plus cyclophosphamide in treatment of extensive small-cell lung cancer: a French Federation of Cancer Institutes multicenter phase III randomized study. *J Natl Cancer Inst.* 2001 Feb 21;93(4):300-8.

[22] Miyamoto H, Nakabayashi T, Isobe H, Akita H, Kawakami Y, Arimoto T, et al. A phase III comparison of etoposide/cisplatin with or without added ifosfamide in small-cell lung cancer. *Oncology.* 1992;49(6):431-5.

[23] Niell HB, Herndon JE, 2nd, Miller AA, Watson DM, Sandler AB, Kelly K, et al. Randomized phase III intergroup trial of etoposide and cisplatin with or without paclitaxel and granulocyte colony-stimulating factor in patients with extensive-stage small-cell lung cancer: Cancer and Leukemia Group B Trial 9732. *J Clin Oncol.* 2005 Jun 1;23(16):3752-9.

[24] Ardizzoni A, Boni L, Tiseo M, Fossella FV, Schiller JH, Paesmans M, et al. Cisplatin-versus carboplatin-based chemotherapy in first-line treatment of advanced non-small-cell lung cancer: an individual patient data meta-analysis. *J Natl Cancer Inst.* 2007 Jun 6;99(11):847-57.

[25] Hotta K, Matsuo K, Ueoka H, Kiura K, Tabata M, Tanimoto M. Meta-analysis of randomized clinical trials comparing Cisplatin to Carboplatin in patients with advanced non-small-cell lung cancer. *J Clin Oncol.* 2004 Oct 1;22(19):3852-9.

[26] Arriagada R, Bergman B, Dunant A, Le Chevalier T, Pignon JP, Vansteenkiste J. Cisplatin-based adjuvant chemotherapy in patients with completely resected non-small-cell lung cancer. *N Engl J Med.* 2004 Jan 22;350(4):351-60.

[27] Douillard JY, Rosell R, De Lena M, Carpagnano F, Ramlau R, Gonzales-Larriba JL, et al. Adjuvant vinorelbine plus cisplatin versus observation in patients with completely resected stage IB-IIIA non-small-cell lung cancer (Adjuvant Navelbine International Trialist Association [ANITA]): a randomised controlled trial. *Lancet Oncol.* 2006 Sep;7(9):719-27.

[28] Winton T, Livingston R, Johnson D, Rigas J, Johnston M, Butts C, et al. Vinorelbine plus cisplatin vs. observation in resected non-small-cell lung cancer. *N Engl J Med.* 2005 Jun 23;352(25):2589-97.

[29] Pignon JP, Tribodet H, Scagliotti GV, Douillard JY, Shepherd FA, Stephens RJ, et al. Lung adjuvant cisplatin evaluation: a pooled analysis by the LACE Collaborative Group. *J Clin Oncol.* 2008 Jul 20;26(21):3552-9.

[30] Strauss GM, Herndon JE, 2nd, Maddaus MA, Johnstone DW, Johnson EA, Harpole DH, et al. Adjuvant paclitaxel plus carboplatin compared with observation in stage IB non-small-cell lung cancer: CALGB 9633 with the Cancer and Leukemia Group B, Radiation Therapy Oncology Group, and North Central Cancer Treatment Group Study Groups. *J Clin Oncol.* 2008 Nov 1;26(31):5043-51.

[31] Albain KS, Crowley JJ, Turrisi AT, 3rd, Gandara DR, Farrar WB, Clark JI, et al. Concurrent cisplatin, etoposide, and chest radiotherapy in pathologic stage IIIB non-small-cell lung cancer: a Southwest Oncology Group phase II study, SWOG 9019. *J Clin Oncol.* 2002 Aug 15;20(16):3454-60.

[32] Hanna N, Neubauer M, Yiannoutsos C, McGarry R, Arseneau J, Ansari R, et al. Phase III study of cisplatin, etoposide, and concurrent chest radiation with or without consolidation docetaxel in patients with inoperable stage III non-small-cell lung cancer: the Hoosier Oncology Group and U.S. *Oncology. J Clin Oncol.* 2008 Dec 10;26(35):5755-60.

[33] Schiller JH, Harrington D, Belani CP, Langer C, Sandler A, Krook J, et al. Comparison of four chemotherapy regimens for advanced non-small-cell lung cancer. *N Engl J Med.* 2002 Jan 10;346(2):92-8.

[34] Belani CP, Lee JS, Socinski MA, Robert F, Waterhouse D, Rowland K, et al. Randomized phase III trial comparing cisplatin-etoposide to carboplatin-paclitaxel in advanced or metastatic non-small cell lung cancer. *Ann Oncol.* 2005 Jul;16(7):1069-75.

[35] Cooper JS, Pajak TF, Forastiere AA, Jacobs J, Campbell BH, Saxman SB, et al. Postoperative concurrent radiotherapy and chemotherapy for high-risk squamous-cell carcinoma of the head and neck. *N Engl J Med.* 2004 May 6;350(19):1937-44.

[36] Bernier J, Domenge C, Ozsahin M, Matuszewska K, Lefebvre JL, Greiner RH, et al. Postoperative irradiation with or without concomitant chemotherapy for locally advanced head and neck cancer. *N Engl J Med.* 2004 May 6;350(19):1945-52.

[37] Hitt R, Lopez-Pousa A, Martinez-Trufero J, Escrig V, Carles J, Rizo A, et al. Phase III study comparing cisplatin plus fluorouracil to paclitaxel, cisplatin, and fluorouracil induction chemotherapy followed by chemoradiotherapy in locally advanced head and neck cancer. *J Clin Oncol.* 2005 Dec 1;23(34):8636-45.

[38] Lorch JH, Goloubeva O, Haddad RI, Cullen K, Sarlis N, Tishler R, et al. Induction chemotherapy with cisplatin and fluorouracil alone or in combination with docetaxel in locally advanced squamous-cell cancer of the head and neck: long-term results of the TAX 324 randomised phase 3 trial. *Lancet Oncol.* 2011 Feb;12(2):153-9.

[39] Posner MR, Hershock DM, Blajman CR, Mickiewicz E, Winquist E, Gorbounova V, et al. Cisplatin and fluorouracil alone or with docetaxel in head and neck cancer. *N Engl J Med.* 2007 Oct 25;357(17):1705-15.

[40] Vermorken JB, Remenar E, van Herpen C, Gorlia T, Mesia R, Degardin M, et al. Cisplatin, fluorouracil, and docetaxel in unresectable head and neck cancer. *N Engl J Med.* 2007 Oct 25;357(17):1695-704.

[41] Paccagnella A, Ghi MG, Loreggian L, Buffoli A, Koussis H, Mione CA, et al. Concomitant chemoradiotherapy versus induction docetaxel, cisplatin and 5 fluorouracil (TPF) followed by concomitant chemoradiotherapy in locally advanced head and neck cancer: a phase II randomized study. *Ann Oncol.* 2010 Jul;21(7):1515-22.

[42] Clavel M, Vermorken JB, Cognetti F, Cappelaere P, de Mulder PH, Schornagel JH, et al. Randomized comparison of cisplatin, methotrexate, bleomycin and vincristine (CABO) versus cisplatin and 5-fluorouracil (CF) versus cisplatin (C) in recurrent or metastatic squamous cell carcinoma of the head and neck. A phase III study of the EORTC Head and Neck Cancer Cooperative Group. *Ann Oncol.* 1994 Jul;5(6):521-6.

[43] Forastiere AA, Metch B, Schuller DE, Ensley JF, Hutchins LF, Triozzi P, et al. Randomized comparison of cisplatin plus fluorouracil and carboplatin plus fluorouracil versus methotrexate in advanced squamous-cell carcinoma of the head and neck: a Southwest Oncology Group study. *J Clin Oncol.* 1992 Aug;10(8):1245-51.

[44] Browman GP, Cronin L. Standard chemotherapy in squamous cell head and neck cancer: what we have learned from randomized trials. Semin Oncol. 1994 Jun;21(3):311-9.

[45] Gibson MK, Li Y, Murphy B, Hussain MH, DeConti RC, Ensley J, et al. Randomized phase III evaluation of cisplatin plus fluorouracil versus cisplatin plus paclitaxel in advanced head and neck cancer (E1395): an intergroup trial of the Eastern Cooperative Oncology Group. *J Clin Oncol.* 2005 May 20;23(15):3562-7.

[46] Keys HM, Bundy BN, Stehman FB, Muderspach LI, Chafe WE, Suggs CL, 3rd, et al. Cisplatin, radiation, and adjuvant hysterectomy compared with radiation and adjuvant

hysterectomy for bulky stage IB cervical carcinoma. *N Engl J Med.* 1999 Apr 15;340(15):1154-61.

[47] Morris M, Eifel PJ, Lu J, Grigsby PW, Levenback C, Stevens RE, et al. Pelvic radiation with concurrent chemotherapy compared with pelvic and para-aortic radiation for high-risk cervical cancer. *N Engl J Med.* 1999 Apr 15;340(15):1137-43.

[48] Rose PG, Bundy BN, Watkins EB, Thigpen JT, Deppe G, Maiman MA, et al. Concurrent cisplatin-based radiotherapy and chemotherapy for locally advanced cervical cancer. *N Engl J Med.* 1999 Apr 15;340(15):1144-53.

[49] Carey MS, Gawlik C, Fung-Kee-Fung M, Chambers A, Oliver T. Systematic review of systemic therapy for advanced or recurrent endometrial cancer. *Gynecol Oncol.* 2006 Apr;101(1):158-67.

[50] Humber CE, Tierney JF, Symonds RP, Collingwood M, Kirwan J, Williams C, et al. Chemotherapy for advanced, recurrent or metastatic endometrial cancer: a systematic review of Cochrane collaboration. *Ann Oncol.* 2007 Mar;18(3):409-20.

[51] Fleming GF, Brunetto VL, Cella D, Look KY, Reid GC, Munkarah AR, et al. Phase III trial of doxorubicin plus cisplatin with or without paclitaxel plus filgrastim in advanced endometrial carcinoma: a Gynecologic Oncology Group Study. *J Clin Oncol.* 2004 Jun 1;22(11):2159-66.

[52] Covens A, Carey M, Bryson P, Verma S, Fung Kee Fung M, Johnston M. Systematic review of first-line chemotherapy for newly diagnosed postoperative patients with stage II, III, or IV epithelial ovarian cancer. *Gynecol Oncol.* 2002 Apr;85(1):71-80.

[53] du Bois A, Luck HJ, Meier W, Adams HP, Mobus V, Costa S, et al. A randomized clinical trial of cisplatin/paclitaxel versus carboplatin/paclitaxel as first-line treatment of ovarian cancer. *J Natl Cancer Inst.* 2003 Sep 3;95(17):1320-9.

[54] Ozols RF, Bundy BN, Greer BE, Fowler JM, Clarke-Pearson D, Burger RA, et al. Phase III trial of carboplatin and paclitaxel compared with cisplatin and paclitaxel in patients with optimally resected stage III ovarian cancer: a Gynecologic Oncology Group study. *J Clin Oncol.* 2003 Sep 1;21(17):3194-200.

[55] Piccart MJ, Bertelsen K, James K, Cassidy J, Mangioni C, Simonsen E, et al. Randomized intergroup trial of cisplatin-paclitaxel versus cisplatin-cyclophosphamide in women with advanced epithelial ovarian cancer: three-year results. *J Natl Cancer Inst.* 2000 May 3;92(9):699-708.

[56] Alberts DS, Liu PY, Hannigan EV, O'Toole R, Williams SD, Young JA, et al. Intraperitoneal cisplatin plus intravenous cyclophosphamide versus intravenous cisplatin plus intravenous cyclophosphamide for stage III ovarian cancer. *N Engl J Med.* 1996 Dec 26;335(26):1950-5.

[57] Armstrong DK, Bundy B, Wenzel L, Huang HQ, Baergen R, Lele S, et al. Intraperitoneal cisplatin and paclitaxel in ovarian cancer. *N Engl J Med.* 2006 Jan 5;354(1):34-43.

[58] Markman M, Bundy BN, Alberts DS, Fowler JM, Clark-Pearson DL, Carson LF, et al. Phase III trial of standard-dose intravenous cisplatin plus paclitaxel versus moderately high-dose carboplatin followed by intravenous paclitaxel and intraperitoneal cisplatin in small-volume stage III ovarian carcinoma: an intergroup study of the Gynecologic Oncology Group, Southwestern Oncology Group, and Eastern Cooperative Oncology Group. *J Clin Oncol.* 2001 Feb 15;19(4):1001-7.

[59] Yano T, Itoh Y, Matsuo M, Kawashiri T, Egashira N, Oishi R. Involvement of both tumor necrosis factor-alpha-induced necrosis and p53-mediated caspase-dependent apoptosis in nephrotoxicity of cisplatin. *Apoptosis.* 2007 Oct;12(10):1901-9.

[60] Meijer S, Sleijfer DT, Mulder NH, Sluiter WJ, Marrink J, Koops HS, et al. Some effects of combination chemotherapy with cis-platinum on renal function in patients with nonseminomatous testicular carcinoma. *Cancer.* 1983 Jun 1;51(11):2035-40.

[61] Gonzales-Vitale JC, Hayes DM, Cvit-kovic E, Sternberg SS. The renal pathology in clinical trials of cis-platinum (II) diamminedichloride. *Cancer.* 1977;39(4):1362-71.

[62] Berghmans T. Hyponatremia related to medical anticancer treatment. *Support Care Cancer.* 1996 Sep;4(5):341-50.

[63] Hutchison FN, Perez EA, Gandara DR, Lawrence HJ, Kaysen GA. Renal salt wasting in patients treated with cisplatin. *Ann Intern Med.* 1988 Jan;108(1):21-5.

[64] el Weshi A, Thieblemont C, Cottin V, Barbet N, Catimel G. Cisplatin-induced hyponatremia and renal sodium wasting. *Acta Oncol.* 1995;34(2):264-5.

[65] Levin L, Sealy R, Barron J. Syndrome of inappropriate antidiuretic hormone secretion following dis-dichlorodiammineplatinum II in a patient with malignant thymoma. *Cancer.* 1982 Dec 1;50(11):2279-82.

[66] Porter AT. Syndrome of inappropriate antidiuretic hormone secretion during cis-dichlorodiammineplatinum therapy in a patient with an ovarian carcinoma. *Gynecol Oncol.* 1985 May;21(1):103-5.

[67] Bissett D, Cornford EJ, Sokal M. Hyponatraemia following cisplatin chemotherapy. *Acta Oncol.* 1989;28(6):823.

[68] Ritch PS. Cis-dichlorodiammineplatinum II-induced syndrome of inappropriate secretion of antidiuretic hormone. *Cancer.* 1988 Feb 1;61(3):448-50.

[69] Goldstein RS, Mayor GH. Minireview. The nephrotoxicity of cisplatin. *Life Sci.* 1983 Feb 14;32(7):685-90.

[70] Madias NE, Harrington JT. Platinum nephrotoxicity. *Am J Med.* 1978 Aug;65(2):307-14.

[71] Heidemann HT, Gerkens JF, Jackson EK, Branch RA. Attenuation of cisplatinum-induced nephrotoxicity in the rat by high salt diet, furosemide and acetazolamide. *Naunyn Schmiedebergs Arch Pharmacol.* 1985 Apr;329(2):201-5.

[72] Pera MF, Jr., Zook BC, Harder HC. Effects of mannitol or furosemide diuresis on the nephrotoxicity and physiological disposition of cis-dichlorodiammineplatinum-(II) in rats. *Cancer Res.* 1979 Apr;39(4):1269-78.

[73] Lehane D, Winston A, Gray R, Daskal Y. The effect of diuretic pre-treatment on clinical, morphological and ultrastructural cis-platinum induced nephrotoxicity. *Int J Radiat Oncol Biol Phys.* 1979 Aug;5(8):1393-9.

[74] Al-Sarraf M, Fletcher W, Oishi N, Pugh R, Hewlett JS, Balducci L, et al. Cisplatin hydration with and without mannitol diuresis in refractory disseminated malignant melanoma: a southwest oncology group study. *Cancer Treat Rep.* 1982 Jan;66(1):31-5.

[75] Santoso JT, Lucci JA, 3rd, Coleman RL, Schafer I, Hannigan EV. Saline, mannitol, and furosemide hydration in acute cisplatin nephrotoxicity: a randomized trial. *Cancer Chemother Pharmacol.* 2003 Jul;52(1):13-8.

[76] Salem P, Khalyl M, Jabboury K, Hashimi L. Cis-diamminedichloroplatinum (II) by 5-day continuous infusion. A new dose schedule with minimal toxicity. *Cancer.* 1984 Feb 15;53(4):837-40.

[77] Haas A, Anderson L, Lad T. The influence of aminoglycosides on the nephrotoxicity of cis-diamminedichloroplatinum in cancer patients. *J Infect Dis.* 1983 Feb;147(2):363.

[78] Hodgkinson E, Neville-Webbe HL, Coleman RE. Magnesium depletion in patients receiving cisplatin-based chemotherapy. *Clin Oncol* (R Coll Radiol). 2006 Nov;18(9):710-8.

[79] Cohen L, de Moor CA, Eisenberg P, Ming EE, Hu H. Chemotherapy-induced nausea and vomiting: incidence and impact on patient quality of life at community oncology settings. *Support Care Cancer.* 2007 May;15(5):497-503.

[80] Hesketh PJ. Chemotherapy-induced nausea and vomiting. *N Engl J Med.* 2008 Jun 5;358(23):2482-94.

[81] del Giglio A, Soares HP, Caparroz C, Castro PC. Granisetron is equivalent to ondansetron for prophylaxis of chemotherapy-induced nausea and vomiting: results of a meta-analysis of randomized controlled trials. *Cancer. 2000* Dec 1;89(11):2301-8.

[82] Jordan K, Hinke A, Grothey A, Schmoll HJ. Granisetron versus tropisetron for prophylaxis of acute chemotherapy-induced emesis: a pooled analysis. *Support Care Cancer.* 2005 Jan;13(1):26-31.

[83] Aapro MS, Grunberg SM, Manikhas GM, Olivares G, Suarez T, Tjulandin SA, et al. A phase III, double-blind, randomized trial of palonosetron compared with ondansetron in preventing chemotherapy-induced nausea and vomiting following highly emetogenic chemotherapy. *Ann Oncol.* 2006 Sep;17(9):1441-9.

[84] Hesketh PJ, Grunberg SM, Gralla RJ, Warr DG, Roila F, de Wit R, et al. The oral neurokinin-1 antagonist aprepitant for the prevention of chemotherapy-induced nausea and vomiting: a multinational, randomized, double-blind, placebo-controlled trial in patients receiving high-dose cisplatin--the Aprepitant Protocol 052 Study Group. *J Clin Oncol.* 2003 Nov 15;21(22):4112-9.

[85] Poli-Bigelli S, Rodrigues-Pereira J, Carides AD, Julie Ma G, Eldridge K, Hipple A, et al. Addition of the neurokinin 1 receptor antagonist aprepitant to standard antiemetic therapy improves control of chemotherapy-induced nausea and vomiting. Results from a randomized, double-blind, placebo-controlled trial in Latin America. *Cancer.* 2003 Jun 15;97(12):3090-8.

[86] Schmoll HJ, Aapro MS, Poli-Bigelli S, Kim HK, Park K, Jordan K, et al. Comparison of an aprepitant regimen with a multiple-day ondansetron regimen, both with dexamethasone, for antiemetic efficacy in high-dose cisplatin treatment. *Ann Oncol.* 2006 Jun;17(6):1000-6.

[87] Ithimakin S, Runglodvatana K, Nimmannit A, Akewanlop C, Srimuninnimit V, Keerativitayanan N, et al. Randomized, double-blinded, placebo-controlled trial of ondansetron plus dexamethasone with or without metoclopramide as antiemetic prophylaxis in patients receiving high-dose cisplatin in medical practice. *Support Care Cancer.* 2011 Apr 20.

[88] Kris MG, Hesketh PJ, Somerfield MR, Feyer P, Clark-Snow R, Koeller JM, et al. American Society of Clinical Oncology guideline for antiemetics in oncology: update 2006. *J Clin Oncol.* 2006 Jun 20;24(18):2932-47.

[89] Ito Y, Arahata Y, Goto Y, Hirayama M, Nagamutsu M, Yasuda T, et al. Cisplatin neurotoxicity presenting as reversible posterior leukoencephalopathy syndrome. *AJNR Am J Neuroradiol.* 1998 Mar;19(3):415-7.

[90] von Schlippe M, Fowler CJ, Harland SJ. Cisplatin neurotoxicity in the treatment of metastatic germ cell tumour: time course and prognosis. Br J Cancer. 2001 Sep 14;85(6):823-6.

[91] Albers JW, Chaudhry V, Cavaletti G, Donehower RC. Interventions for preventing neuropathy caused by cisplatin and related compounds. Cochrane Database Syst Rev. 2011(2):CD005228.

[92] Reddel RR, Kefford RF, Grant JM, Coates AS, Fox RM, Tattersall MH. Ototoxicity in patients receiving cisplatin: importance of dose and method of drug administration. *Cancer Treat Rep.* 1982 Jan;66(1):19-23.

[93] Bertolini P, Lassalle M, Mercier G, Raquin MA, Izzi G, Corradini N, et al. Platinum compound-related ototoxicity in children: long-term follow-up reveals continuous worsening of hearing loss. *J Pediatr Hematol Oncol.* 2004 Oct;26(10):649-55.

[94] Fouladi M, Chintagumpala M, Ashley D, Kellie S, Gururangan S, Hassall T, et al. Amifostine protects against cisplatin-induced ototoxicity in children with average-risk medulloblastoma. *J Clin Oncol.* 2008 Aug 1;26(22):3749-55.

[95] Marina N, Chang KW, Malogolowkin M, London WB, Frazier AL, Womer RB, et al. Amifostine does not protect against the ototoxicity of high-dose cisplatin combined with etoposide and bleomycin in pediatric germ-cell tumors: a Children's Oncology Group study. *Cancer.* 2005 Aug 15;104(4):841-7.

[96] Paulino AC, Lobo M, Teh BS, Okcu MF, South M, Butler EB, et al. Ototoxicity after intensity-modulated radiation therapy and cisplatin-based chemotherapy in children with medulloblastoma. *Int J Radiat Oncol Biol Phys.* 2010 Dec 1;78(5):1445-50.

[97] Rossof AH, Slayton RE, Perlia CP. Preliminary clinical experience with cis-diamminedichloroplatinum (II) (NSC 119875, CACP*). Cancer.* 1972 Dec;30(6):1451-6.

[98] Ithimakin S, Srimuninnimit V. Cancer anemia survey in Division of Medical Oncology at Siriraj Hospital (CAS). *J Med Assoc Thai.* 2009 Mar;92 Suppl 2:S110-8.

[99] Von Hoff DD, Schilsky R, Reichert CM, Reddick RL, Rozencweig M, Young RC, et al. Toxic effects of cis-dichlorodiammineplatinum(II) in man. *Cancer Treat Rep.* 1979 Sep-Oct;63(9-10):1527-31.

[100] Ludwig H, Van Belle S, Barrett-Lee P, Birgegard G, Bokemeyer C, Gascon P, et al. The European Cancer Anaemia Survey (ECAS): a large, multinational, prospective survey defining the prevalence, incidence, and treatment of anaemia in cancer patients. *Eur J Cancer.* 2004 Oct;40(15):2293-306.

[101] Bohlius J, Wilson J, Seidenfeld J, Piper M, Schwarzer G, Sandercock J, et al. Recombinant human erythropoietins and cancer patients: updated meta-analysis of 57 studies including 9353 patients. *J Natl Cancer Inst.* 2006 May 17;98(10):708-14.

[102] Vansteenkiste J, Pirker R, Massuti B, Barata F, Font A, Fiegl M, et al. Double-blind, placebo-controlled, randomized phase III trial of darbepoetin alfa in lung cancer patients receiving chemotherapy. *J Natl Cancer Inst.* 2002 Aug 21;94(16):1211-20.

[103] Littlewood TJ, Bajetta E, Nortier JW, Vercammen E, Rapoport B. Effects of epoetin alfa on hematologic parameters and quality of life in cancer patients receiving nonplatinum chemotherapy: results of a randomized, double-blind, placebo-controlled trial. *J Clin Oncol.* 2001 Jun 1;19(11):2865-74.

[104] Henke M, Laszig R, Rube C, Schafer U, Haase KD, Schilcher B, et al. Erythropoietin to treat head and neck cancer patients with anaemia undergoing radiotherapy:

randomised, double-blind, placebo-controlled trial. *Lancet.* 2003 Oct 18;362(9392):1255-60.

[105] Smith RE, Jr., Aapro MS, Ludwig H, Pinter T, Smakal M, Ciuleanu TE, et al. Darbepoetin alpha for the treatment of anemia in patients with active cancer not receiving chemotherapy or radiotherapy: results of a phase III, multicenter, randomized, double-blind, placebo-controlled study. *J Clin Oncol.* 2008 Mar 1;26(7):1040-50.

[106] Thomas G, Ali S, Hoebers FJ, Darcy KM, Rodgers WH, Patel M, et al. Phase III trial to evaluate the efficacy of maintaining hemoglobin levels above 12.0 g/dL with erythropoietin vs above 10.0 g/dL without erythropoietin in anemic patients receiving concurrent radiation and cisplatin for cervical cancer. *Gynecol Oncol.* 2008 Feb;108(2):317-25.

[107] Wright JR, Ung YC, Julian JA, Pritchard KI, Whelan TJ, Smith C, et al. Randomized, double-blind, placebo-controlled trial of erythropoietin in non-small-cell lung cancer with disease-related anemia. *J Clin Oncol.* 2007 Mar 20;25(9):1027-32.

[108] Leyland-Jones B, Semiglazov V, Pawlicki M, Pienkowski T, Tjulandin S, Manikhas G, et al. Maintaining normal hemoglobin levels with epoetin alfa in mainly nonanemic patients with metastatic breast cancer receiving first-line chemotherapy: a survival study. *J Clin Oncol.* 2005 Sep 1;23(25):5960-72.

[109] Bennett CL, Silver SM, Djulbegovic B, Samaras AT, Blau CA, Gleason KJ, et al. Venous thromboembolism and mortality associated with recombinant erythropoietin and darbepoetin administration for the treatment of cancer-associated anemia. *JAMA.* 2008 Feb 27;299(8):914-24.

[110] Bohlius J, Schmidlin K, Brillant C, Schwarzer G, Trelle S, Seidenfeld J, et al. Recombinant human erythropoiesis-stimulating agents and mortality in patients with cancer: a meta-analysis of randomised trials. *Lancet.* 2009 May 2;373(9674):1532-42.

[111] Tonelli M, Hemmelgarn B, Reiman T, Manns B, Reaume MN, Lloyd A, et al. Benefits and harms of erythropoiesis-stimulating agents for anemia related to cancer: a meta-analysis. *CMAJ.* 2009 May 26;180(11):E62-71.

In: Cisplatin: Pharmacology, Clinical Uses and Adverse Effects ISBN: 978-1-61942-359-6
Editors: Toshiko Kojima and Yoko Morita

Chapter IV

INTERACTIONS BETWEEN CISPLATIN AND PROTEINS, AND THEIR PHARMACOLOGICAL IMPLICATIONS

Xianchan Li,[1] Zhilong Zhao,[2] Wenbing Hu[1] and Fuyi Wang[1,*]

[1]Beijing National Laboratory for Molecular Sciences, CAS Key Laboratory of Analytical Chemistry for Living Biosystems, Institute of Chemistry, the Chinese Academy of Sciences (CAS), Beijing, China

[2]The Affiliated Zhongshan Hospital of Dalian University, Dalian, China

ABSTRACT

Cisplatin, (cis- diamminedichloroplatinum, CDDP)), has been widely used over the last 30 years for chemotherapy of various solid tumors, including testicular and ovarian, bladder, oral, head and neck and small cell lung and bladder cancers. [1-3] It has been thought for long time that the formation of intra-stranded and inter-stranded crosslinked DNA adducts triggers apoptosis signaling by high mobility group box 1 (HMGB1) protein recognition and the consequent blocking of nucleotide excision repair (NER). [4-7] However, both *in vivo* and *in vitro* researches have suggested that only a very modest fraction of the administered cisplatin reacts with nuclear DNA and produces cytotoxic lesions, and the largest amount reacts with various types of proteins outside and inside of cells *via* coordinating to cysteine, methionine, histidine and tyrosine residues. [8,9] For instance, following intravenous administration cisplatin can bind extensively to serum proteins [9-11] such as albumin, [10,12] transferrin8, [13] and hemoglobin; [11,14,15] and transport proteins such as the organic cation transporters (OCTs) [16] and the copper transporters Ctr1. [17] And inside cells cisplatin can also bind to various polypeptides and proteins, including Cu-transporting ATPases ATP7B and ATP7A, [18] the copper chaperone Atox1, [19-21] insulin, [22] metallothioniens, [15,23-25] cytochrome *c*, [15,26-29] superoxide dismutase, [29-32] ubiquitin, [29,33] and etc. Such interactions may have a crucial effect on the bioavailability, transport and metabolism of cisplatin, and some are thought to be associated with undesired side effects and acquired resistance of the drug. [9]

[*] Email: fiui.wang@iccas.ac.cn.

On the other hand, a number of cellular proteins and enzymes are implicated in the cellular responses to the formation of platinated DNA adducts, in particular, inter-stranded crosslinked DNA adducts, including those involved in regulating the signaling of DNA damage, cell-cycle checkpoints and arrest, DNA repair and cell death. [5,7] However, this chapter is mainly focused on highlighting the update advances on the research of directly interactions between cisplatin and proteins which are thought to be associated with the cellular uptake, transport, efflux and distribution of cisplatin, looking to future directions of development of platinum-based anticancer agents.

1. Plasma Protein

As cisplatin is administrated *via* intravenous injection, cisplatin firstly encounters plasma proteins, and extensively binds to plasma proteins, [34] for example, albumin, transferrin and macroglobulin, through the coordination of the "soft" metal platinum to the sulfur atoms in cysteine and methionine, and the nitrogen atom in the imidazole ring of histidine residues. [35] A most recent *in vitro* study on the protein binding of cisplatin in human plasma indicates that 95% of platinum was protein-bound [24] h after the addition of cisplatin to plasma, whereas 40% of platinum was protein-bound in the case of carboplatin, the less toxic platinum-based anticancer drug which is also widely used in clinic as a replacement of cispaltin. [11]

The distribution of cisplatin-protein adducts in human blood plasma has been extensively investigated by various analytical methods, including ultrafiltration fractionation coupled with electrothermal atomic absorption spectrometry (ETAAS) and inductively coupling plasma – atomic emission spectrometry (ICP-AES) or ICP-MS (mass spectrometry) detection, which demonstrated that the highest percentage of platinum is bound to the fraction with the largest molecular mass (*MW* > 100 kDa). [11,36,37] Some studies have revealed the following reaction activity of cisplatin towards different plasma proteins: hemoglobin > albumin > immunoglobulin. [38] A centrifuging filtration method was used to compare the binding percentages of cisplatin to serum proteins *in vitro*, with the result of 72.3% ± 6.5% for albumin, 39.5% ± 2.5% for α_1-acid glycoprotein, and 49.2%±1.9% for γ-globulin. [39]

1.1. Albumin

Human serum albumin (HSA) is the most abundant serum protein (about 52%) with a serum concentration of 40–45 g L^{-1} in healthy humans (ca. 0.6 mM). It (*MW* 66-67 kDa) comprises a single-chain with 585 amino acids organized in three similar domains (I, II, and III), each consisting of two subdomains (IA, IB, etc.). HSA contains 17 disulfide bridges, one free thiol group at Cys-34, and one tryptophan residue at Try-214, which are located in hydrophobic cavities in subdomains IIA and IIIA, with the mutual binding potential toward many types of compounds, for example, fatty acids, bilirubin, metal ions, steroid hormones, vitamins, and pharmaceuticals, including metallodrugs. HSA performs as a transport protein responsible for the transport of metals, fatty acids, thyroid hormones and drugs. [40-42] Binding of drugs to serum albumin affects their metabolism, efficacy, and body distribution. [43] It has been reported [44,45] that the cell toxicity of the complex of cisplatin-HSA was decreased seriously or even lost in *in vitro* studies. Yet a few researchers thought that some cisplatin linked to specific sites on HSA could be released or substituted, and the cytotoxicity of cisplatin would be recovered inside cells. In other words, HSA services as the reservoir of cisplatin in blood. [46] Therefore, increasing interest has been drawn in the investigation on the coordinative chemistry of the interaction of cisplatin and HSA.

Although numerous studies on the interaction of cisplatin with albumin have been reported, few Pt binding sites have been characterized unambiguously. The cysteine-34 residue, sterically accessible for drug molecules, is one of the most likely places for platinum attachment.

However, bovine serum albumin with no free SH group still bound substantial amounts of cisplatin, [47] which suggested there should be additional binding sites on the protein that participate in adduct formation. According to NMR spectroscopic study by Sadler et al, [48] the Met298 S,N macrochelate was the major cisplatin binding site, and monofunctional adducts involving Cys34 and surface histidine residues were also observed. Recently, using multidimensional liquid chromatograph coupled with tandem mass spectrometry (LC-MS/MS), Sheldrick et. al. identified Cys34, Met329, Tyr150 (or Tyr148) and Asp375 (or Glu376) residues as the cisplatin binding sites in albumin after incubating cisplatin with blood serum for 3h. [49]

According to their FTIR study, [50] Neault et. al. concluded that cisplatin binds to human serum albumin through the polypeptide C–N, C=O and sulfur donor groups. At high cisplatin contents, drug–protein binding occurs with the participation of the tyrosine residues and major alterations of the protein secondary structure from that of the α-helix to β-sheet conformation. In a most recent work, applying LC-MS/MS approach to analyze the tryptic digestion of recombinant human albumin (rHA)-cispaltin complex, we found that cisplatin binds to surface residues His67, His 128, His247 and Met298 in albumin, involving an inter-domain crosslinking of His67 and His247 by platinum (Figure 1). [51] Since residues His67 and His247 form part of the proposed major zinc-binding site on albumin, the crosslinking of His67 and His247 indicates that cisplatin coordination to rHA may disturb Zn transport *via* HSA binding (Figure 2), and perhaps account for hyperzincuria and hypozincemia developed in patients treated with cisplatin. [52]

As was demonstrated in a number of subsequent reports, platinum-based drugs could react with oxidized glutathione (GSSG) and induce the cleavage of the disulfide bond of GSSG. [53-55] As mentioned above, HSA contains 17 disulfide bridges, some of which could be broken during platinum binding possibly followed by intramolecular cross-linking of protein molecules. [56,57]

As reported by Yotsuyanagi et al, 1 mol of disulfide bond was cleaved upon binding every 5.3 mol of cisplatin, which totals the overall disulfide-bond cleavage of HSA up to four during cisplatin binding. [56]

As a consequence, the protein's biological activity may be subject to changes since disulfide bonds play an important role in maintaining the structure and the biological function of the proteins. In our most recent study, [51] cisplatin is shown to be able to induce the cleavage of the disulfide bond Cys124-Cys169 of HSA, [51] which may change the hydrophobicity of the binding cavities of heme and bilirubin in subdomains IIA and IIIA of HSA, and hinder the binding of these types of endogenous molecules to albmin.

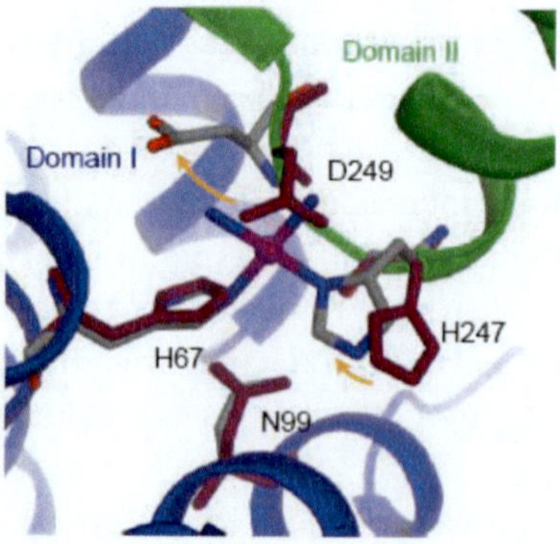

Figure 1. Superposition of a model of the His67-His247 adduct of human albumin with cis-$\{(NH_3)_2Pt\}^{2+}$ (energy-minimized, $\{(NH_3)_2Pt\}$ in CPK coloring) and the X-ray structure of unliganded rHA (PDB ID 1bm0, magenta) showing crosslinking of domains I and II by Pt. Orange arrows indicate direction of rotation of side chains of His247 and Asp249 induced by Pt coordination. Figure is prepared using PyMol Ver 0.99rc6 (Reproduced with permission from reference 20. Copyright 2011 RSC).

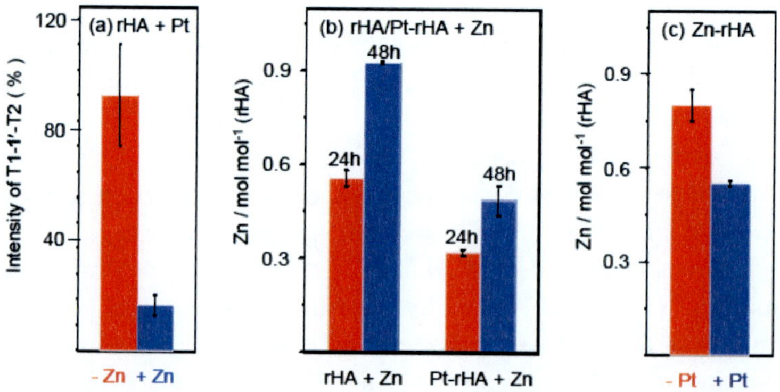

Figure 2. Competitive binding of cisplatin and zinc to human albumin. (a) Relative intensities (%) of cis-$\{(NH_3)_2Pt\}^{2+}$ (**1′**) His67-His247 crosslinked platinated peptide ion $\{$T1-**1′**-T2$\}^{5+}$ (T1 = (65)SLH*TLFGDK(73), T2 = (241)VHTECCH*GDLLECADDR(257); * represents platniated histidine residue) in the tryptic digests of Pt-rHA adducts formed in the absence or presence of Zn^{2+} (rHA:cPt:Zn = 1:5:5, cPt = cisplatin) in 20 mM TEAA buffer at 310 K for 80 h. The average value (n = 3) of the relative signal intensity of $\{$T1-**1′**-T2$\}^{5+}$ in the absence of Zn was set as 100%; (b) Zinc bound to rHA determined from reaction mixtures of zinc acetate with native rHA or Pt-rHA complex in 20 mM TEAA buffer at 310 K for 24 h or 48 h (rHA:Zn or Pt-rHA:Zn = 0.05:0.05 mM); (c) Zinc bound to rHA in 20 mM TEAA buffer (pH 7.4) incubated in the absence or presence of 10-fold excess of cisplatin at 310 K for 80 h. Zn content is the mean from three independent determinations. (Reproduced with permission from reference 20. Copyright 2011 RSC.).

1.2. Transferrin

Human serum transferrin (Tf) with a molecular mass of approximately 80 kDa is found in blood plasma at a concentration of about 2.5 g L^{-1} (35 μM) in healthy humans. [8,58] The Tf molecule is stabilized by 19 intra-chain disulfide bonds and is protected by three carbohydrate side chains of which two are N-linked (Asn-413 and Asn-611) and the third is O-linked (Ser-

32). As one kind of iron-transport glycoproteins, transferrin is capable of binding two iron ions in oxidation state +3. Transferrin arranged two similar lobes (N- and C-terminal lobe), each containing one iron binding site consisting of two tyrosines, one histidine, one aspartate and a bicarbonate anion bound in an adjacent pocket. Tf binds to iron(Ⅲ) in blood and delivers it to cells through the Tf receptor (TfR). When Tf is internalized by cells, the iron is released, and the protein is recirculated. Certain diseased cells, for instance cancer cells, have a high iron(Ⅲ) requirement, in order to facilitate rapid cell growth, which is satisfied by the increasing expression of TfR on the cell surface and thereby sequestering a greater amount of the circulating metal-loaded Tf. [59,60] Under physiological conditions, only 30% of Tf is bound to iron, there is potential use in diagnosis and therapy because Tf can bind strongly to a range of other metal ions and many heterometal-transferrin complexes are still recognized by transferrin receptor (TfR). [8,61] The efficient binding of cisplatin to transferrin has been recognized as the important route for cisplatin input and transport of cancer cells.

During the past decades, there has been a large body of reports about the binding sites of cisplatin to transferrin. Sadler and co-workers confirmed that the preferred binding site in Tf for cisplatin analog [Pt(en)Cl_2] appears to be Met256 according to NMR spectroscopic data. [58,62] Dyson et al suggested that the surface threonine Thr457, which is involved in the coordination with iron, was likely the only specific coordination site of cisplatin in human transferrin. [13] Their UV spectroscopic data and molecular modeling indicated that there is a competition between cisplatin and iron for the iron binding site, as a consequence, cisplatin binding retards coordination of iron to Tf. Sheldrick and co-workers reported that apart from Thr457, O-donor side chains of Y314, E265, E385 on Tf were also kinetically preferred binding sites for cisplatin. [49] According to one of our ongoing studies, formation of cisplatin-Tf adduct appears to hinder the interactions of Tf and TfR (unpublished data), implying that cisplatin may substitute iron binding to Tf. On the other hand, we also found that both the cellular uptake and nuclear uptake levels of cisplatin conjugating to Tf significantly decreased compared to those of cisplatin alone. These finding suggest that it is not a rational strategy to apply transferrin as the drug carrier for cisplatin.

1.3. Hemoglobin

Hemoglobin is perhaps the most thoroughly studied protein with respect to structure and function because of its importance in biological system. It posses a heterotetrameric structure composed of four subunits having similar three-dimensional (3D) structures, two identical α-chains of 141 amino acid residues (15126.4 Da) each referred to as α_1 and α_2 subunits, and two identical β-chains, β_1 and β_2, of 146 amino acid residues (15867.2 Da) each. Each subunit has a heme-binding pocket. The heme group, which is deeply buried in the hydrophobic pockets of Hb, coordinated to the proximal histidine (His F8) and abutted upon the distal histidine (His E7) with a gap to bind oxygen, is a five-coordinate high-spin complex.

Structure changes of hemoglobin induced by cisplatin, as well as the second generation of platinum-based anticancer drugs oxaliplatin and carboplatin, were studied using both nanoelectrospray mass spectrometry (nanoESI-MS) and a combination of size exclusion high performance liquid chromatography with inductively coupled plasma mass spectrometry (HPLC-ICP-MS). [63-65] Nanospray MS analyses of reaction mixtures of cisplatin with Hb demonstrated that the ion at *m/z* 616.5 corresponding to the heme group increased in content with an increase of cisplatin concentration, indicating the loss of heme groups from the protein.

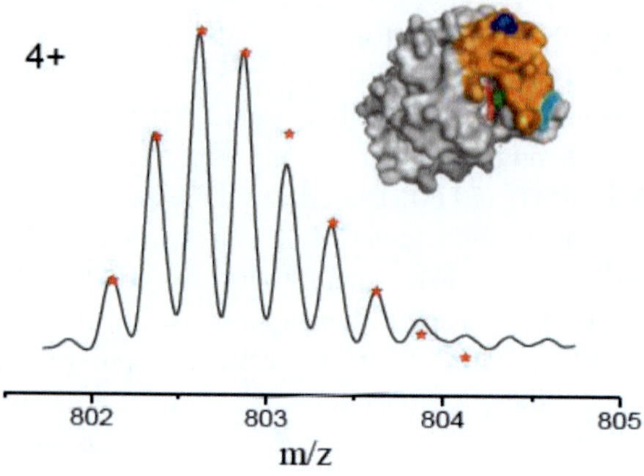

Figure 3. Isotopic models (pentacle) and mass spectra (lines) for mono-platinated peptide: (62)VADALTNAVAHVDDMPNALSALSDLHAHK(90) detected from the tryptic digestion of cisplatin-Hb adduct (unpublished data).

Concerning the place of coordination, size-exclusion HPLC separation of free and protein-bound cisplatin followed by simultaneous monitoring of [195]Pt and [57]Fe by ICP-MS demonstrated the presence of Hb-bound Pt complexes, and the platinum moiety is mainly attached to an intact protein molecule. Participating in a supplementary but a weaker binding were the pockets accommodating the heme groups which could be released from the protein subject to platinum coordination.

Nanospray quadrupole time-of-flight mass spectrometry (NonoESI-TOF-MS) studies of the Hb–cisplatin complexes further demonstrated the specific binding of cisplatin to the α-chain, heme-α, β-chain, and heme-β units of hemoglobin. The findings of the cisplatin interaction with Hb and the dissociation of heme from Hb are helpful to a better understanding of the toxicity and side effects of cisplatin as well as to optimize treatment strategies. In our recent work, LC-ESI-QTOF-MS analysis enables to identify six platinated peptides from the tryptic digestions of cisplatin-Hb adducts, of which one platinated peptide is consist of amino acid residues AA62 – AA90 which contains His87 coordinated with heme group on α chain of intact Hb (Figure 3, unpublished data).

Our results also show that the reactivity of cisplatin towards Hb is higher than that of ruthenium-based metal anticancer complexes. [66,67] Further studies to characterize the exactly binding site is being undertaken.

2. Transport Proteins

Cisplatin is a polar compound, and its cellular accumulation generally occurs at a slower rate than that of other small-molecule anticancer drugs. Krieger et al found that in ovarian cancer cell lines cisplatin delivered in liposomes displayed high efficacy compared with in monophasic aqueous solution, [68] demonstrating that cisplatin does not readily traverse the lipid bilayer.

Therefore, uptake and efflux of cisplatin by cells must be facilitated by membrane transport proteins including organic cation transporter (OCTs) and copper transporters.

2.1. Organic Cation Transporters (OCTs)

OCTs mediates the transport of organic cations having MW < 400 Da across the cell membrane. [69] OCT1-3 are believed to play a role in platinum drug uptake. [16,70] Cisplatin has been shown to compete for uptake with the tetraethylammonium (TEA), an OCTs substrate, [71] indicating that cispaltin binds to OCT in a similar way to that of TEA. Besides cisplatin, OCTs had been found to mediate the uptake of other platinum compounds, such as oxaliplatin [71] and $[Pt(NH_3)_2(pyridine)Cl]^+$, [69] but not carboplatin and nedaplatin. [71].

2.2. Copper Transporter-1(Ctr1)

Ctr1 is not only essential for high-affinity copper uptake but also responsible for making copper available in the cytosol utilization by various cellular proteins and further efflux in mammalian cells. Ctr1 is a homotrimer, in which each of the monomer composites four key domains: an extracellular N-terminus; three transmembrane (TM) helices; an intracellular loop connecting the first and second TM helices and an intracellular C-terminal tail. Of these domains, the extracellular N-terminus contains two Met-rich sequences, M1 (M^7GMSYM^{12}) and M2 ($M^{40}MMMPM^{45}$) and two His-rich sequences, H1 (H^3SHH^6) and H2 ($H^{22}HH^{24}$), some of which have been reported to be implicated in copper binding.

The important role of Ctr1 in the process of the cisplatin uptake has been particularly documented by Howell et al, [17] although the molecular mechanism is far from being clear. There are a number of reports correlating the expression level of Ctr1 with cisplatin resistance of cancer cells. Knockout of yCtr1 in yeast results in 50% reduction of cisplatin accumulation and the cells exhibit an 8-fold higher resistance to cisplatin compared with wild-type strain. The similar results were obtained in mammalian cells. And a moderate increase in intracellular platinum content was induced by overexpression of Ctr1 in an ovarian carcinoma cell line. [72]

However, a few of reports are inconsistent with the mechanism that Ctr1 facilitates cisplatin uptake directly. For example, Sinani et al reported in 2007 that the complete loss of Ctr1 function only induced a 10-15% decrease of cisplatin uptake. [73] In 2008, Dolan and co-workers showed that overexpression of Ctr1 had no effect on the intracellular concentration of cisplatin. [74].

Copper and cisplatin compete for binding to Ctr1 and reduce one another uptake in yeast. [17] However, current reports indicate that cisplatin interact with Ctr1 at distinct sites from those of copper as evidenced by FRET study, [73] which showed that cisplatin binding yielded yCtr1 conformation change which was different from copper binding. And Met127 to Ala substitution in yCTR1 influenced copper uptake, but has little effect on cisplatin uptake. In HEK293 cells, cisplatin treatment resulted in a stable trimer, while copper treatment resulted in a dimer on a gel. [75] These results suggest that cisplatin possibly bind to the extracellular N-terminus of Ctrl and crosslink the Ctrl monomers without blocking copper binding and copper-induced endocytosis. [76]

Although a lot of experiments attempting to understand the role of copper transporters in cisplatin uptake and resistance have been done, the precise mechanism still needs further investigations.

2.3. Copper-Transporting ATPases

Human cells express two homologous copper transporting ATPases: ATP7A and ATP7B, known as Menkes disease-associated protein and Wilson disease-associated protein, respectively. [77-80] ATP7B, strongly expressed in the liver and kidneys, plays a key role in the excretion of excess copper from the cells, while ATP7A plays a critical role in copper uptake into blood in the small intestine. They both transport copper in the reduced Cu(I) form with ATP supplying the energy. ATP7A and ATP7B, having 55% sequence similarity, are 160-170 kDa multidomain membrane proteins with 8 transmembrane (TM) segments and several cytosolic domains. [18] The N-terminal domain contains 6 copper binding sites formed by GMxCxxC, where the two cysteines bind a single Cu (I) in a linear coordination environment. [81-84].

The important role of copper-transporting ATPases, ATP7B and ATP7A in modulating cell resistance to cisplatin was suggested by a series of observations that ATP7B expression change, overexpression or low expression induced higher or lower resistance to cisplatin. [85-92] ATP7B seems to play a main role for cisplatin resistance, while ATP7A probably a minor role. [92] It is thought that the ATP7B-mediated cell resistance to cisplatin was attributed to the cisplatin or its derivatives efflux from cells catalyzed by ATP7B *in vivo*. [85,92,93] Interestingly, the researches reported recently showed [94-96] that the ATP-dependent cisplatin transport catalyzed by ATP7B is pH independence and the rate is very low, inconsistent with the mechanism stated above. Using a simple *in vivo* assay in bacterial culture,

Dmitrlev and co-workers proposed that ATP7B confers resistance to cisplatin by sequestering the drug in its N-terminal metal-binding repeats (MBRs) without active drug extrusion from the cells. [97] Cisplatin could bind to the CxxC motifs of MBRs of ATP7B and result in cross-linking of two MBRs, as observed for a number of other proteins. [21,48,98-100] Although ATP7B has at least 6 potential platinum-binding sites, the low abundance of ATP7B may be insufficient to effectively lower the concentration of active platinum derivatives in the cells, which proposes a hypothesis that ATP7B traps platinum derivatives transiently with a high affinity and hand them to other more abundant proteins or small molecular, for example, metallothionien and GSH in a less toxic form. The precise mechanism for ATP7B induced cisplatin resistance is still unclear and further investigations are needed.

2.4. Copper Chaperone Atox1

The soluble cytosolic Cu chaperone Atox1 (antioxidant-1, 68 amino acids), previously known as Hah1 (human atx1 homologue 1), mediates Cu(I) delivery to the Cu-transporting

ATPases ATP7A and ATP7B, was shown recently to act as a Cu-dependent transcription factor. It has been reported that loss of Atox1 increased Cu accumulation and reduced efflux. In contrast, loss of Atox1 reduced the influx of cisplatin, probably due to blocking the cisplatin-induced down regulation of Ctr1, and subsequent accumulation in vesicular compartments and in DNA.101 Atox1 has a β1α1β2β3α2β4 ferredoxin-like structure. The metal-binding site, CxxC, is located in the loop between secondary structure elements β1 and α1 and is highly conserved among metallochaperones and soluble domains of Cu-transporting ATPases.

Therefore, the coordination mode of cisplatin to Atox1 is likely similar to that to ATPases, i.e. coordinating to the MBR motif. Indeed, a recently crystallographic study shows definitively that cisplatin binds to the CXXC motif in Atox1 (Figure 4).21 Most recently, two groups independently investigated the interactions between cisplatin and Atox1, gaining similar results. Using spectroscopic methods to probe the interaction of cisplatin and purified Atox1 in solution in vitro,

Wittung-Stafshede and co-workers found that cisplatin binds to Atox1's metal-binding site regardless of the presence of Cu or not.20 Their NMR data indicate that cisplatin initially bound to the folded protein, but the cisplatin-bound Atox1 is not stable over time and the bound protein began to unfold and aggregate. By binding to Atox1 in the cytoplasm, cisplatin transport to DNA may be blocked, in agreement with author's cell line studies which demonstrate a correlation between Atox1 expression levels and cisplatin resistance. Natile and co-workers applied both solution and in-cell NMR spectroscopy approaches to explore the intracellular drug delivery and interaction of cisplatin with Atox1. Their results show that a mono-platinated adduct is first formed, and at longer reaction time protein dimerization and loss of the ammines in cisplatin were observed. Such a process is resemble to the copper-promoted formation of Atox1 dimers which have been proposed to be able to cross the nuclear membrane and act as a transcription factor. The overexpression of Atox1 in E. coli was also shown to reduce the amount of DNA platination and, consequently, the degree of cell filamentation. [102].

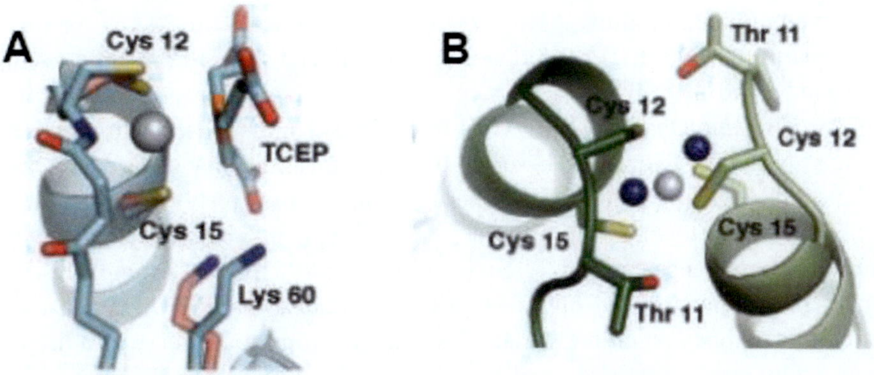

Figure 4. (A) Superposition of the metal binding sites in the Crystal structures of cisplatin bound to an Atox1 monomer (Pt-Atox1, light blue) and Cu bound to an Atox1 monomer (Cu(I)-Atox1, salmon). (B) Crystal structure of cisplatin bound to an Atox1 dimer. The Pt(II) ion is shown as a gray sphere, and the ammine nitrogens are shown as blue spheres. (Reproduced from reference 21, permission is needed from ACS).

3. METALLOTHIONIENS

Metallothioneins (MTs) are a group of low molecular weight (6-7kDa) non-enzymatic polypeptides characterized by distinctive amino acid composition (no aromatic amino acids, high cysteine content, 30% in mammals) and a high content of sulfur and metals in the form of metal-thiolate clusters. [103,104] MTs, of which the gene transcription can be induced by a variety of stimuli including hormones, cytokines and metal ions, have important biological functions such as storage, trafficking and homeostasis of metal ions, detoxification of heavy metals, resistance to ionizing radiation, scavenging hydroxyl radical, etc.

Four isoforms of mammalian MTs have been identified (MT-I–IV), of which MT-I and MT-II, ubiquitously existing in mammalian cells with high amounts, are the best characterized MT proteins. Under physiological conditions, mammalian MTs mostly contain 7 zinc ions which coordinate to cysteine residues to form two metal thiolate clusters located in the C-terminal α-domain (Zn_4S_{11}-cluster) and N-terminal β-domain (Zn_3S_9-cluster), respectively. [105]

The metal thiolate clusters make the proteins highly stable. In cancer cells, basal MT levels are often significantly increased resulting in an even stronger Pt(II) scavenging effect.Because of the strong reactivity of Pt(II) compounds with sulfur-donor molecules and high stability of Pt–S bonds, intracellular thiols, which are glutathione (GSH) and metallothionien (MT) existing with high concentration in the cells, confer resistance to antitumor platinum drugs through their competition with DNA.

Although MT is not the most abundant intracellular thiol, its reactivity with Pt(II) compounds is ~50-times higher than that observed with GSH, the most abundant intracellular thiol. [106] This makes MTs a highly effective intracellular scavenger of Pt(II) drugs which may explain the dramatic resistance to anticancer metallodrug increase in cancer cells. In order to deeply understand the resistance mechanism of cancer cells to metallodrugs, the interactions between MTs and platinum-based anticancer drugs, in particularly cisplatin, have been extensively studied during the past decades. [106-111]

It has been found that besides terminal thiolates, bridging thiolates in the MT structure are also involved in metal binding. And cisplatin reacted slower with MT-II than its inactive isoform transplatin, the cis-Pt(II) compounds released Zn(II) slower compared to their trans-Pt(II) compounds, and that all the ligands in cis-Pt(II) compounds including cisplatin were replaced by cysteine thiolates of MT-II, while trans-Pt(II) compounds, for instance transplatin retained their N-donor ligands. These results demonstrate that steric hindrance and electrophilicity of the Pt(II) center represents the major factor responsible for the different reactivity of Pt(II) drugs towards MT-II.

In addition, no evidence for Pt(II) transfer from *trans*-Pt(II)MT-II complexes to plasmid DNA, single- or double-stranded oligodeoxyribonucleotides, or GMP was obtained, which demonstrated that it appeared unlikely that Pt-MT interactions could serve as a drug reservoir affording an additional pathway toward platination of DNA. In our recent work, [25] we presented a comparative study on interactions between MTs and cisplatin and ruthenium arene anticancer complexes using MALDI-TOF-MS.

The results showed that cisplatin coordinated to MT-I and MT-II at either pH 3.0 or 7.4, and exhibited a higher affinity to MT-II than to MT-I. The MT–Pt complexes increased significantly in content with decrease in pH values of solutions, indicating that cisplatin competed with zinc for coordination to cysteine residues on MTs and interfered with the binding of zinc to the proteins.

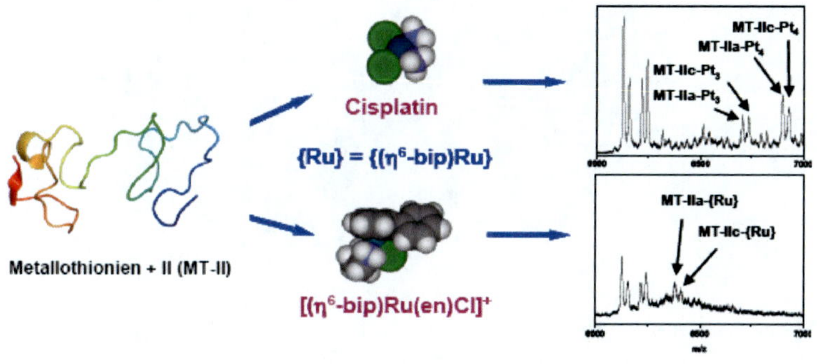

Figure 5. A comparison on the reactivity towards MT-II of cispaltin and ruthenium arene anticancner complexes at pH 7.4. (Reproduced from reference 26 with permission from Elsevier.).

Whereas the ruthenium arene anticancer complexes $[(\eta^6\text{-arene})Ru(en)Cl]PF_6$ (arene = benzene or biphenyl, en = ethylenediamine) hardly bind to MTs at acidic pH and coordinate to MTs at a much lower level than cisplatin at pH 7.4 (Figure 5), which may account for the less toxicity and lack of cross-resistance to cisplatin for this class of ruthenium anticancer complexes. [66,67].

4. OTHER PROTEINS

Additional studies have been carried out on a few other proteins such as SOD, [112] ubiquitin, [113] cytochrome c, [114] myoglobin, [115] and glutathione-S-transferase, [116] insulin, [22] in most cases, serving as model proteins to study the interactions between cisplatin and proteins.

4.1. Superoxide Dismutase (SOD)

SOD is a class of enzymes that catalyze the dismutation of superoxide into oxygen and hydrogen peroxide. As such, they are an important antioxidant defense in nearly all cells exposed to oxygen. Bovine erythrocyte copper–zinc superoxide dismutase (beSOD; EC 1.15.1.1) was selected as the model protein for the interaction study with cisplatin for several reasons: [117,118] its crystal structure is available at high resolution; it is a medium-sized protein with several potential binding sites for platinum; it’s good solubility; and it is commercially available and so on.

In 2005, Calderone et al. [112] obtained the first X-ray crystal structure of beSOD-cispaltin complex which unambiguously demonstrated that His19 is the primary binding site for cisplatin, and that cisplatin, upon protein binding, releases its two ammonia ligands rather than losing the two chlorine atoms (Figure 6).

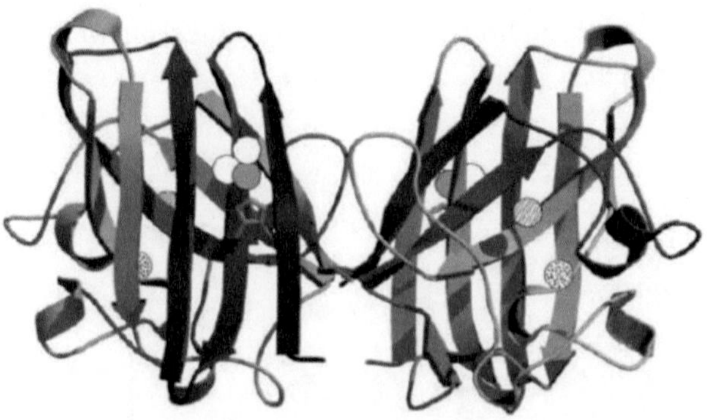

Figure 6. Schematic representation of the asymmetric unit containing the physiological dimer of the cisplatin-bound beSOD complex; the side chain of His19 is shown along with Cu (hatched), Zn (dotted), Pt (gray), and Cl (white). (Reproduced from reference 112, permission is needed from Wiley-VCH Verlag GmbH and Co.).

Such a result raises the possibility that reactions of cisplatin with beSOD may follow an unusual pathway in which ammonia release from platinum is readily promoted, possibly induced by the high trans effect of protein S-ligands. Later Sadler's group studied the platination of beSOD by cisplatin using FT-ICR MS with high resolving power in 2007. Interestingly, the mass spectrum showed that up to two cisplatin fragments could bind per monomer beSOD, as shown in Figure 7.

The possible binding sites are His19 and His41 considering of space-filling models of beSOD. Meanwhile, the cisplatin fragment binding to beSOD was $\{PtCl(NH_3)_2\}^+$, i.e. one of the chlorido ligands on platinum being displaced while the two ammine ligands are still present upon the protein binding. [119]

The obvious differences in the results reported by two groups could be explained as: the two used analytical techniques, i.e. X-ray crystallography and MS have rather different solution requirements that might affect in some cases the resulting reactivity and the nature of adducts themselves. X-ray crystallography provides the ''static'' structure of the metallodrug–protein adducts while ESI-MS offers valuable information on the temporal evolution of these adducts in solution.

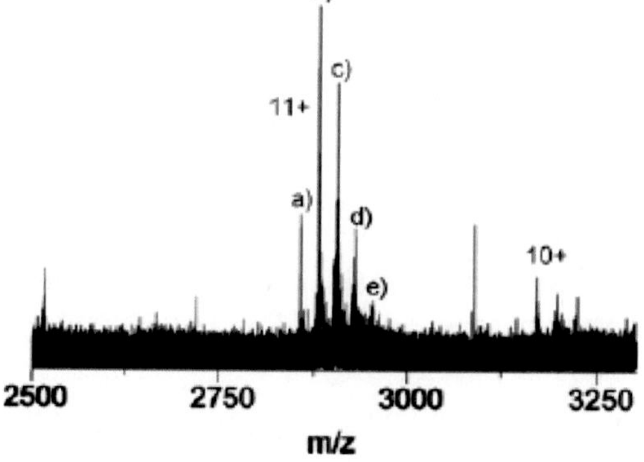

Figure 7. Mass spectrum of beSOD-cisplatin complex formed after reaction of beSOD with cisplatin for 16 h. Labeled peaks refer to 11+ ions of $(beSOD)_2$ (a) unmodified, (b) + $\{PtCl(NH_3)_2\}$, (c) + $\{PtCl(NH_3)_2\}_2$, (d) + $\{PtCl(NH_3)_2\}_3$, (e) + $\{PtCl(NH_3)_2\}_4$. (Reproduced from reference 83, permission is needed from RSC.) .

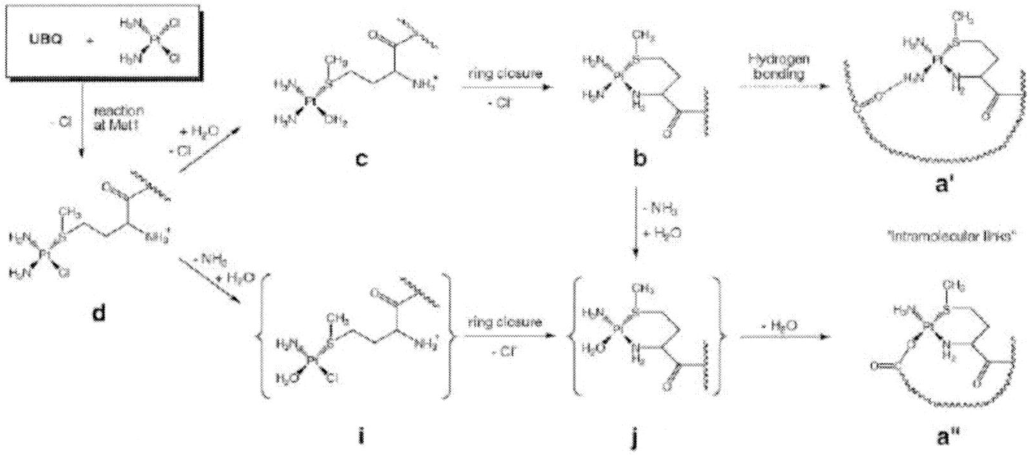

Figure 8. Potential reaction pathways for the formation of mono-platinated adduct observed in the reaction of cisplatin with ubiquitin. (Reproduced from reference 87, permission is needed from Springer.).

4.2. Ubiquitin

Ubiquitin is a small protein that exists in all eukaryotic cells. It performs its myriad functions through conjugation to a large range of target proteins. The ubiquitin protein itself consists of 76 amino acids and has a molecular mass of about 8.5 kDa. Ubiquitin is tightly folded protein whose structure is well characterized by both X-ray crystallography and NMR. Key features include its C-terminal tail and the 7 lysine residues. Bovine erythrocyte ubiquitin was often selected as the model protein for the interaction study between transition metal drugs and proteins because of its small size, high stability in water and low price. [113].The binding of ubiquitin with cisplatin, transplatin, and oxaliplatin was studied with different methods, [120] such as FT-ICR-ESI-MS, NMR spectroscopy, MALDI-TOF-MS, ESI-IT-MS and ESI-QTOF-MS, and a distinctly difference in terms of both binding kinetics and the type of formed adducts was reported. Cisplatin was shown to bind primarily at the Met1 and as a secondary target at His68 to form a variety of mono-, di-, and tri-functional 1:1 adducts, while the transplatin was observed to be attached to the peptide sequence [19]Pro-Ser-Asp-Thr-Ile-Glu [24.33,121] Sadler and Co-workers studied ubiquitin shape changes induced by n-terminal platination by cisplatin with ion-mobility mass spectrometry in 2010. [122] Met1 was also identified as the primary binding site. The potential reaction pathways for the formation of platinated mono-adducts observed in the reaction of cisplatin with ubiquitin was shown in Figure 8. Furthermore, their results indicated that the platinatied ubiquitin's structure is more compact compared with its unmodified counterpart, which may have a significant effect on its function *in vivo*.

4.3. Cytochrome c (Cyt *c*)

Cyt *c* is an important sulfur-containing mitochondrial protein (*M*W 12500 Da) containing one heme group which is covalently linked to the polypeptide chain *via* thioether linkages to Cys-14 and Cys-17, leading to a strong coordinative bond between the heme iron and His18 even under denaturing conditions. It is a component of the electron transport chain in mitochondria and also involved in initiation of apoptosis by binding apoptotic protease activating factor during its release to the cytoplasm from mitochondria.The characterization of interactions between cisplatin and Cyt *c* was reported twenty years ago. [114,123,124] In recent years, Casini et al analyzed the interactions of four classical platinum(II) drugs–cisplatin, its inactive isomer transplatin, carboplatin and oxaliplatin and several novel platinum compounds with horse heart Cyt *c*. [125,126] The four compounds exhibited a roughly similar pattern of reactivity with Cyt *c*, which has little relevance to the stability and reactivity of the four compounds, and Met65 is demonstrated as the major binding site for platinum(II) iminoethers on Cyt *c*. They hypothesized that Cyt *c* should play a major role in enhancing the reactivity of the kinetically stable carboplatin and oxaliplatin compared to cisplatin and transplatin.

4.4. Insulin

Insulin is a small protein which is consist of two peptide chains (A and B) linked by two inter-chain disulfide bonds, containing another intra-chain cystine25. It is synthesized in the pancreatic b-cells and participates in the regulation of blood glucose levels. This protein is applied as a model protein for studying interactions between cisplatin and proteins due to its low molecular mass (5733.51 Da in bovine insulin) and the presence in its sequence of potentially reactive amino acids towards platinum such as histidines and cysteines participating in disulfide bonds.Very recently, Canas and co-workers applied both top-down and bottom-up mass spectrometric methods to characterize the binding reaction of cisplatin to insulin. [22,127] The Top-down analysis through MALDI-TOF MS and nanoelectrospray ionization mass spectrometry using a linear ion trap (nESI-LIT-MS) analysis demonstrated the formation of mono-, di-, and even tri-platinated insulin adducts upon the reactions. [22]

Platinum binding sites were identified by tandem MS as B chain N-terminus, His5, and probably His10 residues, regardless of the incubation conditions. Coordination of Pt to Cys7 in B chain was also observed, indicating that cisplatin can induce cleavage of disulfide bond in insulin as the cisplatin-induced cleavage of the disulfide bond Cys124-Cys169 of albumin. [51] In the later bottom-up MS study of the same group, the nESI-LIT MS analysis of the peptides generated by trypsin digestion allowed more Pt-binding sites in insulin determined, including B Chain N-terminus, His5, His10, Cys7, Cys19 and A Chain Cys6, Cys7, Cys20. These results indicate that more information on metallodrug-protein reactions can be obtained with the bottom-up approach than the top-down method. [127]

Conclusion and Future Outlooks

Cisplatin reacts with various types of proteins outside and inside of cells *via* coordinating to specific residues, such as cysteine, methionine, histidine and tyrosine. In blood, following intravenous administration cisplatin can bind extensively to plasma proteins such as albumin, transferrin and hemoglobin, which may supply a storage pool for cisplatin. During cisplatin transporting across cell membrane, the organic cation transporters (OCTS) and the copper transporters, such as Ctr1, ATP7B and ATP7A as well as the copper chaperone Atox1, play an important role to facilitate the drug to move to DNA. Synchronously, these proteins are likely related to the acquired resistance of cancer cells to cisplatin. And inside cells cisplatin can bind to metallothioniens, cytochrome *c*, superoxide dismutase, ubiquitin, and so on. Such interactions may have a crucial effect on the bioavailability, transport and metabolism of cisplatin, and some are thought to be associated with undesired side effects and acquired resistance of the drug. Although some of the interaction mechanisms are not clear, and some existing reports have yielded contradictory or inconclusive answers, the important role of cisplatin binding to proteins for drug bioavailability, transport, side effects and resistance is unassailable.It is acknowledged that the introduction and refinement of modern analytical techniques, including X-ray crystallography, NMR spectroscopy and mass spectrometry, has greatly facilitated the research on the coordination chemistry and pharmacology of platinum-based anticancer drugs, in particular cisplatin, providing a better understanding on interactions between the metallodrugs and proteins. However, there are still many challenges to be addressed in the years ahead. For instance, the characterization of interactions between cisplatin and proteins in terms of binding constants, stoichiometry and the nature of the metal moiety and protein active sites involved in adduct formation. Another challenge on the way to explore the coordination chemistry and biology of cisplatin with proteins is to elucidate the role and proper functions of platinum-protein binding and to assess its reversibility with respect to relevant intracellular targets, for instance DNA. This requires steering the major research from outside to the interior of the tumor cells where the metallodrug exerts its antiproliferating function in the released active metal species after transport *via* the protein-mediated uptake or in the protein-bound forms. The exact role of metal-protein adducts remains in many cases unclear, and many questions are still to be answered. For example, is there a contribution of albumin-bound species in cisplatin's antiproliferative action? Do the abundant plasma proteins albumin and transferrin really act as a drug reservoir for cisplatin? Do intracellular proteins act only competitors for platinum binding or contribute to the antiproliferative action of cisplatin in some way? These kinds of interactions between cisplatin and proteins as well as their biological and pharmacological implications need to be explored in more detail in order to deeply understand how cisplatin crosses cells and kills the cells.

References

[1] Bruijnincx, P. C. A.; Sadler, P. *J. Curr. Opin. Chem. Biol.,* 2008, *12*, 197-206.
[2] Bruijnincx, P. C. A.; Sadler, P. *J. Adv. Inorg. Chem.,* 2009, *61*, 1-62.
[3] Ronconi, L.; Sadler, P. *J. Coordin. Chem. Rev.,* 2007, *251*, 1633-1648.

[4] Jamieson, E. R.; Lippard, S. *J. Chem. Rev.,* 1999, *99*, 2467-2498.
[5] Jung, Y. W.; Lippard, S. *J. Chem. Rev.,* 2007, *107*, 1387-1407.
[6] Ohndorf, U. M.; Rould, M. A.; He, Q.; Pabo, C. O.; Lippard, S. *J. Nature,* 1999, *399*, 708-712.
[7] Wang, D.; Lippard, S. *J. Nat Rev Drug Discov.,* 2005, *4*, 307-320.
[8] Sun, H. Z.; Li, H. Y.; Sadler, P. *J. Chem. Rev.,* 1999, *99*, 2817-2842.
[9] Timerbaev, A. R.; Hartinger, C. G.; Aleksenko, S. S.; Keppler, B. K. *Chem. Rev.,* 2006, *106*, 2224-2248.
[10] Esposito, B. P.; Najjar, R. *Coordin Chem Rev* 2002, *232*, 137-149.
[11] Sooriyaarachchi, M.; Narendran, A.; Gailer, *J. Metallomics* ,2011, *3*, 49-55.
[12] Hu, W. B.; Luo, Q.; Wu, K.; Li, X. C.; Wang, F. Y.; Chen, Y.; Ma, X. Y.; Wang, J. P.; Liu, J. A.; Xiong, S. X.; Sadler, P. *J. Chem. Commun.,* 2011, *47*, 6006-6008.
[13] Khalaila, I.; Allardyce, C. S.; Verma, C. S.; Dyson, P. *J. Chembiochem.,* 2005, *6*, 1788-1795.
[14] Lemma, T.; Mandal, R.; Li, X. F.; Pawliszyn, J. *J. Sep. Sci.,* 2008, *31*, 1803-1809.
[15] Mandal, R.; Li, X. F. *Rapid. Commun. Mass. Sp.,* 2006, *20*, 48-52.
[16] Choi, M.-K.; Song, I.-S. *Drug Metabolism and Pharmacokinetics,* 2008, *23*, 243-253.
[17] Ishida, S.; Lee, J.; Thiele, D. J.; Herskowitz, I. *P Natl Acad Sci USA* 2002, *99*, 14298-14302.
[18] Lutsenko, S.; Barnes, N. L.; Bartee, M. Y.; Dmitriev, O. Y. *Physiological Reviews,* 2007, *87*, 1011-1046.
[19] Hua, H. Q.; Gunther, V.; Georgiev, O.; Schaffner, W. *Biometals,* 2011, *24*, 445-453.
[20] Palm, M. E.; Weise, C. F.; Lundin, C.; Wingsle, G.; Nygren, Y.; Bjorn, E.; Naredi, P.; Wolf-Watz, M.; Wittung-Stafshede, P. *P. Natl. Acad. Sci. USA,* 2011, *108*, 6951-6956.
[21] Boal, A. K.; Rosenzweig, A. C. *J. Am. Chem. Soc.,* 2009, *131*, 14196-+.
[22] Moreno-Gordaliza, E.; Canas, B.; Palacios, M. A.; Gomez-Gomez, M. M. *Anal. Chem.,* 2009, *81*, 3507-3516.
[23] Waalkes, M. P.; Liu, J.; Kasprzak, K. S.; Diwan, B. A. *Int. J. Cancer,* 2006, *119*, 28-32.
[24] Liu, J.; Liu, Y. P.; Habeebu, S. S. M.; Klaassen, C. D. *Toxicol. Appl. Pharm.,* 1998, *149*, 24-31.
[25] Zhang, G.; Hu, W.; Du, Z.; Lv, S.; Zheng, W.; Luo, Q.; Li, X.; Wu, K.; Han, Y.; Wang, F. *Int. J. Mass. Spectrom.,* 2011, *307*, 79-84.
[26] Chen, C. B.; Zhou, H.; Xu, L. J.; Xu, D.; Wang, Y.; Zhang, Y. M.; Liu, X. G.; Liu, Z. J.; Ma, D. L.; Ma, Q. J.; Chen, Y. Y. *Apoptosis,* 2010, *15*, 805-813.
[27] Liu, L.; Xing, D.; Chen, W. R.; Chen, T. S.; Pei, Y. H.; Gao, X. J. *Int. J. Cancer,* 2008, *122*, 2210-2222.
[28] Dhar, S.; Lippard, S. J. *P Natl. Acad. Sci. USA*, 2009, *106*, 22199-22204.
[29] Casini, A.; Gabbiani, C.; Michelucci, E.; Pieraccini, G.; Moneti, G.; Dyson, P. J.; Messori, L. *J. Biol. Inorg. Chem.,* 2009, *14*, 761-770.
[30] Nishikawa, M.; Nagatomi, H.; Chang, B. J.; Sato, E.; Inoue, M. *Arch. Biochem. Biophys.,* 2001, *387*, 78-84.
[31] Zhang, C. X.; Lippard, S. *J. Curr. Opin. Chem. Biol.,* 2003, *7*, 481-489.
[32] Mansour, H. H.; Hafez, H. F.; Fahmy, N. M. *J. Biochem. Mol. Biol.,* 2006, *39*, 656-661.
[33] Hartinger, C. G.; Tsybin, Y. O.; Fuchser, J.; Dyson, P. *J. Inorg. Chem.,* 2008, *47*, 17-19.

[34] Deconti, R. C.; Toftness, B. R.; Lange, R. C.; Creasey, W. A. *Cancer Res.,* 1973, *33*, 1310-1315.

[35] Reedijk, J. *Chem. Rev.,* 1999, *99*, 2499-2510.

[36] Groessl, M.; Terenghi, M.; Casini, A.; Elviri, L.; Lobinski, R.; Dyson, P. J. *J. Anal. Atom. Spectrom.,* 2010, *25*, 305-313.

[37] Einhauser, T. J.; Galanski, M.; Keppler, B. K. *J. Anal. Atom. Spectrom.,* 1996, *11*, 747-750.

[38] Zhmareva, E. N.; Zegzhda, G. D.; Kas'yan, G. B.; Livenskaya, O. A. *Ukrainskii Biokhimicheskii Zhurnal,* 1996, *68*, 74-79.

[39] Takada, K.; Kawamura, T.; Inai, M.; Masuda, S.; Oka, T.; Yoshikawa, Y.; Shibata, N.; Yoshikawa, H.; Ike, O.; Wada, H.; Hitomi, S. *Biopharm. Drug Dispos.,* 1999, *20*, 421-428.

[40] Blindauer, C. A.; Harvey, I.; Bunyan, K. E.; Stewart, A. J.; Sleep, D.; Harrison, D. J.; Berezenko, S.; Sadler, P. J. *J. Biol. Chem.,* 2009, *284*, 23116-23124.

[41] Lu, J.; Stewart, A. J.; Sadler, P. J.; Pinheiro, T. J. T.; Blindauer, C. A. *Biochem. Soc., T* 2008, *36*, 1317-1321.

[42] Stewart, A. J.; Blindauer, C. A.; Berezenko, S.; Sleep, D.; Sadler, P. J. *P Natl Acad Sci USA* 2003, *100*, 3701-3706.

[43] Herve, F.; Urien, S.; Albengres, E.; Duche, J. C.; Tillement, J. P. *Clinical Pharmacokinetics,* 1994, *26*, 44-58.

[44] Hoshino, T.; Misaki, M.; Yamamoto, M.; Shimizu, H.; Ogawa, Y.; Toguchi, H. *J. Pharm. Sci.,* 1995, *84*, 216-221.

[45] Moller, C.; Tastesen, H. S.; Gammelgaard, B.; Lambert, I. H.; Sturup, S. *Metallomics,* 2010, *2*, 811-818.

[46] Sun, X. S.; Tsang, C. N.; Sun, H. Z. *Metallomics,* 2009, *1*, 25-31.

[47] Sugii, A.; Nishimura, K.; Harada, K.; Nakayama, M.; Masuda, S. *Chem. Pharm. Bull.,* 1991, *39*, 408-410.

[48] Ivanov, A. I.; Christodoulou, J.; Parkinson, J. A.; Barnham, K. J.; Tucker, A.; Woodrow, J.; Sadler, P. J. *J. Biol. Chem.,* 1998, *273*, 14721-14730.

[49] Will, J.; Wolters, D. A.; Sheldrick, W. S. *Chemmedchem.,* 2008, *3*, 1696-1707.

[50] Neault, J. F.; Tajmir-Riahi, H. A. *Bba-Protein Struct., M* 1998, *1384*, 153-159.

[51] Hu, W. B.; Luo, Q.; Ma, X. Y.; Wu, K.; Liu, J. A.; Chen, Y.; Xiong, S. X.; Wang, J. P.; Sadler, P. J.; Wang, F. Y. *Chem.-Eur. J.,* 2009, *15*, 6586-6594.

[52] Sweeney, J. D.; Ziegler, P.; Pruet, C.; Spaulding, M. B. *Cancer-Am. Cancer Soc.,* 1989, *63*, 2093-2095.

[53] Wei, H. Y.; Wang, X. Y.; Liu, Q.; Mei, Y. H.; Lu, Y.; Guo, Z. *J. Inorg. Chem.,* 2005, *44*, 6077-6081.

[54] Fakih, S.; Munk, V. P.; Shipman, M. A.; Murdoch, P. D.; Parkinson, J. A.; Sadler, P. *J. Eur. J. Inorg. Chem.,* 2003, 1206-1214.

[55] Murdoch, P. D.; Kratochwil, N. A.; Parkinson, J. A.; Patriarca, M.; Sadler, P. *J. Angew. Chem. Int. Edit.,* 1999, *38*, 2949-2951.

[56] Ohta, N.; Yotsuyanagi, T.; Chen, D.; Ono, R.; Ito, S.; Ikeda, K. *Int. J. Pharm.,* 1992, *85*, 39-44.

[57] Ohta, N.; Chen, D.; Ito, S.; Futo, T.; Yotsuyanagi, T.; Ikeda, K. *Int. J. Pharm.,* 1995, *118*, 85-93.

[58] Guo, M.; Sun, H.; Sadler, P. J. *J. Inorg. Biochem.,* 1999, *74*, 150-150.

[59] Menter, D. G.; Herrmann, J. L.; Nicolson, G. L. *Clin. Exp. Metastas.,* 1995, *13*, 67-88.

[60] Qian, Z. M.; Li, H. Y.; Sun, H. Z.; Ho, K. *Pharmacol. Rev.,* 2002, *54*, 561-587.

[61] Li, H. Y.; Qian, Z. M. *Med. Res. Rev.,* 2002, *22*, 225-250.

[62] Cox, M. C.; Barnham, K. J.; Frenkiel, T. A.; Hoeschele, J. D.; Mason, A. B.; He, Q. Y.; Woodworth, R. C.; Sadler, P. J. *J. Biol. Inorg. Chem.,* 1999, *4*, 621-631.

[63] Mandal, R.; Kalke, R.; Li, X. F. *Rapid. Commun. Mass. Sp.,* 2003, *17*, 2748-2754.

[64] Mandal, R.; Kalke, R.; Li, X. F. *Chem. Res. Toxicol.,* 2004, *17*, 1391-1397.

[65] Mandal, R.; Teixeira, C.; Li, X. F. *Analyst,* 2003, *128*, 629-634.

[66] Wang, F. Y.; Habtemariam, A.; van der Geer, E. P. L.; Fernandez, R.; Melchart, M.; Deeth, R. J.; Aird, R.; Guichard, S.; Fabbiani, F. P. A.; Lozano-Casal, P.; Oswald, I. D. H.; Jodrell, D. I.; Parsons, S.; Sadler, P. *J. P. Natl. Acad. Sci. USA,* 2005, *102*, 18269-18274.

[67] Aird, R. E.; Cummings, J.; Ritchie, A. A.; Muir, M.; Morris, R. E.; Chen, H.; Sadler, P. J.; Jodrell, D. I. *Brit J Cancer* 2002, *86*, 1652-1657.

[68] Krieger, M. L.; Eckstein, N.; Schneider, V.; Koch, M.; Royer, H.-D.; Jaehde, U.; Bendas, G. *Int. J. Pharm.,* 2010, *389*, 10-17.

[69] Lovejoy, K. S.; Todd, R. C.; Zhang, S.; McCormick, M. S.; D'Aquino, J. A.; Reardon, J. T.; Sancar, A.; Giacomini, K. M.; Lippard, S. J. *P. Natl. Acad. Sci. USA,* 2008, *105*, 8902-8907.

[70] Ciarimboli, G. *Xenobiotica,* 2008, *38*, 936-971.

[71] Yonezawa, A.; Masuda, S.; Yokoo, S.; Katsura, T.; Inui, K.-i. *J. Pharmacol. Exp. Ther.,* 2006, *319*, 879-886.

[72] Holzer, A. K.; Samimi, G.; Katano, K.; Naerdemann, W.; Lin, X. J.; Safaei, R.; Howell, S. B. *Mol. Pharmacol.,* 2004, *66*, 817-823.

[73] Sinani, D.; Adle, D. J.; Kim, H.; Lee, J. *J. Biol. Chem.,* 2007, *282*, 26775-26785.

[74] Rabik, C. A.; Fishel, M. L.; Holleran, J. L.; Kasza, K.; Kelley, M. R.; Egorin, M. J.; Dolan, M. E. *J. Pharmacol. Exp. Ther.,* 2008, *327*, 442-452.

[75] Guo, Y.; Smith, K.; Petris, M. J. *J Biol Chem* 2004, *279*, 46393-46399.

[76] Guo, Y.; Smith, K.; Lee, J.; Thiele, D. J.; Petris, M. J. *J. Biol. Chem.,* 2004, *279*, 17428-17433.

[77] Bull, P. C.; Thomas, G. R.; Rommens, J. M.; Forbes, J. R.; Cox, D. W. *Nature Genetics,* 1993, *5*, 327-337.

[78] Petrukhin, K.; Fischer, S. G.; Pirastu, M.; Tanzi, R. E.; Chernov, I.; Devoto, M.; Brzustowicz, L. M.; Cayanis, E.; Vitale, E.; Russo, J. J.; Matseoane, D.; Boukhgalter, B.; Wasco, W.; Figus, A. L.; Loudianos, J.; Cao, A.; Sternlieb, I.; Evgrafov, O.; Parano, E.; Pavone, L.; Warburton, D.; Ott, J.; Penchaszadeh, G. K.; Scheinberg, I. H.; Gilliam, T. C. *Nature Genetics,* 1993, *5*, 338-343.

[79] Tanzi, R. E.; Petrukhin, K.; Chernov, I.; Pellequer, J. L.; Wasco, W.; Ross, B.; Romano, D. M.; Parano, E.; Pavone, L.; Brzustowicz, L. M.; Devoto, M.; Peppercorn, J.; Bush, A. I.; Sternlieb, I.; Pirastu, M.; Gusella, J. F.; Evgrafov, O.; Penchaszadeh, G. K.; Honig, B.; Edelman, I. S.; Soares, M. B.; Scheinberg, I. H.; Gilliam, T. C. *Nature Genetics,* 1993, *5*, 344-350.

[80] Vulpe, C.; Levinson, B.; Whitney, S.; Packman, S.; Gitschier, J. *Nature Genetics,* 1993, *3*, 7-13.

[81] Lutsenko, S.; LeShane, E. S.; Shinde, U. *Arch. Biochem. Biophys.,* 2007, *463*, 134-148.

[82] Lutsenko, S.; Petrukhin, K.; Cooper, M. J.; Gilliam, C. T.; Kaplan, J. H. *J. Biol. Chem.,* 1997, *272*, 18939-18944.

[83] DiDonato, M.; Narindrasorasak, S.; Forbes, J. R.; Cox, D. W.; Sarkar, B. *J. Biol. Chem.,* 1997, *272*, 33279-33282.

[84] Yatsunyk, L. A.; Rosenzweig, A. C. *J. Biol. Chem.,* 2007, *282*, 8622-8631.

[85] Komatsu, M.; Sumizawa, T.; Mutoh, M.; Chen, Z. S.; Terada, K.; Furukawa, T.; Yang, X. L.; Gao, H.; Miura, N.; Sugiyama, T.; Akiyama, S. *Cancer Res.,* 2000, *60*, 1312-1316.

[86] Nakagawa, T.; Inoue, Y.; Kodama, H.; Yamazaki, H.; Kawai, K.; Suemizu, H.; Masuda, R.; Iwazaki, M.; Yamada, S.; Ueyama, Y.; Inoue, H.; Nakamura, M. *Oncol Rep.,* 2008, *20*, 265-270.

[87] Nakayama, K.; Kanzaki, A.; Ogawa, K.; Miyazaki, K.; Neamati, N.; Takebayashi, Y. *Int. J. Cancer,* 2002, *101*, 488-495.

[88] Nakayama, K.; Kanzaki, A.; Terada, K.; Mutoh, M.; Ogawa, K.; Sugiyama, T.; Takenoshita, S.; Itoh, K.; Yaegashi, N.; Miyazaki, K.; Neamati, N.; Takebayashi, Y. *Clin Cancer Res* 2004, *10*, 2804-2811.

[89] Yoshizawa, K.; Nozaki, S.; Kitahara, H.; Ohara, T.; Kato, K.; Kawashiri, S.; Yamamoto, E. *Oncol. Rep.,* 2007, *18*, 987-991.

[90] Mangala, L. S.; Zuzel, V.; Schmandt, R.; Leshane, E. S.; Haider, J. B.; Armaiz-Pena, G. N.; Spannuth, W. A.; Tanaka, T.; Shahzad, M. M. K.; Lin, Y. G.; Nick, A. M.; Danes, C. G.; Lee, J.-W.; Jennings, N. B.; Vivas-Mejia, P. E.; Wolf, J. K.; Coleman, R. L.; Siddik, Z. H.; Lopez-Berestein, G.; Lutsenko, S.; Sood, A. K. *Clin. Cancer Res.,* 2009, *15*, 3770-3780.

[91] Samimi, G.; Varki, N. M.; Wilczynski, S.; Safaei, R.; Alberts, D. S.; Howell, S. B. *Clin. Cancer Res.,* 2003, *9*, 5853-5859.

[92] Samimi, G.; Safaei, R.; Katano, K.; Holzer, A. K.; Rochdi, M.; Tomioka, M.; Goodman, M.; Howell, S. B. *Clin. Cancer Res.,* 2004, *10*, 4661-4669.

[93] Katano, K.; Safaei, R.; Samimi, G.; Holzer, A.; Rochdi, M.; Howell, S. B. *Mol. Pharmacol.,* 2003, *64*, 466-473.

[94] Zisowsky, J.; Koegel, S.; Leyers, S.; Devarakonda, K.; Kassack, M. U.; Osmak, M.; Jaehde, U. *Biochem. Pharmacol.,* 2007, *73*, 298-307.

[95] Safaei, R.; Otani, S.; Larson, B. J.; Rasmussen, M. L.; Howell, S. B. *Mol. Pharmacol.,* 2008, *73*, 461-468.

[96] Leonhardt, K.; Gebhardt, R.; Moessner, J.; Lutsenko, S.; Huster, D. *J. Biol. Chem.,* 2009, *284*, 7793-7802.

[97] Dolgova, N. V.; Olson, D.; Lutsenko, S.; Dmitrlev, O. Y. *Biochem. J.*, 2009, *419*,51-56.

[98] Roche, P. A.; Jensen, P. E. H.; Pizzo, S. V. *Biochemistry.-Us.,* 1988, *27*, 759-764.

[99] Wells, W. W.; Rocque, P. A.; Xu, D. P.; Yang, Y. F.; Deits, T. L. *Biochem. Bioph. Res. Co.,* 1991, *180*, 735-741.

[100] Prast-Nielsen, S.; Cebula, M.; Pader, I.; Arner, E. S. *J. Free Radical Bio Med.,* 2010, *49*, 1765-1778.

[101] Safaei, R.; Maktabi, M. H.; Blair, B. G.; Larson, C. A.; Howell, S. B. *J Inorg Biochem* 2009, *103*, 333-341.

[102] Arnesano, F.; Banci, L.; Bertini, I.; Felli2, I. C.; Losacco, M.; Natile, G. *J. Am. Chem. Soc.,* 2011, DOI: 10.1021/ja207346p.

[103] Andon, B.; Barbosa, J.; Sanz-Nebot, V. *Electrophoresis,* 2006, *27*, 3661-3670.

[104] Sanz-Nebot, V.; Andon, B.; Barbosa, J. *J. Chromatogr., B* 2003, *796*, 379-393.

[105] Pedersen, M. O.; Larsen, A.; Stoltenberg, M.; Penkowa, M. *Progress in Histochemistry and Cytochemistry,* 2009, *44*, 29-64.

[106] Hagrman, D.; Goodisman, J.; Dabrowiak, J. C.; Souid, A. K. *Drug. Metab. Dispos.,* 2003, *31*, 916-923.

[107] Knipp, M. *Current Medicinal Chemistry,* 2009, *16*, 522-537.

[108] Twentyman, P. R.; Wright, K. A.; Mistry, P.; Kelland, L. R.; Murrer, B. A. *Cancer Res.,* 1992, *52*, 5674-5680.

[109] Mounicou, S.; Polec, K.; Chassaigne, H.; Potin-Gautier, M.; Lobinski, R. *J. Anal. Atom. Spectrom,* 2000, *15*, 635-642.

[110] Karotki, A. V.; Vasak, M. *J. Biol. Inorg. Chem.,* 2009, *14*, 1129-1138.

[111] Knipp, M.; Karotki, A. V.; Chesnov, S.; Natile, G.; Sadler, P. J.; Brabec, V.; Vasak, M. *J. Med. Chem.,* 2007, *50*, 4075-4086.

[112] Calderone, V.; Casini, A.; Mangani, S.; Messori, L.; Orioli, P. L. *Angew. Chem. Int. Edit.,* 2006, *45*, 1267-1269.

[113] Gibson, D.; Costello, C. E. *Eur. Mass Spectrom.,* 1999, *5*, 501-510.

[114] Yang, G.; Miao, R.; Jin, C.; Mei, Y.; Tang, H.; Hong, J.; Guo, Z.; Zhu, L. *Journal of Mass Spectrometry,* 2005, *40*, 1005-1016.

[115] Peleg-Shulman, T.; Najajreh, Y.; Gibson, D. *J. Inorg. Biochem.,* 2002, *91*, 306-311.

[116] Ang, W. H.; Khalaila, I.; Allardyce, C. S.; Juillerat-Jeanneret, L.; Dyson, P. J. *J. Am. Chem. Soc.,* 2005, *127*, 1382-1383.

[117] Fisher, C. L.; Hallewell, R. A.; Roberts, V. A.; Tainer, J. A.; Getzoff, E. D. *Free Radical Research Communications,* 1991, *12-3*, 287-296.

[118] Tainer, J. A.; Getzoff, E. D.; Beem, K. M.; Richardson, J. S.; Richardson, D. C. *J. Mol. Biol.,* 1982, *160*, 181-217.

[119] Weidt, S. K.; Mackay, C. L.; Langridge-Smith, P. R. R.; Sadler, P. J. *Chem. Commun.,* 2007, 1719-1721.

[120] Hartinger, C. G.; Ang, W. H.; Casini, A.; Messori, L.; Keppler, B. K.; Dyson, P. J. *J. Anal. Atom. Spectrom.,* 2007, *22*, 960-967.

[121] Peleg-Shulman, T.; Gibson, D. *J. Am. Chem. Soc.,* 2001, *123*, 3171-3172.

[122] Williams, J. P.; Phillips, H. I. A.; Campuzano, I.; Sadler, P. J. *Journal of the American Society for Mass Spectrometry,* 2010, *21*, 1097-1106.

[123] Treskes, M.; Holwerda, U.; Klein, I.; Pinedo, H. M.; Vandervijgh, W. J. F. *Biochem. Pharmacol.,* 1991, *42*, 2125-2130.

[124] Andersson, A.; Hedenmalm, H.; Elfsson, B.; Ehrsson, H. *J. Pharm. Sci.,* 1994, *83*, 859-862.

[125] Messori, L.; Casini, A.; Gabbiani, C.; Mastrobuoni, G.; Pellicani, R. Z.; Intini, F. P.; Arnesano, F.; Natile, G.; Moneti, G.; Francese, S. *Biochemistry-Us.,* 2007, *46*, 12220-12230.

[126] Casini, A.; Gabbiani, C.; Mastrobuoni, G.; Messori, L.; Moneti, G.; Pieraccini, G. *Chemmedchem.,* 2006, *1*, 413-417.

[127] Moreno-Gordaliza, E.; Canas, B.; Palacios, M. A.; Gomez-Gomez, M. M. *Analyst.,* 2010, *135*, 1288-1298.

[128] Dube, N.; Bourdeau, A.; Heinonen, K. M.; Cheng, A.; Loy, A. L.; Tremblay, N. L. *Cancer Res.,* 2005, *65*, 10088-10095.

[129] Liu, G. *Drugs of the Future,* 2004, *29*, 1245-1259.

[130] Tonks, N. K. *Febs Letters,* 2003, *546*, 140-148.
[131] Wiener, J. R.; Kerns, B. J. M.; Harvey, E. L.; Conaway, M. R.; Iglehart, J. D.; Berchuck, A.; Bast, R. C. *J. Natl. Cancer I.,* 1994, *86*, 372-378.
[132] Dube, N.; Julien, S. G.; Mes-Masson, A.; Muller, W. J.; Saad, F.; Tremblay, M. L.; Univ Mcgill Royal Inst Advancement; Cent Rech Chum.
[133] Johnson, K. J.; Peck, A. R.; Liu, C.; Tran, T. H.; Utama, F. E.; Sjolund, A. B.; Schaber, J. D.; Witkiewicz, A. K.; Rui, H. *Am. J. Pathol.,* 2010, *177*, 2971-2983.

In: Cisplatin: Pharmacology, Clinical Uses and Adverse Effects ISBN: 978-1-61942-359-6
Editors: Toshiko Kojima and Yoko Morita

Chapter V

CISPLATIN: ITS CLINICAL APPLICATION AND THERAPY INDIVIDUALIZATION IN GASTRIC AND ESOPHAGEAL CANCERS

Shouji Shimoyama*
Gastrointestinal Unit, Settlement Clinic, 4-20-7, Towa, Adachi-ku, Tokyo, Japan

ABSTRACT

Cisplatin [cis-diamminedichloroplatinum (II)] is one of several platinum containing compounds used for the treatment of a variety of malignancies. It is generally accepted that cisplatin initiates cell death primarily through the formation of intrastrand cross-links, the majority of which involve neighboring purine bases. Subsequently, cisplatin has been placed as one of the pivotal chemotherapeutic agents in the treatment of gastric and esophageal cancers by combining with fluorouracil, irinotecan, and taxane. During the progress of advanced gastric cancer treatment, cisplatin has usually gained a constituent of several doublet or triplet regimens such as CS (cisplatin and S-1), ECF (epirubicin, cisplatin, and fluorouracil), and DCF (docetaxel, cisplatin, and fluorouracil). In particular, survivals of gastric cancer patients that received CS have been proved to be superior to, or at least equal to, those of the control regimens of S-1 monotherapy (in Japan) or CF (cisplatin and fluorouracil) (in the United States). In esophageal cancer, CF has been recognized as an active regimen in an adjuvant or neoadjuvant setting, or as a powerful partner of radiotherapy (chemoradiation).

Although cisplatin is widely used and promising, a great individual variability in both outcomes and toxicities hamper the wide therapeutic window. Response to platinum is influenced by the detoxification capacity of platinum-DNA adducts. One of the responsible factors relevant to platinum detoxification is glutathione S-transferases (GSTs), and there are interindividual and interethnic variabilities of GSTs activity that are determined by genetic polymorphism of the gene. This chapter highlights the current achievement of gastric and esophageal cancer treatment incorporating cisplatin, as well as

*Address of corresponding author and for reprints: Shouji Shimoyama, M.D., Gastrointestinal Unit, Settlement Clinic, 4-20-7, Towa, Adachi-ku, Tokyo, 120-0003, Japan, Tel: +81-3-3605-7747 Fax: +81-3-3605-0244, e-mail address: shimoyama@apost.plala.or.jp.

current knowledge on molecular differences in pharmacologically relevant genes involved in the metabolism of cisplatin. This knowledge will contribute towards optimizing therapy selection on an individual basis with an anticipation of superior efficacy with a minimal chance of toxicity, and ultimately allowing treatment to be individualized which realizes the maximum patient benefit of the current exciting cisplatin-based regimen.

Keywords: Cisplatin, gastric cancer, esophageal cancer, glutathione S-transferases, polymorphism, individualized therapy

INTRODUCTION

Cisplatin [cis-diamminedichloroplatinum (II)] is one of the several platinum containing compounds used for the treatment of a variety of malignancies. It is generally accepted that cytotoxic effects of cisplatin are exerted primarily through the formation of intrastrand cross-links between platinum compounds and purine DNA bases [1]. For gastric and esophageal cancer treatment, cisplatin was traditionally used alone, but is currently used in combination regimens as a partner of other cytotoxic agents such as fluorouracil, irinotecan, and taxane. However, in a clinical setting, it is also true that there is a great variability in tumor response and patient survival among regimens. In addition, cisplatin can cause significant nephrotoxicity in some patients, which can be severe enough to require discontinuation of therapy. Unfortunately, however, it is difficult to predict precisely the efficacy and toxicity prior to therapy. Therefore, it is urgently needed to explore mechanisms that can explain interindividual differences of efficacy and toxicity of cisplatin. This chapter will provide an overview of the current achievements of gastric and esophageal cancer treatment with the possible involvement of cisplatin, as well as the current knowledge on predictive biomarkers that could allow treatment to be individualized.

GASTRIC CANCER- ADJUVANT SETTING

In an adjuvant treatment of gastric cancer, substantial numbers of clinical trials have been conducted; however, no regimens have been proved to be definitively effective.

There have been several metaanalyses [2-11] involving the extant randomized trials, and the results consistently suggest that the benefit of adjuvant chemotherapy is significant; however, there are several limitations in these metaanalyses due to significant heterogeneity of the involved trials. Against these backgrounds, several new large adjuvant randomized trials have been conducted in Japan [12], the United States (INT0116) [13], and Europe (MAGIC trial [14], FNCLCC94012-FFCD9703 [15], and CRITICS trial [16]). Among these, three randomized trials, from the United Kingdom [14], France [15], and the Netherlands [16], chose cisplatin as one of the perioperative chemotherapeutic agents, and the former two trials [14,15] have provided results (Table 1).

The MAGIC trial (Medical Research Council Adjuvant Gastric Infusional Chemotherapy) [14] was a randomized perioperative chemotherapy trial in the United Kingdom for patients with stage II or higher resectable adenocarcinoma of the stomach, esophagogastric junction, or lower esophagus. The perioperative chemotherapy consisted of three preoperative and three postoperative cycles of epirubicin, cisplatin, and fluorouracil (ECF), which resulted in significantly improved 5-year disease free and 5-year overall survivals. In the French trial (FNCLCC94012-FFCD9703) [15], perioperative cisplatin and 5FU (CF) was compared with surgery only. Although these two trials have demonstrated survival benefits in the chemotherapy arm, there have been some criticisms directed towards these studies.

Table 1. Recent preoperative and adjuvant randomized trials incorporating cisplatin for gastric cancer

Authors	Cunningham [14]		Ychou [15]		CRITICS [16]
Entry stage	stage II or higher		excluding in situ cancer		stageIb-IVa
Arm	Surgery only	ECF+ Surgery+ ECF	Surgery only	ECC+ Surgery+ECC	ECC+Surgery +CRTx
Patients (n)	253	250	111	113	
Relapse free survival rate, % (year)	20* (5y)	30* (5y)	21 (5y)	34 (5y)	
	p<0.001		p=0.003		ongoing
Overall survival rate, % (year)	23 (5y)	36 (5y)	24 (5y)	38 (5y)	
	p=0.009		p=0.02		
Morbidity (%)	45	46	19	26	
Mortality (%)	5.9	5.6	4.5	4.4	

* approximate value.

ECF: epirubicin+cisplatin+fluorouracil, CF: cisplatin+fluorouracil, ECC: epirubicin+cisplatin+ capecitabine, CRTx: chemoradiotherapy.

Curative resection rates in the surgery only arm accounted only for 66% (MAGIC trial) [14] or 87% (FFCD trial) [15] of the patients, suggesting that both were not purely adjuvant chemotherapy trials and likely recruited extremely advanced cases. On the other hand, in the MAGIC trial, pathological T1 disease patients comprised 8% of the surgery only arm, suggesting that preoperative staging was not necessarily accurate and such earlier stage patients received unnecessary ECF, which would be more harmful than beneficial. Furthermore, perioperative ECF may be harsh because of the relatively higher rate (9%) of not completing the three planned cycles of ECF, and of low rates of commencement (55%) and completion (42%) of the postoperative ECF, leading to a relatively higher rate of 30-day mortality (6%) as compared with those (0-5%) of gastrectomy with a second-tier or wider scope of lymphadenectomy in the Japanese and Western dedicated centers.

One randomized chemoradiotherapy trial has been ongoing in the Netherlands [16], in which adjuvant three cycles of chemoradiation (investigational arm) after 3 preoperative cycles of ECC (epirubicin, cisplatin, capecitabine) and surgery (clearance of >15 nodes) were compared with 3 adjuvant cycles of ECC (control arm) after the same preoperative ECC and the same quality of surgery (http://www.critics.nl) [16].

Gastric Cancer- Advanced Setting

Contrary to an adjuvant setting, the roles of cisplatin in an advanced setting seem to be more distinct. In the 1990s, ECF has been recognized as a standard regimen for the treatment of advanced gastric cancer because of the higher response rate (46%), longer median survival time (8.7 months), decreased toxicity, and more favorable cost effectiveness as compared with FAMTX (5FU, adriamycin, methotrexate) [17,18]. In this century, cisplatin has become a partner of several new combination regimens. The combination of docetaxel, cisplatin, and 5FU (DCF) has been developed due to the nonoverlapping toxicity profiles of these agents and synergism among these agents in vitro [19,20]. In Europe, DCF was found to be superior to DC or ECF with regard to the response rate (37% versus 18% or 25%) and median survival time (10.4 months versus 11 months or 8.3 months) [21]. In the United States, the response rate and median survival time of the DCF (37% and 9.2 months) was found to be superior to those of the CF (25% and 8.6 months) [22]. The results of these two studies lead to the recommendation of DCF as an investigational regimen for further clinical trials.

However, a higher incidence of grade 3/4 hematological toxicities (82% of neutropenia, 65% of leucopenia, and 29% of neutropenic fever) of the DCF regimen emphasized a need for careful patient management and monitoring. Against these backgrounds, several modifications of the DCF regimen have been developed to improve tolerability. Since weekly administration of taxane is less toxic while maintaining more antitumor activity than conventional triweekly administration of taxane, several DCF modifications with weekly or split doses of docetaxel, or replacement of 5FU with S-1 (fluoropyrimidine derivative) have been reported [23-28] (Table 2). Among these regimens, GASTRO-TAX-1 trial [27] proved to have a remarkably prolonged median survival time (17.9 months) and median time to progression (9.4 months), with a reduced incidence of toxicity (22% of grade 3/4 neutropenia and 5% of febrile neutropenia). Furthermore, a combination of docetaxel, cisplatin, and S-1 (DCS) yielded a remarkable response rate (84%) and median survival time (23 months) [28].

Another promising regimen incorporating cisplatin is a combination of cisplatin and S-1. JCOG9912 trial [29] proved that infusion of 5FU monotherapy could be replaced by S-1, and the subsequent SPIRITS trial has led to the conclusion that an S-1 plus cisplatin combination (CS) is currently considered a standard regimen in Japan for the treatment of advanced gastric cancer [30]. The efficacy of the CS regimen has been also investigated in the USA (FLAGS trial) [31] and in China (http://www.ClinicalTrial.gov. NCT 01198392) [32]. Unfortunately, in the FLAGS trial, CS failed to prolong median survival time as compared with CF (8.6 months versus 7.9 months), but exhibited significant safety advantages. In the Chinese trial, the S-1 dose is the same (80mg/m^2/day, twice daily) as that of the SPIRITS trial [30] in Japan, but cisplatin is given in four administrations, each being 20mg/m^2.

Table 2. DCF and its modifications for gastric and esophageal cancers

Authors	n	Tumor site	Dose and schedule (mg/m^2)	Cycle	RR (%)	median TTP	MST	Grade 3/4 granulocytopenia/ neutropenia (%)	Neutropenic fever (%)
van Cutsem [22]	221	G	75, triweekly	q3w	37	5.6mo	9.2mo	82	29
			75, triweekly						
			750, 5days						
Overmann [23]	95	G,GEJ,E	20, weekly	q8w	34	4.1mo	8.9mo	4	0
			20, weekly						
			350, weekly						
Tebutt [24]	50	G,GEJ,E	20, weekly	q3w	47	5.9mo	11.2mo	10	6
			20, weekly						
			350, weekly						
Park [25]	47	G	50, triweekly	q3w	40	4.6mo	9.7mo	68	26
			80, triweekly						
			1200, 3days						
Li [26]	45	G	36, weekly	q3w	58	6.8mo	13.9mo	51	4
			30, weekly						
			300, 14days						

Table 2. (Continued)

Authors	n	Tumor site	Dose and schedule (mg/m^2)	Cycle	RR (%)	median TTP	MST	Grade 3/4 granulocytopenia/ neutropenia (%)	Neutropenic fever (%)
Lorenzen [27]	60	G,GEJ	40, biweekly	q8w	47	9.4mo	17.9mo	22	5
			40, biweekly						
			2000, weekly						
Sato [28]	31	G	60, triweekly	q3w	87	226d	687d	77	16
			60, triweekly						
			80, 14days						
Tanaka [60]	18	E	40, monthly	q4w	89	ND	ND	6	28
			40, biweekly						
			400, 5days, biweekly						
Minowa [61]	9	E	75, monthly	q4w	56	ND	ND	78	56
			75, monthly						
			750, 5days						
Minamide [62]	32	E	70, monthly	q4w	50	ND	ND	71	ND
			80, monthly						
			800, 5days						
JCOG0807*	ND	E	30-40, biweekly	q4w	ND	ND	ND	ND	ND
			80, monthly						
			800, 5days						

D: docetaxel, C: cisplatin, F: 5FU, U: UFT, S: S-1, G: gastric cancer, GEJ: gastroesophageal junction cancer, E: esophageal cancer, ND: not described.

* Ongoing trial.

Table 3. Neoadjuvant randomized chemotherapy trials incorporating cisplatin for esophageal cancer

Authors	Year	Histology	Chemotherapy					Surgery alone		Statistics
			Drugs	Dose (mg/m^2)	Schedule	n	MST	n	MST	
Roth [49]	1988	SCC, undif	C	120	1day, 1cycle	19	9mo	20	9mo	NS
			B	10*	4days, 1cycle					
			V	3	4days, 1cycle					
Nygaard [50]	1992	SCC	C	20	5days, 2cycles	56	ND	50	ND	NS
			B	10	5days, 2cycles					
Schlag [51]	1992	SCC	C	20	5days, 3cycles	21	ND	24	ND	NS
			F	1000	5days, 3cycles					
Maipang [52]	1994	SCC	C	100	1day, 2cycles	24	17mo	22	17mo	NS
			B	10	5days, 2cycles					
			V	3	4days, 2cycles					
Law [53]	1997	SCC	C	100	1day, 2cycles	74	16.8mo	73	13mo	NS
			F	500	5days, 2cycles					
Kelsen [54]	1998	SCC, Ad	C	100	1day, 3cycles	233	14.9mo	234	16.1mo	NS
			F	1000	5days, 3cycles					

Table 3. (Continued)

Authors	Year	Histology	Chemotherapy					Surgery alone		Statistics
			Drugs	Dose (mg/m^2)	Schedule	n	MST	n	MST	
Baba [55]	2000	SCC	C	70	1day, 2cycles	21	ND	21	ND	NS
			F	700	5days, 2cycles					
Ancona [56]	2001	SCC	C	100	1day, 2or3cycles	47	25mo	47	24mo	NS
			F	1000	5days, 2or3cycles					
MRC [57]	2002	SCC, Ad	C	80	1day, 2cycles	400	16.8mo	402	13.3mo	0.004
			F	1000	4days, 2cycles					
Cao [58]	2009	SCC	C	20	5days, 1cycle	119	ND	118	ND	NS
			F	500	5days, 1cycle					
			M	10	1day, 1cycle					

C; cisplatin, B; bleomycin, F; 5-fluorouracil, V; vindesine, M; mytomicin C.
SCC; squamous cell cancer, Ad; adenocarcinoma, undif; undifferentiated cancer.
* Unit.
MRC; Medical Research Counsil Esophageal Cancer Working Party.
n: number of patients, ND; not described, NS; not significant, MST; median survival time, mo; months.

Table 4. Neoadjuvant randomized chemoradiotherapy trials incorporating cisplatin for esophageal cancer

Authors	Year	Histology	Chemoradiotherapy					Surgery alone		Statistics
			Drugs	Dose (mg/m²)	Schedule	n	MST	n	MST	
Nygaard [50]	1992	SCC	C	20	5days, 2cycles	53	ND	50	ND	NS
			B	10	5days, 2cycles					
			Rx		35Gy					
LePrise [66]	1994	SCC	C	100	1day, 2cycles	41	ND	45	ND	NS
			F	600	4days, 2cycles					
			Rx		20Gy					
Apinop [67]	1994	SCC	C	100	1day, 2cycles	35	9.7mo	34	7.4mo	NS
			F	1000	4days, 2cycles					
			Rx		40Gy					
Walsh [68]	1996	Ad	C	75	1day, 2cycles	58	16mo	55	11mo	0.01
			F	15*	5days, 2cycles					
			Rx		40Gy					
Bosset [69]	1997	SCC	C	80	3days, 2cycles	143	18.6mo	139	18.6mo	NS
Urba [70]	2001	SCC, Ad	C	20	5days, 2cycles	50	16.9mo	50	17.6mo	NS
			F	300	21days					
			V	1	4days, 2cycles					
			Rx		45Gy					
Lee [71]	2004	SCC	C	60	4days, 1cycle	51	28.2mo	50	27.3mo	NS
			F	1000	2days, 1cycle					
			Rx		45.6Gy					

Table 4. (Continued)

Authors	Year	Histology	Chemoradiotherapy					Surgery alone		Statistics
			Drugs	Dose (mg/m^2)	Schedule	n	MST	n	MST	
Burmeister [72]	2005	SCC, Ad	C	80	1day, 1cycle	128	22.2mo	128	19.3mo	NS
			F	800	4days, 1cycle					
			Rx		35Gy					
Natsugoe [73]	2006	SCC	C	7	5days, 4cycles	22	ND	23	ND	NS
			F	350	5days, 4cycles					
			Rx		40Gy					
Tepper [74]	2008	SCC, Ad	C	100	1day, 2cycles	30	4.48y	26	1.79y	0.002
			F	1000	4days, 2cycles					
			Rx		50.4Gy					
Cao [58]	2009	SCC	C	20	5days, 1cycle	118	ND	118	ND	<0.005
			F	500	5days, 1cycle					
			M	10	1day, 1cycle					
			Rx		40Gy					

C; cisplatin, B; bleomycin, F; 5-fluorouracil, V; vindesine, M; mytomicin C, Rx; radiotherapy.
n: number of patients, SCC; squamous cell cancer, Ad; adenocarcinoma.
ND; not described, NS; not significant, MST; median survival time, mo; months, y; years.
* per kilogram.

Gastric Cancer- Neoadjuvant Setting

The majority of the extant randomized controlled trials for neoadjuvant chemotherapy has failed to provide evidence of the superiority of neoadjuvant chemotherapy as compared with the control [33-38], which is accounted for by the small number of recruited patients (usually less than 200), heterogeneous tumor stage (some studies recruited earlier T1/T2 tumors), heterogeneity in the scope of the lymph node dissection or drug administration route, and allowance of additional postoperative adjuvant therapies. Therefore, the results of the subsequent meta-analyses are unfortunately conflicting [39-41]. Against these backgrounds and with the fact of the promising response rate of the CS regimen, as described above, several neoadjuvant chemotherapy trials using CS are ongoing in Japan. First, JCOG0501 is a randomized controlled trial comparing surgery alone with neoadjuvant CS for type 4 or large type 3 gastric cancer (http://www.ClinicalTrial.gov. NCT00252161) [42]. Second, JCOG0405 is a phase II study investigating the efficacy of neoadjuvant CS for gastric cancer with bulky second-tier nodes or positive paraaortic nodes [43]. The results of this study have been reported very recently as an abstract form, in which the pathological response rate and 3-year survival rate were 51% and 59%, respectively [43]. The third study is a comparison between surgery alone and neoadjuvant CS for stage III gastric cancer, both containing adjuvant S-1 (http://www.ClinicalTrial.gov. NCT00182611) [44]. Finally, the COMPASS study is a comparison between CS and paclitaxel plus S-1, in which two types of preoperative treatment schedules (2 or 4 weeks) are also compared in each arm [45].

Esophageal Cancer-Chemotherapy

Multimodal regimens for esophageal cancer treatment commonly include cisplatin-based chemotherapy; however, they have consistently provided negative results both in adjuvant or neoadjuvant settings. In earlier trials as an adjuvant setting, cisplatin and 5FU [46], or cisplatin and vindesine [47], failed to find any survival benefits as compared with surgery alone. Subsequently, the JCOG9204 trial comparing adjuvant CF with surgery alone [48] provided evidence that adjuvant CF was able to yield significantly improved 5-year disease free survival (p=0.04), which was more evident in node positive patients.

In a neoadjuvant setting, most chemotherapy trials have been developed in the West, but their efficacy has been conflicting (Table 3). The significance of survival prolongation by neoadjuvant cisplatin-based chemotherapy was evident in one largest (n=802) trial [57], allowing a recruitment of both squamous cell cancers and adenocarcinoma, while most of the trials in which the recruited patients were less than 100 in number and squamous cancer cells showed no marginal benefit of neoadjuvant chemotherapy (Table 3). By contrast, JCOG9907 [59] has recently provided evidence that preoperative CF was superior to postoperative CF both in progression free (p=0.044) and overall (p=0.014) survivals in squamous cell cancer.

As described in the gastric cancer section, the DCF regimen has been investigated for the treatment of advanced esophageal cancer [60-62] (Table 2). In these studies, response rates were remarkable (>50%), with 20-30% complete response rates, while toxicity was also severe. Response rates seemed to be positively correlated with toxicity, and such a relationship depended on the schedule of docetaxel, i.e., high dose docetaxel by tri- or monthly administration, or low dose docetaxel by weekly administration. Furthermore, JCOG has conducted the phase I/II trial of this regimen for esophageal cancer treatment (JCOG0807). The results of the DCF regimen are still preliminary and therefore require validation, preferably within the context of a large clinical trial in which treatment selection and patient demographics will be more homogeneous.

Esophageal Cancer-Chemoradiotherapy

In esophageal cancer treatment, most chemoradiotherapy regimens consist of CF with radiation. So far, there have been no randomized controlled trials evaluating adjuvant chemoradiotherapy versus surgery alone [63]; however, several retrospective analyses have demonstrated that adjuvant chemoradiotherapy appeared to prolong survival [64,65].

In a neoadjuvant setting, several randomized chemoradiotherapy trials have been conducted in the West and most individual trials failed to provide survival benefits by neoadjuvant chemoradiotherapy (Table 4). However, metaanalyses involving these trials have elucidated that neoadjuvant chemoradiotherapy can improve the downstaging rate [75], R0 resection rate [76], and 3-year survival rate [75,76]. Such survival benefits in favor of neoadjuvant chemoradiotherapy were observed in both adenocarcinoma and squamous cell cancer [77].

Pharmacogenetics

Cisplatin is the most commonly used chemotherapeutic agent in the treatment of gastric and esophageal cancers, however, individuals exist with low therapeutic indices, in which the chemotherapy doses thought necessary for optimal eradication of malignant cells in turn damage normal cells, which eventually manifests adverse events. One of the responsible factors for this phenomenon is the interindividual variation in activation of the glutathione metabolic pathway, which directly involves the detoxification or inactivation of platinum drugs. Consequently, genotypes corresponding to decreased enzymatic activity resulting in reduced detoxification may predict better treatment outcomes and severe adverse events. The following section describes currently available evidence of variations in genes involved in the glutathione pathway influencing drug detoxification or adverse events. Although a definitive role of the glutathione pathway in cisplatin treatment for gastric and esophageal cancers needs to be elucidated, the potential application of glutathione system polymorphic genetic markers is most profound in identifying patients who may respond favorably, balancing drug efficacy and toxicity, and ultimately, differentiating patients who receive the best benefit of cisplatin-containing regimens from those who should not receive the drugs due to the predicted severe adverse events.

Table 5. GSTs polymorphism and treatment outcome by platinum-based chemotherapy

Cancer site	GSTP1 exon5 codon105		GSTP1 exon 6 codon114		GSTT1null		GSTM1null	
	Efficacy*	References	Efficacy*	References	Efficacy*	References	Efficacy*	References
Stomach	↑	[88]			→	[88]	→	[88]
Esophagus	→	[91,92]	↓	[91]	→	[90]	→	[90]
	↓	[90]						
Colorectal	↑	[93-95]	↑	[94]	→	[93,97]	→	[93,97]
	→	[97,98]						
Pancereas	↑	[96]	→	[96]				
Breast					↑	[99]	↑	[99]

* clinical benefit in polymorphism; ↑ : increased, ↓ :decreased, →:no correlation.
GSTs; glutathione S-transferase.

Table 6. Frequencies of GSTP1, T1, and M1 polymorphism in each ethnicity

Ethnicity	GSTP1 exon5 codon105		GSTP1 exon 6 codon114		GSTT1		GSTM1	
	Val/Val	references	Val/Val	references	null	references	null	references
Caucasians	2-16% (around10%)	[101,102]	0-1%	[83,91,94,96,100]	0-36% (mostly<25%)	[102,105,106]	21-74% (around 50%)	[102,107,108,111]
Asians	1-20% (around 5%)	[101,102]	0.3-1%	[109]	18-62% (mostly>40%)	[102,105,110]	26-78% (around 50%)	[102,107,108,110]
African Americans, Black	17-20%	[83,93, 100]	0%	[83,100]	20-40%	[99,106, 111]	34-52% (mostly<40%)	[99,106, 111]
Hispanic	7-33%	[93,100]	0%	[100]	ND		ND	

ND: not described.

Glutathione S-Transferase

The glutathione conjugate pathway is one mechanism by which platinum compounds can be detoxified either by the conjugation of free cisplatin or by binding DNA-cisplatin, thus preventing cytotoxic DNA cross-link formation. This process is mediated by glutathione S-transferases (GSTs) to form less toxic and more water-soluble glutathione conjugates. Glutathione conjugates are subsequently removed from cells by the GS-X pump, representing the final elimination process of the detoxification system [78]. Overexpression of GSTs and the GS-X pump has been correlated closely with cisplatin resistance [79]. Therefore, drug metabolizing GSTs are responsible for the inactivation and detoxification of cisplatin; however, they are highly genetically polymorphic and such polymorphism is attributable to an altered exposure to cisplatin and a wide interindividual variability in efficacy and toxicity of cisplatin.

Human GSTs are subdivided into eight separate subclasses designated alpha, kappa, mu, pi, sigma, theta, zeta, and omega [80]. Several types of allelic variation have been identified [81] and among these, polymorphism of pi, theta, and mu classes has been extensively investigated. The pi class GSTP1 variants are A1404G resulting in amino acid substitution of isoleucine by valine at codon 105 (Ile105Val), and C2294T encoding an alanine to valine exchange at codon 114 (Ala114Val), both conferring lower enzymatic activity [82] [83]. By a combination of these two types of amino acid substitution, there are currently four haplotypes identified (GSTP1*A, *B, *C, and *D), arising from nucleotide transitions that change codon 105 from Ile to Val, and codon 114 from Ala to Val: (i) 105Ile/114Ala (GSTP1*A); (ii) 105Val/114Ala (GSTP1*B); (iii) 105Val/114Val (GSTP1*C); and (iv) 105Ile/114Val (GSTP1*D) [83,84]. The theta class enzyme GSTT1 and the mu class enzyme GSTM1 exhibit gene deletion polymorphism, leading to an absence of enzymatic activity [85]. Therefore, it is conceivable that polymorphism in GSTP1 (Ile105Val, Ala114Val), GSTT1null, and GSTM1null may result in increased response to cisplatin leading to prolonged survival, and at the same time, an increased risk of adverse events.

Taking into account that GSTP1 and GSTT1, and to a lesser extent GSTM1, are widely distributed in the human gastrointestinal tract [86,87], researches on polymorphism of these enzymes provides important knowledge on responses to cisplatin treatment against gastric and esophageal cancers. A number of studies reporting an association between GSTP1, GSTT1, or GSTM1 polymorphism and cancer therapy outcomes or adverse events have been published; however, the existing evidence is seemingly conflicting concerning efficacy of cisplatin-based chemotherapy in gastric and esophageal cancers (Table 5). In gastric cancer, patients harboring the GSTP1 105 Val/Val allele exhibited a better clinical outcome after CF treatment than those with wild type GSTP1 [88]. On the contrary, in esophageal cancer, increased expression of GSTP1 mRNA was correlated with poorer survival after neoadjuvant chemoradiotherapy consisted of CF and radiation [89]. Similarly, a poorer outcome was found in esophageal cancer patients carrying a GSTP1 105Val genotype [90] or 114Val genotype [91] by platinum-based chemotherapy, while other investigators failed to find such an association [92]. On the other hand, GSTT1 null or GSTM1 null rendered no significant survival impact of these cancers [88,90]. In other malignancies, GSTP1, M1, and T1 polymorphism also rendered divergent results concerning clinical outcomes or adverse events. The GSTP1 105Val phenotype could provide favorable prognostic significance in colorectal [93-95] and pancreas [96] cancers, but other studies failed to find such an association [97,98]. Prognostic significance of the null phenotype of GSTT1 and GSTM1 was positive in breast cancer [99] while null in colorectal cancer [93,97]. With regard to adverse events, risks of adverse events in the GSTP1 105Val phenotype were increased [97], neutral [98], and decreased [94], as compared with those in wild type GSTP1 105Ile/Ile carriers. These inconsistent results are attributable to differences in enzymatic activity in various tissues, sequence variations in genes encoding each member in the glutathione system, genetic complexity and differences in key metabolic enzymes for a given chemotherapy regimen, and heterogeneity in terms of treatment modalities.

In addition to such a paradoxical relationship between GSTP1, GSTT1, and GSTM1 polymorphism and clinical outcomes, the polymorphism frequencies are different by ethnicities (Table 6). Frequencies of GSTP1 105Val/Val tended to be higher in African Americans (17-20%) and Hispanics (7-33%) [83,93,100], followed by Caucasians (mostly around 10%) and Asians (mostly around 5%) [101,102]. On the other hand, GSTP1 114Val/Val is a rare occurance (<1%) in all ethnicities. The null genotype of GSTT1 is found in half of Asians while it occurs less frequently in Caucasians and in African Americans. On the other hand, no marked differences are found in the frequencies of GSTM1null between Caucasians and Asians, and they seem to be higher than those of Africans. Previous literature reviews also demonstrated that [103,104] allele frequency in GSTT1 deletion was 0.47-0.58 in Asians, which was two or three times higher than those in Caucasians (0.11-0.20) and in Africans (0.24-0.38). Allele frequencies in GSTM1 deletion were similar in Asians (0.33-0.63), Caucasians (0.38-0.67), and Hispanics (0.49-0.53), which were doubled as compared with those (0.22-0.35) in Africans. Pacific islanders showed the highest (0.64-1.0) GSTM1 deletion frequencies. In other words, GSTT1null and GSTM1null both occur relatively frequently in Asians, less frequently in Africans, while in Caucasians, GSTM1null is dominant as opposed to GSTT1null.

Future Perspectives

In clinical fields, substantial interpatient differences in both clinical response and toxicity are common with many cancer chemotherapy regimens. For example, some tumors are sensitive to chemotherapy while, at the other extreme, some tumors develop de novo resistance to chemotherapy with poor survival. The dose prescribed is close to the dose likely to produce unacceptable toxicity in one patient while being less toxic in another. Pharmacogenetics, the rapidly evolving field of research, holds great promise for assisting the selection of patient-individualized treatment regimens and dosages. Although platinum drugs continue to be a member in the combination chemotherapy regimens for gastric and esophageal cancers, it is less common that gastric and esophageal cancer patients are treated by a single usage of cisplatin. Since two- or three drug regimens are more common in gastric and esophageal cancer treatments, interindividual variations of response and toxicity of these regimens may be defined by the polymorphism in the genes encoding the drug metabolizing enzymes for the all given agents. Such polymorphism may potentially have relevance in decreasing the intracellular enzyme concentrations or structurally altering the enzymes with consequent increases or decreases in functional or dysfunctional proteins. Furthermore, it is also a fact that a significant gap sometimes exists between the discovery of pharmacogenetically relevant markers in basic science laboratories and the results of tests for their clinical values in patient populations. Since the ultimate goal of the application of pharmacogenetics in gastric and esophageal cancer treatment is to diminish adverse events without compromising anticancer activities of chemotherapeutic agents, the focus of future studies may lie in more exploratory pathway-based and comprehensive genome-wide association studies. Therefore, most potential markers are in the discovery phase waiting to undergo clinical validation. Advancing our understanding of the clinical experiences in collaboration with laboratory findings could potentially accelerate our efforts toward decreasing morbidity and mortality of gastric and esophageal cancers.

Conclusion

Cisplatin has been used for the treatment of gastric and esophageal cancers in combination with several anticancer agents. Attempts have been made to establish the effective regimens incorporating cisplatin, and several recent randomized trials have demonstrated the promising results. Since the efficacy of chemotherapy should be evaluated by balancing antitumor effects and toxicities, recent research has explored the pharmacologically relevant genes responsible for cisplatin metabolism and detoxification. Although the most clinically relevant genes have not been definitively determined, one of the candidate genes on this topic is GSTs, and individuals who are carriers of decreased activity of this enzyme may have an impaired ability to metabolize cisplatin, and may therefore be at an increased risk of toxicities. Furthermore, differences in frequencies of polymorphism of GSTs among ethnicities should be taken into account for planning global clinical trials of cisplatin recruiting different ethnicities. The investigation of such gene activities prior to administration will contribute to therapy individualization, i.e., maximizing drug efficacy with minimizing adverse events.

References

[1] Zlatanova, J., Yaneva, J., & Leuba, S.H. (1998). Proteins that specifically recognize cisplatin-damaged DNA: a clue to anticancer activity of cisplatin. *FASEB J.* 12, 791-799.

[2] Hermans, J., Bonenkamp, J.J., Boon, M.C., Bunt, A.M., Ohyama, S., Sasako, M., & Van de Velde, C.J. (1993). Adjuvant therapy after curative resection for gastric cancer: meta-analysis of randomized trials. *J Clin Oncol.* 11, 1441-1447.

[3] Earle, C.C. & Maroun, J.A. (1999). Adjuvant chemotherapy after curative resection for gastric cancer in non-Asian patients: revisiting a meta-analysis of randomised trials. *Eur J Cancer.* 35, 1059-1064.

[4] Mari, E., Floriani, I., Tinazzi, A., Buda, A., Belfiglio, M., Valentini, M., Cascinu, S., Barni, S., Labianca, R., & Torri, V. (2000). Efficacy of adjuvant chemotherapy after curative resection for gastric cancer: a meta-analysis of published randomised trials. A

study of the GISCAD (Gruppo Italiano per lo Studio dei Carcinomi dell'Apparato Digerente). *Ann Oncol.* 11, 837-843.

[5] Panzini, I., Gianni, L., Fattori, P.P., Tassinari, D., Imola, M., Fabbri, P., Arcangeli, V., Drudi, G., Canuti, D., Fochessati, F., & Ravaioli, A. (2002). Adjuvant chemotherapy in gastric cancer: a meta-analysis of randomized trials and a comparison with previous meta-analyses. *Tumori.* 88, 21-27.

[6] Janunger, K.G., Hafström, L., & Glimelius, B. (2002). Chemotherapy in gastric cancer: a review and updated meta-analysis. *Eur J Surg.* 168, 597-608.

[7] Hu, J.K., Chen, Z.X., Zhou, Z.G., Zhang, B., Tian, J., Chen, J.P., Wang,L., Wang, C.H., Chen, H.Y., & Li, Y.P. (2002). Intravenous chemotherapy for resected gastric cancer: meta-analysis of randomized controlled trials. *World J Gastroenterol.* 8, 1023-1028.

[8] Oba, K., Morita, S., Tsuburaya, A., Kodera, Y., Kobayashi, M., & Sakamoto, J. (2006). Efficacy of adjuvant chemotherapy using oral fluorinated pyrimidines for curatively resected gastric cancer: a meta-analysis of centrally randomized controlled clinical trials in Japan. *J Chemother.* 18, 311-317.

[9] Liu, T.S., Wang, Y., Chen, S.Y., & Sun, Y.H. (2008). An updated meta-analysis of adjuvant chemotherapy after curative resection for gastric cancer. *Eur J Surg Oncol.* 34, 1208-1216.

[10] Zhao, SL. & Fang, JY. (2008). The role of postoperative adjuvant chemotherapy following curative resection for gastric cancer: a meta-analysis. *Cancer Invest.* 26, 317-325.

[11] GASTRIC (Global Advanced/Adjuvant Stomach Tumor Research International Collaboration) Group. Paoletti, X., Oba, K., Burzykowski, T., Michiels, S., Ohashi, Y., Pignon, J.P., Rougier, P., Sakamoto, J., Sargent, D., Sasako, M., Van Cutsem, E., & Buyse, M. (2010). Benefit of adjuvant chemotherapy for resectable gastric cancer: a meta-analysis. *JAMA.* 303, 1729-1737.

[12] Sakuramoto, S., Sasako, M., Yamaguchi, T., Kinoshita, T., Fujii, M., Nashimoto, A., Furukawa, H., Nakajima, T., Ohashi, Y., Imamura, H., Higashino, M., Yamamura, Y., Kurita, A., & Arai, K.; ACTS-GC Group. (2007). Adjuvant chemotherapy for gastric cancer with S-1, an oral fluoropyrimidine. *N Engl J Med.* Vol.357, No.18, pp1810-1820.

[13] Macdonald, J.S., Smalley, S.R., Benedetti, J., Hundahl, S.A., Estes, N.C., Stemmermann, G.N., Haller, D.G., Ajani, J.A., Gunderson, L.L., Jessup, J.M., & Martenson, J.A. (2001). Chemoradiotherapy after surgery compared with surgery alone for adenocarcinoma of the stomach or gastroesophageal junction. *N Engl J Med.* 345, 725-730.

[14] Cunningham, D., Allum, W.H., Stenning, S.P., Thompson, J.N., Van de Velde, C.J., Nicolson, M., Scarffe, J.H., Lofts, F.J., Falk, S.J., Iveson, T.J., Smith, D.B., Langley, R.E., Verma, M., Weeden, S., & Chua, Y.J., MAGIC Trial Participants. (2006). Perioperative chemotherapy versus surgery alone for resectable gastroesophageal cancer. *N Engl J Med.* 355, 11-20.

[15] Ychou, M., Boige, V., Pignon, J.P., Conroy, T., Bouché, O., Lebreton, G., Ducourtieux, M., Bedenne, L., Fabre, J.M., Saint-Aubert, B., Genève, J., Lasser, P., Rougier, P. (2011) Perioperative chemotherapy compared with surgery alone for resectable gastroesophageal adenocarcinoma: an FNCLCC and FFCD multicenter phase III trial. *J Clin Oncol.* 29, 1715-1721.

[16] http://www.critics.nl, Accessed April, 2011.

[17] Waters, J.S., Norman, A., Cunningham, D., Scarffe, J.H., Webb, A., Harper, P., Joffe, J.K., Mackean, M., Mansi, J., Leahy, M., Hill, A., Oates, J., Rao, S., Nicolson, M., & Hickish, T. (1999). Long-term survival after epirubicin, cisplatin and fluorouracil for gastric cancer: results of a randomized trial. *Br J Cancer*. 80, 269-272.

[18] Webb, A., Cunningham, D., Scarffe, J.H., Harper, P., Norman, A., Joffe, J.K., Hughes, M., Mansi, J., Findlay, M., Hill, A., Oates, J., Nicolson, M., Hickish, T., O'Brien, M., Iveson, T., Watson, M., Underhill, C., Wardley, A., & Meehan, M. (1997). Randomized trial comparing epirubicin, cisplatin, and fluorouracil versus fluorouracil, doxorubicin, and methotrexate in advanced esophagogastric cancer. *J Clin Oncol*. 15, 261-267.

[19] Maeda, S., Sugiura, T., Saikawa, Y., Kubota, T., Otani ,Y., Kumai, K., & Kitajima, M. (2004). Docetaxel enhances the cytotoxicity of cisplatin to gastric cancer cells by modification of intracellular platinum metabolism. *Cancer Sci*. 95, 679-684.

[20] Kodera, Y., Fujiwara, M., Yokoyama, H., Ohashi, N., Miura, S., Ito, Y., Koike, M., Ito, K., & Nakao, A. (2005). Combination of oral fluoropyrimidine and docetaxel: reappraisal of synergistic effect against gastric carcinoma xenografts. *In Vivo*. 19, 861-866.

[21] Roth, A.D., Fazio, N., Stupp, R., Falk, S., Bernhard, J., Saletti, P., Köberle, D., Borner, M.M., Rufibach, K., Maibach, R., Wernli, M., Leslie, M., Glynne-Jones, R., Widmer, L., Seymour, M., & de Braud ,F.; Swiss Group for Clinical Cancer Research. (2007). Docetaxel, cisplatin, and fluorouracil; docetaxel and cisplatin; and epirubicin, cisplatin, and fluorouracil as systemic treatment for advanced gastric carcinoma: a randomized phase II trial of the Swiss Group for Clinical Cancer Research. *J Clin Oncol*. 25, 3217-3223.

[22] van Cutsem, E., Moiseyenko, V.M., Tjulandin, S., Majlis, A., Constenla, M., Boni, C., Rodrigues, A., Fodor, M., Chao, Y., Voznyi, E., Risse, M.L., & Ajani, J.A.; V325 Study Group. (2006). Phase III study of docetaxel and cisplatin plus fluorouracil compared with cisplatin and fluorouracil as first-line therapy for advanced gastric cancer: a report of the V325 Study Group. *J Clin Oncol*. 24, 4991-4997.

[23] Overman, M.J., Kazmi, S.M., Jhamb, J., Lin, E., Yao, J.C., Abbruzzese, J.L., Ho, L., Ajani, J., & Phan, A. (2010). Weekly docetaxel, cisplatin, and 5-fluorouracil as initial therapy for patients with advanced gastric and esophageal cancer. *Cancer*. 116, 1446-1453.

[24] Tebbutt, N.C., Cummins, M.M., Sourjina, T., Strickland, A., Van Hazel, G., Ganju, V., Gibbs, D., Stockler, M., Gebski, V., & Zalcberg, J.; Australasian Gastro-Intestinal Trials Group. (2010). Randomised, non-comparative phase II study of weekly docetaxel with cisplatin and 5-fluorouracil or with capecitabine in oesophagogastric cancer: the AGITG ATTAX trial. *Br J Cancer*. 102, 475-481.

[25] Park, S.R., Chun, J.H., Kim, Y.W., Lee, J.H., Choi, I.J., Kim, C.G., Lee, J.S., Bae, J.M., & Kim, H.K. (2005). Phase II study of low-dose docetaxel/fluorouracil/cisplatin in metastatic gastric carcinoma. *Am J Clin Oncol*. 28, 433-438.

[26] Li, C.P., Chen, J.S., Chen, L.T., Yen, C.J., Lee, K.D., Su, W.P., Lin, P.C., Lu, C.H., Tsai, H.J., & Chao, Y. (2010). A phase II study of weekly docetaxel and cisplatin plus oral tegafur/uracil and leucovorin as first-line chemotherapy in patients with locally advanced or metastatic gastric cancer. *Br J Cancer*. 103, 1343-1348.

[27] Lorenzen, S., Hentrich, M., Haberl, C., Heinemann, V., Schuster, T., Seroneit, T., Roethling, N., Peschel, C., & Lordick, F. (2007). Split-dose docetaxel, cisplatin and leucovorin/ fluorouracil as first-line therapy in advanced gastric cancer and adenocarcinoma of the gastroesophageal junction: results of a phase II trial. *Ann Oncol.* 18, 1673-1679.

[28] Sato, Y., Takayama, T., Sagawa, T., Takahashi, Y., Ohnuma, H., Okubo, S., Shintani, N., Tanaka, S., Kida, M., Sato, Y., Ohta, H., Miyanishi, K., Sato, T., Takimoto, R., Kobune, M., Yamaguchi, K., Hirata, K., Niitsu, Y., & Kato, J. (2010). Phase II study of S-1, docetaxel and cisplatin combination chemotherapy in patients with unresectable metastatic gastric cancer. *Cancer Chemother Pharmacol.* 66, 721-728.

[29] Boku, N., Yamamoto, S., Fukuda, H., Shirao, K., Doi, T., Sawaki, A., Koizumi, W., Saito, H., Yamaguchi, K., Takiuchi, H., Nasu, J., & Ohtsu, A.; Gastrointestinal Oncology Study Group of the Japan Clinical Oncology Group. (2009). Fluorouracil versus combination of irinotecan plus cisplatin versus S-1 in metastatic gastric cancer: a randomised phase 3 study. *Lancet Oncol.* 10, 1063-1069.

[30] Koizumi, W., Narahara, H., Hara, T., Takagane, A., Akiya, T., Takagi, M., Miyashita, K., Nishizaki, T., Kobayashi, O., Takiyama, W., Toh, Y., Nagaie, T., Takagi, S., Yamamura, Y., Yanaoka, K., Orita, H., & Takeuchi, M. (2008). S-1 plus cisplatin versus S-1 alone for first-line treatment of advanced gastric cancer (SPIRITS trial): a phase III trial. *Lancet Oncol.* 9, 215-221.

[31] Ajani, J.A., Rodriguez, W., Bodoky, G., Moiseyenko, V., Lichinitser, M., Gorbunova, V., Vynnychenko, I., Garin, A., Lang, I., & Falcon, S. (2010). Multicenter phase III comparison of cisplatin/S-1 with cisplatin/infusional fluorouracil in advanced gastric or gastroesophageal adenocarcinoma study: the FLAGS trial. *J Clin Oncol.* 28, 1547-1553.

[32] http://www.ClinicalTrial.gov. NCT 01198392, Accessed April, 2011

[33] Schuhmacher, C., Gretschel, S., Lordick, F., Reichardt, P., Hohenberger, W., Eisenberger, C.F., Haag, C., Mauer, M.E., Hasan, B., Welch, J., Ott, K., Hoelscher, A., Schneider, P.M., Bechstein, W., Wilke, H., Lutz, M.P., Nordlinger, B., Cutsem, E.V., Siewert, J.R., & Schlag, P.M. (2010). Neoadjuvant chemotherapy compared with surgery alone for locally advanced cancer of the stomach and cardia: European Organisation for Research and Treatment of Cancer randomized trial 40954. *J Clin Oncol.* 28, 5210-5218.

[34] Hartgrink, H.H., van de Velde, C.J., Putter, H., Songun, I., Tesselaar, M.E., Kranenbarg, E.K., de Vries, J.E., Wils, J.A., van der Bijl, J., & van Krieken, J.H.; Cooperating Investigators of The Dutch Gastric Cancer Group. (2004). Neo-adjuvant chemotherapy for operable gastric cancer: long term results of the Dutch randomised FAMTX trial. *Eur J Surg Oncol.* 30, 643-649.

[35] Imano, M., Itoh, T., Satou, T., Sogo, Y., Hirai, H., Kato, H., Yasuda, A., Peng, Y.F., Shinkai, M., Yasuda, T., Imamoto, H., Okuno, K., Shiozaki, H., & Ohyanagi, H. (2010). Prospective randomized trial of short-term neoadjuvant chemotherapy for advanced gastric cancer. *Eur J Surg Oncol.* 36, 963-968.

[36] Zhang, C.W., Zou, S.C., Shi, D., & Zhao, D.J. (2004). Clinical significance of preoperative regional intra-arterial infusion chemotherapy for advanced gastric cancer. *World J Gastroenterol.* 10, 3070-3072.

[37] Nio, Y., Koike, M., Omori, H., Hashimoto, K., Itakura, M., Yano, S., Higami, T., & Maruyama, R. (2004). A randomized consent design trial of neoadjuvant chemotherapy with tegafur plus uracil (UFT) for gastric cancer--a single institute study. *Anticancer Res*. 24, 1879-1887.

[38] Yonemura, Y., Sawa, T., Kinoshita, K., Matsuki, N., Fushida, S., Tanaka, S., Ohoyama, S., Takashima, T., Kimura, H., Kamata, T., Fujimura, T., Sugiyama, K., Shima, K., & Miyazaki, I. (1993). Neoadjuvant chemotherapy for high-grade advanced gastric cancer. *World J Surg*. 17, 256-261.

[39] Li, W., Qin, J., Sun, Y.H., & Liu, T.S. (2010). Neoadjuvant chemotherapy for advanced gastric cancer: a meta-analysis. *World J Gastroenterol*. 16, 5621-5628.

[40] Li, H., Zhu, F., Cao, Y., Zhai, L., & Lin, T. (2010). Meta-analyses of randomized trials assessing the effect of neoadjuvant chemotherapy in locally advanced gastric cancer. *Proc ASCO*. Abs 4042.

[41] Wu, A.W., Xu, G.W., Wang, H.Y., Ji, J.F., & Tang, J.L. (2007). Neoadjuvant chemotherapy versus none for resectable gastric cancer. *Cochrane Database Syst Rev*. 18, CD005047.

[42] http://www.ClinicalTrial.gov. NCT00252161, Accessed April, 2011.

[43] Yoshikawa, T., Nakamura, K., Tsuburaya, A., Sano, T., Mizusawa, J., Katai,H., Kurita, A., Uyama, I., Nomura, E., Sasako, M. (2011). A phase II study of preoperative chemotherapy with S-1 (S) and cisplatin (P) followed by D3 gastrectomy for gastric cancer (GC) with extensive lymph node metastasis (ELM): Survival results of JCOG0405. *J Clin Oncol*. 29: suppl 4; abstr 70.

[44] http://www.ClinicalTrial.gov. NCT00182611, Accessed April, 2011

[45] Yoshikawa, T., Tsuburaya, A., Morita, S., Kodera, Y., Ito, S., Cho, H., Miyashita, Y., Sakamoto, J. (2010). A comparison of multimodality treatment: two or four courses of paclitaxel plus cisplatin or S-1 plus cisplatin followed by surgery for locally advanced gastric cancer, a randomized Phase II trial (COMPASS). *Jpn J Clin Oncol*. 40, 369-372.

[46] Pouliquen, X., Levard, H., Hay, J.M., McGee, K., Fingerhut, A., & Langlois-Zantin, O. (1996). 5-Fluorouracil and cisplatin therapy after palliative surgical resection of squamous cell carcinoma of the esophagus. A multicenter randomized trial. French Associations for Surgical Research. *Ann Surg*. 223, 127-33.

[47] Ando, N., Iizuka, T., Kakegawa, T., Isono, K., Watanabe, H., Ide, H., Tanaka, O., Shinoda, M., Takiyama, W., Arimori, M., Ishida, K., & Tsugane, S. (1997). A randomized trial of surgery with and without chemotherapy for localized squamous carcinoma of the thoracic esophagus: the Japan Clinical Oncology Group Study. *J Thorac Cardiovasc Surg*. 114, 205-209.

[48] Ando, N., Iizuka, T., Ide, H., Ishida, K., Shinoda, M., Nishimaki, T., Takiyama, W., Watanabe, H., Isono, K., Aoyama, N., Makuuchi, H., Tanaka, O., Yamana, H., Ikeuchi, S., Kabuto, T., Nagai, K., Shimada, Y., Kinjo, Y., & Fukuda, H.; Japan Clinical Oncology Group. (2003). Surgery plus chemotherapy compared with surgery alone for localized squamous cell carcinoma of the thoracic esophagus: a Japan Clinical Oncology Group Study--JCOG9204. *J Clin Oncol*. 21, 4592-4596.

[49] Roth, J.A., Pass, H.I., Flanagan, M.M., Graeber, G.M., Rosenberg, J.C., & Steinberg, S. (1988). Randomized clinical trial of preoperative and postoperative adjuvant chemotherapy with cisplatin, vindesine, and bleomycin for carcinoma of the esophagus. *J Thorac Cardiovasc Surg*. 96, 242-248.

[50] Nygaard, K., Hagen, S., Hansen, H.S., Hatlevoll, R., Hultborn, R., Jakobsen, A., Mäntyla, M., Modig, H., Munck-Wikland, E., Rosengren, B., et al. (1992) Pre-operative radiotherapy prolongs survival in operable esophageal carcinoma: a randomized, multicenter study of pre-operative radiotherapy and chemotherapy. The second Scandinavian trial in esophageal cancer. *World J Surg*. 16, 1104-1109.

[51] Schlag, P.M. (1992). Randomized trial of preoperative chemotherapy for squamous cell cancer of the esophagus. The Chirurgische Arbeitsgemeinschaft Fuer Onkologie der Deutschen Gesellschaft Fuer Chirurgie Study Group. *Arch Surg*. 127, 1446-1450.

[52] Maipang, T., Vasinanukorn, P., Petpichetchian, C., Chamroonkul, S., Geater, A., Chansawwaang, S., Kuapanich, R., Panjapiyakul, C., Watanaarepornchai, S., & Punperk, S. (1994). Induction chemotherapy in the treatment of patients with carcinoma of the esophagus. *J Surg Oncol*. 56, 191-197.

[53] Law, S., Fok, M., Chow, S., Chu, K.M., & Wong, J. (1997). Preoperative chemotherapy versus surgical therapy alone for squamous cell carcinoma of the esophagus: a prospective randomized trial. *J Thorac Cardiovasc Surg*. 114, 210-217.

[54] Kelsen, D.P., Ginsberg, R., Pajak, T.F., Sheahan, D.G., Gunderson, L., Mortimer, J., Estes, N., Haller, D.G., Ajani, J., Kocha, W., Minsky, B.D., & Roth, J.A. (1998). Chemotherapy followed by surgery compared with surgery alone for localized esophageal cancer. *N Engl J Med*. 339, 1979-1984.

[55] Baba, M., Natsugoe, S., Shimada, M., Nakano, S., Kusano, C., Fukumoto, T., Aikou, T., & Akazawa, K. (2000). Prospective evaluation of preoperative chemotherapy in resectable squamous cell carcinoma of the thoracic esophagus. *Dis Esophagus*. 13, 136-141.

[56] Ancona, E., Ruol, A., Santi, S., Merigliano, S., Sileni, V.C., Koussis, H., Zaninotto, G., Bonavina, L., & Peracchia, A. (2001). Only pathologic complete response to neoadjuvant chemotherapy improves significantly the long term survival of patients with resectable esophageal squamous cell carcinoma: final report of a randomized, controlled trial of preoperative chemotherapy versus surgery alone. *Cancer*. 91, 2165-2174.

[57] Medical Research Council Oesophageal Cancer Working Group. Surgical resection with or without preoperative chemotherapy in oesophageal cancer: a randomised controlled trial. (2002). *Lancet*. 359, 1727-1733.

[58] Cao, X.F., He, X.T., Ji, L., Xiao, J., & Lv, J. (2009). Effects of neoadjuvant radiochemotherapy on pathological staging and prognosis for locally advanced esophageal squamous cell carcinoma. *Dis Esophagus*. 22, 477-481.

[59] Ando, N., Kato, H., Shinoda, M., Ozawa, S., Shimizu, H., Nakamura, T., Yabuzaki, Y., Aoyama, N., Kurita, A., & Fukuda, H. (2008). A randomized trial of postoperative adjuvant chemotherapy with cisplatin and 5-fluorouracil versus neoadjuvant chemotherapy for localized squamous cell carcinoma of the thoracic esophagus (JCOG 9907). *Gastrointestinal Cancers Symposium*, Abs10.

[60] Tanaka, Y., Yoshida, K., Sanada, Y., Osada, S., Yamaguchi, K., & Takahashi, T. (2010). Biweekly docetaxel, cisplatin, and 5-fluorouracil (DCF) chemotherapy for advanced esophageal squamous cell carcinoma: a phase I dose-escalation study. *Cancer Chemother Pharmacol*. 66, 1159-1165.

[61] Minowa, M., Kinoshita, Y., Hasebe, S., Ito, T., Ogawa, M., Takebayashi, K., Ehara, K., Ueno, M., Udagawa, H., & Hayashi, M. (2011). Evaluation of efficacy and safety of

first-line docetaxel/cisplatin/5-FU combined therapy for advanced esophageal cancer. *Gan To Kagaku Ryoho*. 38, 393-397.

[62] Minamide, J., Aoyama, N., Takada, K., & Oota, Y. (2007). Evaluation of docetaxel, CDDP and 5-FU combined therapy as second-line chemotherapy for esophagus cancer. *Gan To Kagaku Ryoho*. 34, 49-52.

[63] Malthaner, R.A., Wong, R.K., Rumble, R.B., & Zuraw, L.; Members of the Gastrointestinal Cancer Disease Site Group of Cancer Care Ontario's Program in Evidence-based Care. (2004). Neoadjuvant or adjuvant therapy for resectable esophageal cancer: a systematic review and meta-analysis. *BMC Med*. Vol.2, p35. [Ongoing]

[64] Bédard, E.L., Inculet, R.I., Malthaner, R.A., Brecevic, E., Vincent, M., & Dar, R. (2001). The role of surgery and postoperative chemoradiation therapy in patients with lymph node positive esophageal carcinoma. *Cancer*. 91, 2423-2430.

[65] Rice, T.W., Adelstein, D.J., Chidel, M.A., Rybicki, L.A., DeCamp, M.M., Murthy, S.C., & Blackstone, E.H. (2003). Benefit of postoperative adjuvant chemoradiotherapy in locoregionally advanced esophageal carcinoma. *J Thorac Cardiovasc Surg*. 126, 1590-1596.

[66] Le Prise, E., Etienne, P.L., Meunier, B., Maddern, G., Ben Hassel, M., Gedouin, D., Boutin, D., Campion, J.P., & Launois, B. (1994). A randomized study of chemotherapy, radiation therapy, and surgery versus surgery for localized squamous cell carcinoma of the esophagus. *Cancer*. 73, 1779-1784.

[67] Apinop, C., Puttisak, P., & Preecha, N. (1994). A prospective study of combined therapy in esophageal cancer. *Hepatogastroenterology*. 41, 391-393.

[68] Walsh, T.N., Noonan, N., Hollywood, D., Kelly, A., Keeling, N., & Hennessy, T.P. (1996). A comparison of multimodal therapy and surgery for esophageal adenocarcinoma. *N Engl J Med*. 335, 462-467.

[69] Bosset, J.F., Gignoux, M., Triboulet, J.P., Tiret, E., Mantion, G., Elias, D., Lozach, P., Ollier, J.C., Pavy, J.J., Mercier, M., & Sahmoud, T. (1997). Chemoradiotherapy followed by surgery compared with surgery alone in squamous-cell cancer of the esophagus. *N Engl J Med*. 337, 161-167.

[70] Urba, S.G., Orringer, M.B., Turrisi, A., Iannettoni, M., Forastiere, A., & Strawderman, M. (2001). Randomized trial of preoperative chemoradiation versus surgery alone in patients with locoregional esophageal carcinoma. *J Clin Oncol*. 19, 305-313.

[71] Lee, J.L., Park, S.I., Kim, S.B., Jung, H.Y., Lee, G.H., Kim, J.H., Song, H.Y., Cho, K.J., Kim, W.K., Lee, J.S., Kim, S.H., & Min, Y.I. (2004). A single institutional phase III trial of preoperative chemotherapy with hyperfractionation radiotherapy plus surgery versus surgery alone for resectable esophageal squamous cell carcinoma. *Ann Oncol*. 15, 947-954.

[72] Burmeister, B.H., Smithers, B.M., Gebski, V., Fitzgerald, L., Simes, R.J., Devitt, P., Ackland, S., Gotley, D.C., Joseph, D., Millar, J., North, J., Walpole, E.T., & Denham, J.W.; Trans-Tasman Radiation Oncology Group; Australasian Gastro-Intestinal Trials Group. (2005). Surgery alone versus chemoradiotherapy followed by surgery for resectable cancer of the oesophagus: a randomised controlled phase III trial. *Lancet Oncol*. 6, 659-668.

[73] Natsugoe, S., Okumura, H., Matsumoto, M., Uchikado, Y., Setoyama, T., Yokomakura, N., Ishigami, S., Owaki, T., & Aikou, T. (2006). Randomized controlled study on

preoperative chemoradiotherapy followed by surgery versus surgery alone for esophageal squamous cell cancer in a single institution. *Dis Esophagus*. 19, 468-472.

[74] Tepper, J., Krasna, M.J., Niedzwiecki, D., Hollis, D., Reed, C.E., Goldberg, R., Kiel, K., Willett, C., Sugarbaker, D., & Mayer, R. (2008). Phase III trial of trimodality therapy with cisplatin, fluorouracil, radiotherapy, and surgery compared with surgery alone for esophageal cancer: CALGB 9781. *J Clin Oncol*. 26, 1086-1092.

[75] Fiorica, F., Di Bona, D., Schepis, F., Licata, A., Shahied, L., Venturi, A., Falchi, A.M., Craxì, A., & Cammà, C. (2004). Preoperative chemoradiotherapy for oesophageal cancer: a systematic review and meta-analysis. *Gut*. 53, 925-930.

[76] Urschel, JD. & Vasan, H. (2003). A meta-analysis of randomized controlled trials that compared neoadjuvant chemoradiation and surgery to surgery alone for resectable esophageal cancer. *Am J Surg*. 185, 538-543.

[77] Gebski, V., Burmeister, B., Smithers, B.M., Foo, K., Zalcberg, J., & Simes, J.; Australasian Gastro-Intestinal Trials Group. (2007). Survival benefits from neoadjuvant chemoradiotherapy or chemotherapy in oesophageal carcinoma: a meta-analysis. *Lancet Oncol*. 8, 226-324.

[78] Ishikawa, T., & Ali-Osman, F. (1993). Glutathione-associated cis-diammine-dichloroplatinum(II) metabolism and ATP-dependent efflux from leukemia cells. Molecular characterization of glutathione-platinum complex and its biological significance. *J Biol Chem*. 268, 20116-20125.

[79] Kartalou, M., & Essigmann, J.M. (2001). Mechanisms of resistance to cisplatin. *Mutat Res*. 478, 23-43.

[80] Strange, R.C., Spiteri, M.A., Ramachandran, S., & Fryer, A.A. (2001). Glutathione-S-transferase family of enzymes. *Mutat Res*. 482, 21-26.

[81] Hayes, J.D., & Strange, R.C. (2000). Glutathione S-transferase polymorphisms and their biological consequences. *Pharmacology*. 61, 154-166.

[82] Srivastava, S.K., Singhal, S.S., Hu, X., Awasthi, Y.C., Zimniak, P., & Singh, S.V. (1999). Differential catalytic efficiency of allelic variants of human glutathione S-transferase Pi in catalyzing the glutathione conjugation of thiotepa. *Arch Biochem Biophys*. 366, 89-94.

[83] Watson, M.A., Stewart, R.K., Smith, G.B., Massey, T.E., & Bell, D.A. (1998). Human glutathione S-transferase P1 polymorphisms: relationship to lung tissue enzyme activity and population frequency distribution. *Carcinogenesis*. 19, 275-280.

[84] Ali-Osman, F., Akande, O., Antoun, G., Mao, J.X., & Buolamwini, J. (1997). Molecular cloning, characterization, and expression in Escherichia coli of full-length cDNAs of three human glutathione S-transferase Pi gene variants. Evidence for differential catalytic activity of the encoded proteins. *J Biol Chem*. 272, 10004-100012.

[85] London, S.J., Yuan, J.M., Chung, F.L. Gao, Y.T., Coetzee, G.A., Ross, R.K., & Yu, M.C. (2000). Isothiocyanates, glutathione S-transferase M1 and T1 polymorphisms, and lung-cancer risk: a prospective study of men in Shanghai, China. *Lancet*. 356, 724-729.

[86] de Bruin, W.C., Wagenmans, M.J., & Peters, W.H. (2000). Expression of glutathione S-transferase alpha, P1-1 and T1-1 in the human gastrointestinal tract. *Jpn J Cancer Res*. 91, 310-316.

[87] Peters, W.H., Roelofs, H.M., Hectors, M.P., Nagengast, F.M., & Jansen, J.B. (1993). Glutathione and glutathione S-transferases in Barrett's epithelium. *Br J Cancer*. 67, 1413-1417.

[88] Goekkurt, E., Hoehn, S., Wolschke, C., Wittmer, C., Stueber, C., Hossfeld, D.K., & Stoehlmacher, J. (2006). Polymorphisms of glutathione S-transferases (GST) and thymidylate synthase (TS)--novel predictors for response and survival in gastric cancer patients. *Br J Cancer*. 94, 281-286.

[89] Joshi, M.B., Shirota, Y., Danenberg, K.D., Conlon, D.H., Salonga, D.S., Herndon, JE 2nd., Danenberg, P.V., & Harpole, D.H. Jr. (2005). High gene expression of TS1, GSTP1, and ERCC1 are risk factors for survival in patients treated with trimodality therapy for esophageal cancer. *Clin Cancer Res*. 11, 2215-2221.

[90] Lee, J.M., Wu, M.T., Lee, Y.C., Yang, S.Y., Chen, J.S., Hsu, H.H., Huang, P.M., Kuo, S.W., Lee, C.J., & Chen, C.J. (2005). Association of GSTP1 polymorphism and survival for esophageal cancer. *Clin Cancer Res*. 11, 4749-4753.

[91] Wu, X., Gu, J., Wu, T.T., Swisher, S.G., Liao, Z., Correa, A.M., Liu, J., Etzel, C.J., Amos, C.I., Huang, M., Chiang, S.S., Milas, L., Hittelman, W.N., & Ajani, J.A. (2006). Genetic variations in radiation and chemotherapy drug action pathways predict clinical outcomes in esophageal cancer. *J Clin Oncol*. 24, 3789-3798.

[92] Okuno, T., Tamura, T., Yamamori, M., Chayahara, N., Yamada, T., Miki, I., Okamura, N., Kadowaki, Y., Shirasaka, D., Aoyama, N., Nakamura, T., Okumura, K., Azuma, T., Kasuga, M., & Sakaeda, T. (2007). Favorable genetic polymorphisms predictive of clinical outcome of chemoradiotherapy for stage II/III esophageal squamous cell carcinoma in Japanese. *Am J Clin Oncol*. 30, 252-257.

[93] Stoehlmacher, J., Park, D.J., Zhang, W., Groshen, S., Tsao-Wei, D.D., Yu, M.C., & Lenz, H.J. (2002). Association between glutathione S-transferase P1, T1, and M1 genetic polymorphism and survival of patients with metastatic colorectal cancer. *J Natl Cancer Inst*. 94, 936-942.

[94] Lecomte, T., Landi, B., Beaune, P., Laurent-Puig, P., & Loriot, M.A. (2006). Glutathione S-transferase P1 polymorphism (Ile105Val) predicts cumulative neuropathy in patients receiving oxaliplatin-based chemotherapy. *Clin Cancer Res*. 12, 3050-3056.

[95] Chen, Y.C., Tzeng, C.H., Chen, P.M., Lin, J.K., Lin, T.C., Chen, W.S., Jiang, J.K., Wang, H.S., & Wang, W.S. (2010). Influence of GSTP1 I105V polymorphism on cumulative neuropathy and outcome of FOLFOX-4 treatment in Asian patients with colorectal carcinoma. *Cancer Sci*. 101, 530-535.

[96] Jiao, L., Bondy, M.L., Hassan, M.M., Chang, D.Z., Abbruzzese, J.L., Evans, D.B., Smolensky, M.H., & Li, D. (2007). Glutathione S-transferase gene polymorphisms and risk and survival of pancreatic cancer. *Cancer*. 109, 840-848.

[97] Ruzzo, A., Graziano, F., Loupakis, F., Rulli, E., Canestrari, E., Santini, D., Catalano, V., Ficarelli, R., Maltese, P., Bisonni, R., Masi, G., Schiavon, G., Giordani, P., Giustini, L., Falcone, A., Tonini, G., Silva, R., Mattioli, R., Floriani, I., & Magnani, M. (2007). Pharmacogenetic profiling in patients with advanced colorectal cancer treated with first-line FOLFOX-4 chemotherapy. *J Clin Oncol*. 25, 1247-1254.

[98] Kweekel, D.M., Gelderblom, H., Antonini, N.F., Van der Straaten, T., Nortier, J.W., Punt, C.J., & Guchelaar, H.J. (2009). Glutathione-S-transferase pi (GSTP1) codon 105 polymorphism is not associated with oxaliplatin efficacy or toxicity in advanced colorectal cancer patients. *Eur J Cancer*. 45, 572-578.

[99] Ambrosone, C.B., Sweeney. C., Coles. B.F., Thompson, P.A., McClure, G.Y., Korourian, S., Fares, M.Y., Stone, A., Kadlubar, F.F., & Hutchins, L.F. Polymorphisms

in glutathione S-transferases (GSTM1 and GSTT1) and survival after treatment for breast cancer. *Cancer Res*. 61, 7130-7135.

[100] Lu, C., Spitz, M.R., Zhao, H., Dong, Q., Truong, M., Chang, J.Y., Blumenschein, G.R. Jr., Hong, W.K., & Wu, X. (2006). Association between glutathione S-transferase pi polymorphisms and survival in patients with advanced nonsmall cell lung carcinoma. *Cancer*. 106, 441-447

[101] Zhou, Y., Li, N., Zhuang, W., Yin, Y.Q., Liu, G.J., Wu, T.X., Yao, X., Du, L., Wei, M.L., & Wu, X.T. (2009). Glutathione S-transferase P1 gene polymorphism associated with gastric cancer among Caucasians. *Eur J Cancer*. 45, 1438-1442.

[102] Yang, C.X., Matsuo, K., Wang, Z.M., & Tajima, K. (2005). Phase I/II enzyme gene polymorphisms and esophageal cancer risk: a meta-analysis of the literature. *World J Gastroenterol*. 11, 2531-2538.

[103] Rebbeck, T.R. (1997). Molecular epidemiology of the human glutathione S-transferase genotypes GSTM1 and GSTT1 in cancer susceptibility. *Cancer Epidemiol Biomarkers Prev*. 6, 733-743.

[104] Bolt, H.M., & Their, R. (2006). Relevance of the deletion polymorphisms of the glutathione S-transferases GSTT1 and GSTM1 in pharmacology and toxicology. *Curr Drug Metab*. 7, 613-628.

[105] Chen, B., Cao, L., Zhou, Y., Yang, P., Wan, H.W., Jia, G.Q., Liu, L., & Wu, X.T. (2010). Glutathione S-transferase T1 (GSTT1) gene polymorphism and gastric cancer susceptibility: a meta-analysis of epidemiologic studies. *Dig Dis Sci*. 55, 1831-1838.

[106] Chen, C.L., Liu, Q., & Relling, M.V. (1996). Simultaneous characterization of glutathione S-transferase M1 and T1 polymorphisms by polymerase chain reaction in American whites and blacks. *Pharmacogenetics*. 6, 187-191.

[107] Chen, B., Zhou, Y., Yang, P., & Wu, X.T. (2010). Glutathione S-transferase M1 gene polymorphism and gastric cancer risk: an updated analysis. *Arch Med Res*. 41, 558-566.

[108] Wang, H., Zhou, Y., Zhuang, W., Yin, Y.Q., Liu, G.J., Wu, T.X., Yao, X., Du, L., Wei, M.L., & Wu, X.T. Glutathione S-transferase M1 null genotype associated with gastric cancer among Asians. *Dig Dis Sci*. 55, 1824-1830.

[109] Wang, J., Jiang, J., Zhao, Y., Gajalakshmi, V., Kuriki, K., Suzuki, S., Nagaya, T., Nakamura, S., Akasaka, S., Ishikawa, H., & Tokudome, S. (2011). Genetic polymorphisms of glutathione S-transferase genes and susceptibility to colorectal cancer: a case-control study in an Indian population. *Cancer Epidemiol*. 35, 66-72.

[110] Lee, E.J., Wong, J.Y., Yeoh, P.N., & Gong, N.H. (1995). Glutathione S transferase-theta (GSTT1) genetic polymorphism among Chinese, Malays and Indians in Singapore. *Pharmacogenetics*. 5, 332-334.

[111] Bailey, L.R., Roodi, N., Dupont, W.D., & Parl, F.F. (1998). Association of cytochrome P450 1B1 (CYP1B1) polymorphism with steroid receptor status in breast cancer. *Cancer Res*. 58, 5038-5041.

In: Cisplatin: Pharmacology, Clinical Uses and Adverse Effects ISBN: 978-1-61942-359-6
Editors: Toshiko Kojima and Yoko Morita

Chapter VI

CISPLATIN NEUROTOXICITY INDUCES CELL DEATH *IN VIVO* AND *IN VITRO*

Maria Grazia Bottone,[1,2,*] Giada Santin,[2] Valeria Maria Piccolini,[1] Veronica Dal Bo[1] and Graziella Bernocchi[1,2]

[1]Dipartimento di Biologia Animale, Laboratorio di Biologia Cellulare e Neurobiologia, Università di Pavia, via Ferrata 1, Pavia, Italy

[2]Istituto di Genetica Molecolare del CNR, Università di Pavia, via Ferrata 1, Pavia, Italy

ABSTRACT

It is known that cisplatin is one of the most effective and widely used cytotoxic agents in the treatment of a variety of malignancies, in both childish and adult patients. Cisplatin cytotoxicity originates from its binding to DNA that causes significant distortion of helical structure and results in the inhibition of DNA replication and transcription. Although its effectiveness, the continued clinical use of cisplatinum is limited by the onset of severe side effects (e.g. nephrotoxicity, ototoxicity and neurotoxicity) and drug resistance.

Bcl-2 and Bax are apoptotic regulating proteins belonging to Bcl-2 family. The first one is an anti-apoptotic member, involved in a cellular pro-survival function. Recent findings show that Bcl-2 plays an important role in the regulation of mitochondrial fusion, phenomenon noticed during cisplatin-resistance. Bax, a pro-apoptotic factor, provokes after death stimulus the perturbation of mitochondrial membrane potential with the externalization of apoptotic factors such as cytochrome c and AIF (Apoptosis Inducing Factor). Consequently, both Bcl-2 and Bax are involved in the mitochondrial apoptotic caspase-dependent and -independent pathway. The purpose of this work is to summarize our recent results about cisplatin treatment both *in vivo* and *in vitro*.

In vivo studies were carried out on postnatally developing rat cerebellum and hippocampus, after a single injection of 5 μg/g or 10 μg/g b.w.; the attention was focused on immunocytochemical changes of pro-apoptotic and antiapoptotic proteins.

In vitro, 20/48h 40μM cisplatin is used on B50 neuroblastoma rat cells in order to investigate the activation of mitochondrial apoptotic pathways by means of

*E-mail: bottone@unipv.it.

immunolabelling and western blotting of cytochrome c and AIF and the apoptotic regulation through immunocytochemical analysis of the Bcl-2 and Bax opposite function.

Keywords: Cell death; central nervous system; B50 neuroblastoma rat cells; cisPt; immunohistochemistry

CISPLATIN AND NEUROTOXICITY

i. General Remarks and Mechanisms of Cisplatin Action

Cisplatin (cisPt), that is the most common therapy drugs [1], is a highly effective anticancer drug and has important role also in the treatment of childish malignancies as neuroblastoma, osteosarcoma and some brain tumours [2]. However, chronic ototoxicity, neurotoxicity and nephrotoxicity have encouraged the development of several less toxic platinum analogues, such as carboplatin [3, 4] or oxaliplatin [5].

Mechanisms of action of cisPt are principally based on interaction with DNA of mitotic cells [6, 7]. In proliferating cells, platinum atoms form covalent bonds to purine bases whose result is a blockage of DNA synthesis. The resulting DNA damage triggers cell-cycle arrest, activation of the tumour-suppressor p53 and apoptosis [8]. Moreover cisPt toxicity can also induce death in non mitotic cells by interacting with cytoplasmic proteins [9].

CisPt is commonly administered by an endovenous injection through which it can reach the cell and spread in the cellular membrane by two main mechanisms: (a) passive diffusion [10]; (b) thought the active copper carrier Ctr1p [11]. Inside the cytoplasm it undergoes aquation, and the result of this hydrolysis (loss of $2Cl^-$) is the formation of a positive charged molecule [$(NH_3)_2Pt^{2+}$] that forms inter- and intra-strand crossing links between adjacent guanine residues in the DNA molecule [12, 13].

Unfortunately, the benefit of this frequently prescribed drug is compromised by severe side effects, including neurotoxicity, that leads to neurodegeneration, and chemoresistance [14, 15].

CisPt neurotoxicity is first characterized by painful paresthesias and numbness that typically occurs during the first few drug cycles. The loss of vibration sense, paraesthesia and ataxia can become apparent after several treatment cycles. The loss of motor functions has also been reported in patients treated with cisPt: as a matter of facts platinum-based agents have the propensity to enter the dorsal root ganglia and peripheral nerves as these structures are not protected by the blood brain barrier [14]. Levels of platinum have been shown to be significantly higher in the dorsal root ganglia than in the brain and in the spinal cord, which are protected by the barrier [16].

At a cellular level, due to the distortion of the DNA molecule, cisPt seems to affect the axons, myelin sheath, neuronal cell body, and the glial structures of the neurons, by inhibiting the regular processes or transcription and replication [17]. Moreover, an additional complex composed of platinum-DNA-protein cross-links is able to disrupt nuclear metabolism and spatial organization of chromatin as well as to inhibit DNA replication and repair [14]. Crossing links can be formed also between small molecules as glutathione to DNA, and if the DNA repair machine is unable to repair efficiently the damage, cells will die for apoptosis [18].

In the last years, several morphological and molecular changes have demonstrated the vulnerability to a single injection of cisPt of the postnatally developing cerebellum, including the degeneration of proliferating and postmitotic neurons [19, 20, 21, 22, 23, 24]. Numerous haemorrhagic foci were found in the whole cerebellar cortex, mainly seven days after treatment performed at postnatal day 10 [15]. Recently, decreased immunoreactivity for most of neurotransmitter receptor markers was found after cisPt treatment in the hippocampal formation [25], that is a brain area associated with neurological disorders in which aberrant activation of neurotransmitter systems may occur and lead to neuronal death [26]. CisPt treatment produces a loss of GABAergic interneurons in some hippocampal layers and a significant decrease of some distinctive neurons, such as hilar mossy cells. However, cisPt-induced functional damages of neural circuits found in hippocampus were different from cerebellum: no robust recovery and morphological remodeling was detectable within hippocampus, likely due to the more restricted postnatal neurogenesis [25].

ii. Aim of this Paper

This paper aims to be a review of findings obtained in our laboratory *in vivo* and *in vitro* to document changes of molecular markers of the apoptotic process. In the researches *in vivo*, two areas of rat developing central nervous system (CNS), i.e. the cerebellum and hippocampal formation will be investigated; in particular, new results recently obtained on hippocampal formation will be added. Neuroblastoma cultured cells will be very useful to underline the apoptotic mechanisms of cisPt action.

Cisplatin and Cell Death

i. Morphological and Molecular Aspects of Cell Death

The progressive transformation of normal cells to malignant derivatives is a complex multi-step process, which requires dynamic alterations of the genome and successful breaching of intracellular checkpoints [27]. It is well known that apoptosis is an actively mediated cell suicide process and that defective or inefficient apoptosis is an acquired hallmark of cancer cells. From this viewpoint, apoptosis is the final goal of chemotherapy.

Apoptosis is characterized by cell shrinkage, blebbing of plasma membrane, maintenance of organelle integrity, condensation and fragmentation of DNA, followed by ordered removal of phagocytes [28]. This allows that no inflammation is induced, without damage at near cells or tissues.

There are different apoptotic pathways with the engagement of several molecular factors. Two main classes are distinguishable by the activation/not-activation of caspases, a family of cysteinyl-aspartate-specific proteases executioners of apoptotic cell death. The extrinsic pathway belongs to caspase-dependent apoptosis and it entails a cooperation between the death receptors found on the surface of the cell membranes and their respective ligands [29]. This leads to receptor oligomerization and intracellular recruitment of proteins into a death-inducing signalling complex (DISC), which then activates an initiator caspase, procaspase 8.

Then, activated caspase 8 triggers the execution phase of apoptosis via the activation of the downstream effector caspase 3. The result is the detrimental modifications at the cytosol, membrane and nucleus [30]. The mitochondrial pathway of apoptosis is also generally known as the intrinsic pathway and it allows to the permeabilization of the mitochondrial outer membrane (MOMP); consequently, proteins usually confined to intermembrane space, as cytochrome c and apoptosis inducing factors (AIF) are released into the cytosol [31]. Once the proteins are translocated in the cytosol, it can be distinguished between the intrinsic caspase-dependent pathway and the intrinsic caspase-independent pathway, basing on the apoptotic factor released. Cytochrome c belongs to the first category, because in the cytosol it recruits procaspase 9 in a complex called Apaf-1 (Apoptosis Activator Factor 1) in which it is activated to caspase 9 and effector caspase 3 is triggered as consequence. AIF moves through the cytosol but finally goes into the nucleus, where it cooperate with endonuclease G in the DNA degradation [32]. AIF does not start caspases cascade activation, so this pathway is defined caspase-independent pathway. Endoplasmic Reticulum (ER) is another organelle involved in an intrinsic pathway. Evidence is accumulating that defective folding and rapid degradation of mutant proteins is one of the causes of various disease including amyloidosis, cystic fibrosis and neurodegenerative disorders such as prion disease, Alzheimer's disease and Parkinson's disease [33]. Therefore, proper function of the ER is essential to cell survival and any perturbation of its function induces cellular damage and results in apoptosis. UPR (Unfolded Protein Response) usually activates in order to balance this defect, but when ER stress is prolonged also UPR is not able to work correctly and CHOP and JNK signalling transduction pathways are started with the triggering of initiator caspase 12 [34]. ER-mediating apoptosis can be defined caspase-dependent pathway.

ii. Cisplatin and Apoptotic Molecules (Bax and Bcl2)

Paying attention to the programmed cell death, that has a critical role during normal brain development and cellular homeostasis, it has been equated with apoptosis, although non-apoptotic forms of cell death also exist, e.g. autophagy [35]. A major role in regulating neuronal death in the CNS was assumed by the pro-apoptotic molecule Bax, during development and after injury [36, 37]. Bcl-2 (B-cell lymphoma gene 2) is an antiapoptotic protein expressed at high level during development of CNS and down regulated after birth; Bcl-2 is crucial in the maintenance of neuronal survival [38].

Bcl-2 mitochondrial proteins are involved in regulation of programmed cell death and are divided into two groups: anti-apoptotic and pro-apoptotic factors. Their location changes depending on the function: Bcl-2 protein belongs to the first group, it is located mainly at the mitochondrial membrane and it is involved in the preservation of mitochondrial integrity: it exerts an inhibitory effect on the membrane permeability [39, 40]; Bax belongs to the second group and it is located in the cytosol as inactive form, when it is activated after an apoptotic stimulus it moves into the mitochondria starting off the intrinsic apoptotic pathway [41].

CISPLATIN NEUROTOXICITY *IN VIVO*

i. Adult CNS

Severe neurotoxic effects have been noted [1, 42]. Implications for clinical neuropsychology arising from neurological disruption associated with cisPt based therapy have been reported [43]. Platinum drugs appear to affect the axons, myelin sheath, neuronal cell bodies and the glial structures of the neural tissue [44]. At the cellular level, the chemotherapy interferes not only with DNA replication but also with metabolic function of the neurons [45]. In the mature brain, platinum-based agents have the propensity to enter the dorsal root ganglia and peripheral nerves [46, 47] but not the brain, due to poor penetration through the Brain-Blood Barrier (BBB) [48]. Nevertheless, toxicity of direct infusion of cisPt to the CNS of male rabbit has been reported [49] as well as damages of mammalian brain vessels [19, 49].

ii. Developing CNS

Development of the mammalian CNS does not end at birth but continues in the postnatal life. In humans, the morphological and functional maturation extends through infancy, childhood, and adolescence [50, 51]. Because developmental processes are vulnerable to disruption by agents that may not be toxic to mature systems, it is reasonable to expect that the later stages of brain development present special risks. It is interesting to note that recent studies on cisPt have identified a large number of long-term behavioural issues (such as depression, anxiety and antisocial behavior) in pediatric oncology patients, especially those treated for CNS tumors [52]. The benefit of cisPt is compromised by severe side effects including neurotoxicity [1]; central neurodegeneration with cerebellar cell loss [53] and hippocampal cell death [54] are described. One of the critical factors for cisPt chemotherapy in very young children is linked to the BBB. The developing brain is distinguished by the absence or incomplete BBB. The development of BBB is a gradual process beginning *in utero* terminating around six months in humans [55], while in the rat, the BBB is mature 21 days after birth [56], but achieves full functionality between 33-40 days of age [57].

Nevertheless, the BBB associated to brain tumors is poorly developed leading to increased vascular permeability [58, 59]; in addition, in pathologic conditions or other forms of brain injury a number of chemical mediators are released that increased BBB permeability [59].

iii. Postnatal Development of Rat Cerebellum and Apoptotic Molecules

The complex layered architecture of cerebellum, like the cerebral cortex and hippocampus, add cells over a long period and cell production creates numbers of neurons in excess of the number actually needed [60, 61]. The overproduction is normally followed by a wave of cell death (programmed cell death) to establish the proper final number of neurons [62, 63]. As regards the rodent postnatally developing cerebellum, a germinative matrix

(EGL) persists until the third week [61]. The matrix origins the granule cells only [64] of the IGL, after their migration through Bergmann radial glia fibres. Moreover, the maturation of the largest neurons of cerebellar cortex continues until the third and fourth postnatal week [65].

Several morphological and molecular changes have shown the vulnerability of developing cerebellum to a single injection of cisPt (5 μg/g b.w.) at PD10, mainly due to the degeneration/death of proliferating and postmitotic neurons.

CisPt exerts its neurotoxic action on proliferating cells leading to a dramatic death of immature granule cells of the EGL at early developmental stages, one day (PD11) after treatment [22]. This decrease is to a large extent attributable to induction of apoptosis as shown by TUNEL reaction. Comparing with control rats, there were evident changes of Bax and Bcl-2 immunoreactivities after cisPt treatment, not only in the EGL but also in the Purkinje cell layer. In particular, at PD11, comparing with control rats, the intense immunoreactivity for Bax was observed in the immature neurons of the EGL; a high dose of cisPt revealed nests of cells that are Bax intensely labelled and Bcl-2 immunonegative. In the differentiating Purkinje cells, Bax immunoreactivity was more intense, while the labelling for Bcl-2 lowered after cisPt [66]. Seven days after cisPt injection, i.e. at PD17, we provided evidence that, following a drastic early cell death, the EGL may regenerate and the Bcl-2 anti-apoptotic protein increased. However, the late increase that finally allows to recovery of neural cytoarchitecture, could be responsible of some damages as the altered dendrite growth of Purkinje cells and synaptogenesis [21, 23]. Hence, cisPt prevents an early counterbalance of the increased Bax expression maintaining the Bcl-2 steady state of controls, in both the EGL proliferating cells and the Purkinje cells. The unbalance does not assure a limited cell death in the EGL germinative layer and cell alteration in the Purkinje layer. The recovery occurs only with the late over-expression of Bcl-2 anti-apoptotic protein. Apoptotic cell death in the EGL and concomitant alteration of migratory process was clearly detected [22]. These findings may represent throphic factors influencing the Purkinje cell differentiation and formation of synaptic contacts within the cerebellum neural circuits [19, 20, 21, 24]. However, repair and reorganization with remodelling of the cerebellar cortex cytoarchitecture occurred in the developing cerebellum after the acute cisPt-induced injury. They include recovery of proliferation activity in the EGL, granule cell ectopia in the molecular layer (ML), presence of compartment of the ML linked to reorientation of Purkinje cell dendrite branches, and distribution of GABA-positive inhibitory interneurons [21] and fibre synaptic contacts [23].

iv. Postnatal Development of Rat Hippocampal Formation and Apoptotic Molecules

Critical steps in the histogenesis of the hippocampal formation have been previously reported in detail by Altman and Bayer [67, 68, 69] and more recently by Danglot et al. [70]. While pyramidal cells and major interneurons arise during the prenatal period, granule cells originate at E16 but continue to proliferate and migrate during postnatal development until they reach their final destination [71, 72]. Indeed, synaptogenesis and migration are postnatal events of all the principal cell types of the hippocampal formation [70].

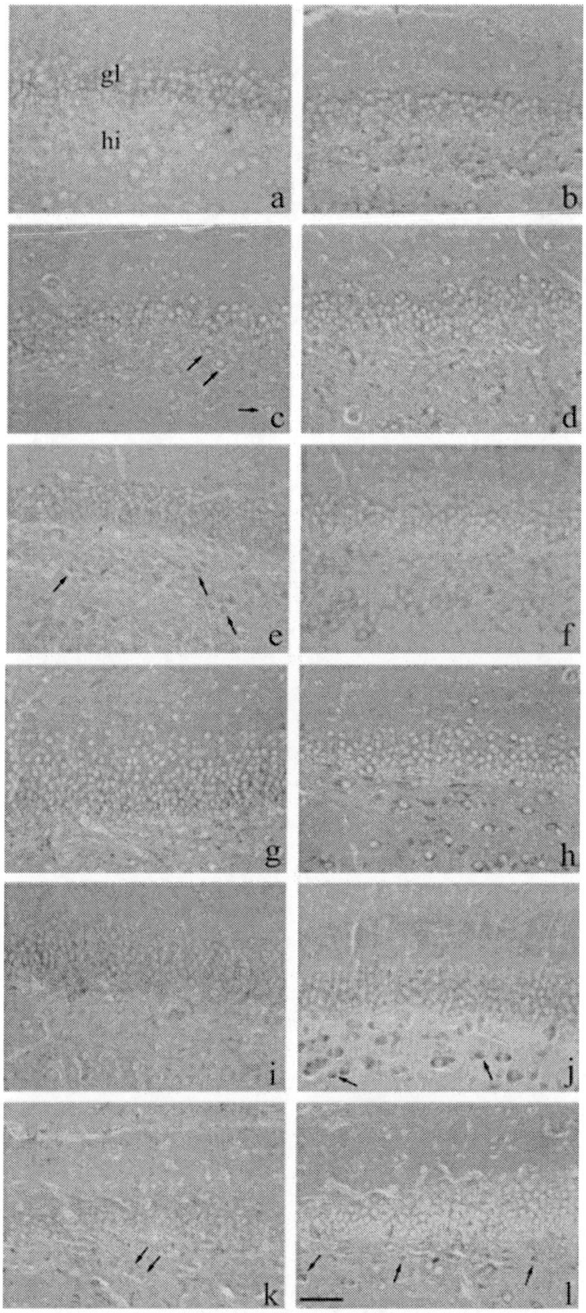

Figure 1. *Bax and Bcl-2 immunoreactions in DG*. PD11: in comparison with control rats (a), Bax immunoreactivity, after cisPt 5 μg/g b.w. treatment, was evident in the cytoplasm of DG granule cells and a moderate immunopositivity was present in the cytoplasm of some hilar cells (c, arrows). In comparison with controls (b) no Bcl2 changes were observed after the treatment (d). After cisPt at the higher dose, Bax immunopositivity increased in the hilar cells (e); Bcl-2 staining decreased in the granular layer while it was similar to controls in the hilar neurons (f). Degenerating cells were observed in the hilus of DG (e, arrows). PD17: in respect to control animals (g), after treatment with both doses, Bax immunoreactivity results unchanged (i, k). Compared to control rats (h), Bcl-2 staining decreased (j, l). Degenerative patterns were present (j, k, l arrows). gl = granular layer; hi =hilus, Scale bar = 50 μm.

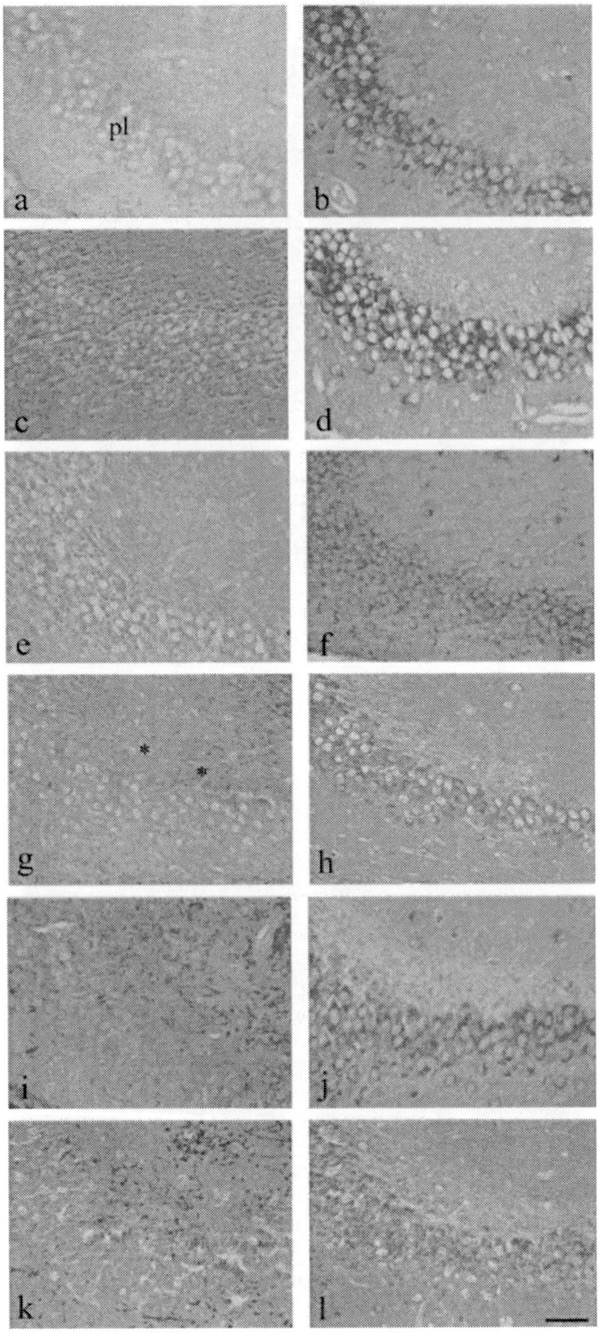

Figure 2. *Bax and Bcl-2 immunoreactions in CA3*. PD11: in comparison with controls (a), Bax immunostaining, after cisPt 5 µg/g, was evident in particular in small elements below the pyramidal layer (c); compared to control animals (b), Bcl-2 labelling resulted increased (d). After cisPt 10 µg/g Bax immunopositivity did not change (e) while Bcl-2 immunoreactivity was lower (f). PD17: after cisPt 5 µg/g (i) Bax immunoreactivity was similar to controls (g), where some fibers appeared non specifically stained (asterisks). In respect to control animals (h) Bcl-2 immunostaining increased (j). After cisPt 10 µg/g Bax immunopositive elements or fibers are evident (k); Bcl-2 immunostaining appeared weak than in controls (l). pl= pyramidal layer, Scale bar = 50 µm.

Dentate Gyrus (DG)

At PD11 in control rats, after Bax immunostaining, DG granule cells showed a weak cytoplasmic immunoreactivity; small immunopositive elements (cells or cell fragments) were strongly labelled within the granular layer while hilar cells had immunonegative cytoplasm (Figure 1.a). Bcl-2 immunolabelling was noticed in the cytoplasm of neurons mainly located in the external side of granular layer. Hilar neurons were intensely labelled, too (Figure 1.b). Following cisPt 5 μg/g, some reactivity for Bax was evident in the cytoplasm, or in cytoplasmic fragments, of DG granule cells; these cells were localized mainly in the external side of granular layer. No Bcl-2 changes were observed. A moderate Bax immunopositivity characterized the cytoplasm of some hilar cells (Figure 1.c); the same staining is observable after Bcl-2 (Figure 1.d). After cisPt 10 μg/g, the intensity of Bax immunopositivity increased in the hilar cells (Figure 1.e). Bcl-2 staining was weak in the granular layer; however, hilar neurons had an immunolabelling similar to control rats, although degenerating cells were observed. (Figure 1.f).

At PD17 in control rats, the immunostaining for Bax revealed cytoplasmic immunopositivity in neurons of the inner part of the granular layer while hilar cells appear immunonegative (Figure 1.g). The immunoreactivity for Bcl-2 was detectable in granular layer neurons and was intense in the hilar ones where some degenerating cells were observed. (Figure 1.h). After treatment with both doses, on one hand Bax immunoreactivity results unchanged (Figure 1.i, k), on the other hand Bcl-2 staining appears decreased, also in the hilar zone where degenerative patterns are present (Figure 1.j, l).

Cornu Ammonis (CA3)

At PD11 in control rats, the immunolabelling trend of CA3 region was almost similar to DG pattern: weak Bax immunopositivity (Figure 2.a) and intense Bcl-2 immunoreactivity in the cytoplasm of pyramidal neurons (Figure 2.b). After cisPt 5 μg/g CA3 area shows Bax immunostaining, in particular in small elements mainly localized below the pyramidal layer (Figure 2.c); Bcl-2 labelling, instead, resulted increased (Figure 2.d). After cisPt 10 μg/g on the contrary, while Bax immunopositivity did not change (Figure 2.e), Bcl-2 immunoreactivity was lower than in controls (Figure 2.f). At PD17 in controls, Bax immunoreactivity in CA3 region was negative (Figure 2.g) while Bcl-2 immunoreactivity was intense in the cytoplasm of pyramidal neurons (Figure 2.h). Some fibers appeared non specifically stained. CisPt lower dose treatment (Figure 2.i) did not induce Bax immunoreactivity in the cytoplasms of CA3 cells. After cisPt 10 μg/g, there were Bax immunopositive elements or fibers (Figure 2.k). After the lower dose, Bcl-2 immunostaining appeared increased, although it did not result homogeneously distributed (Figure 2.j). After cisPt 10 μg/g injection, in comparison with control, Bcl-2 immunolabelling appeared weak then in controls (Figure 2.l). As in the cerebellum, the increase of Bax immunoreactivity was balanced by an increased Bcl-2 immunoreactivity in the DG and CA3 of hippocampal formation after cisPt injection at the dose of 5 μg/g. The strong immunolabelling for Bcl-2 of hilar cells of DG and CA3 pyramidal cells prevents cell damage, at least of some of these cells. Instead, at the dose of 10 μg/g , the high labelling intensity concern only a part of the DG hilar cells and the most of CA3 piramidal cells. The loss of the antiapoptotic, protective Bcl-2 may act on the cells to undergo degeneration.

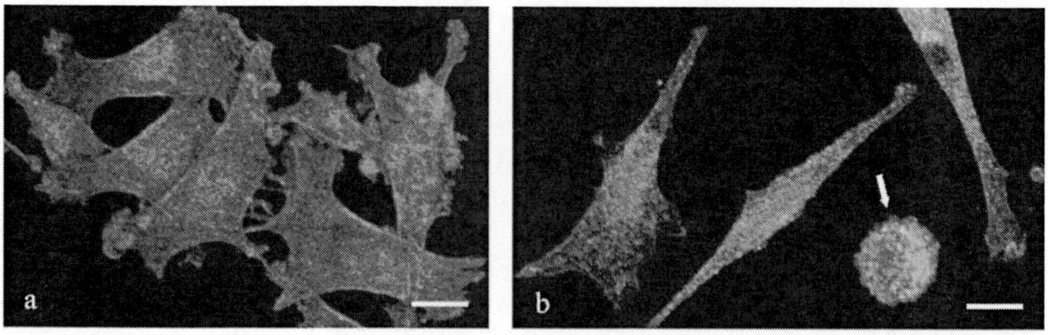

Figure 3. *Confocal images of rat B50 neuroblastoma cell after treatment with 40 μM cisPt for 48h.* (a) in non apoptotic cells, the immunolabelling for Bax (green fluorescence) is located in the cytoplasm and in the nucleus; (b) in early apoptotic cells and in late apoptosis (arrow), Bax is located in the mitochondria cytoplasm. Cytoskeleton was labelled with Alexa 594-conjugated phalloidin (red fluorescence), DNA was stained with Hoechst 33258 (blue fluorescence). Scale bar = 20 μm.

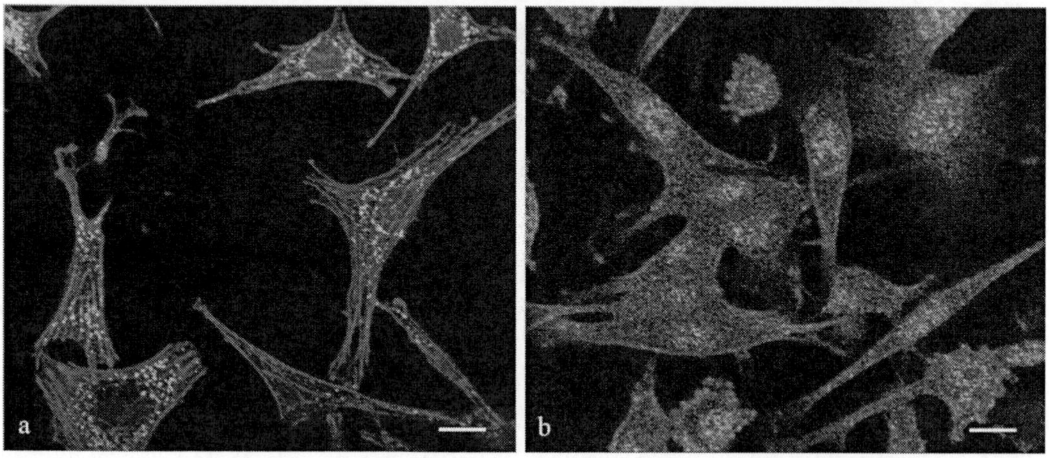

Figure 4. *Confocal images of rat B50 neuroblastoma cell after treatment with 40 μM cisPt for 48h.* In control cells (a) the immunolabelling for Bcl-2 (green fluorescence) is in mitochondria only. After cisPt treatment (b), Bcl-2 protein levels increased significantly in the nucleus. The cytoskeleton was labelled with Alexa 594-conjugated phalloidin (red fluorescence). DNA was counterstained with Hoechst 33258. Scale bar = 20 μm.

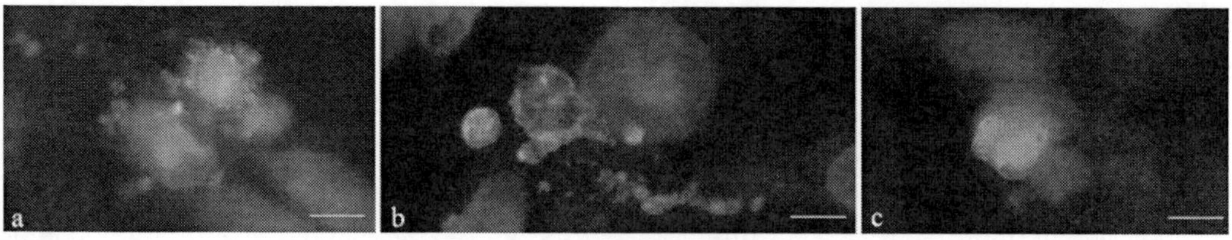

Figure 5. *Fluorescence microscopy.* Immunocytochemical detection of activated caspase 9 (a), caspase 12 (b) and caspase 3 (c) (green fluorescence) in cisPt-treated cells. DNA counterstained Hoechst 33258 and cytoplasm stained with Trypan Blue. Scale bar = 20 μm.

CISPLATIN AND NEUROTOXICITY *IN VITRO*

The primary cytotoxic mechanism of cisPt and other DNA-binding antitumor drugs is DNA damage and subsequent induction of apoptosis [73]. CisPt induces the mitochondria-mediated death in different cell lines [74, 75]. Recently, Bottone et al. [76], have shown that cisPt induces the mitochondria-mediated death in B50 neuroblastoma rat cells in continuous exposure to a single dose of cisPt (40 μM) for–20h or 48h. Mitochondria play an important role in the induction and regulation of apoptosis [77, 78]: pro- and anti-apoptotic molecules, such as Bax and Bcl-2, are present within them [79]. After cisPt treatment, the translocation of Bax (Figure 3), pro-apoptotic protein, to the mitochondrial intermembrane space causes the release of cytochrome c [80], with the implementation of the apoptotic pattern leading to activation of caspase 9, subsequent activation of caspase 3 [81], degradation of many proteins and the final DNA fragmentation. These data are confirmed by changes in mitochondrial membrane permeability that precede the apoptotic typical morphological changes and by the release of cytochrome c. On the contrary, Bcl-2 prevents cell death by blocking the release of cytochrome c [80]. In Figure 4, Bcl-2 localizes in the mitochondria according to physiological condition in control cells, while after treatment it moves from mitochondria to the nucleus. The diffuse labeling in the nucleus, a feature of neural cell lines, indicates an initial resistance to apoptosis with blocking the release of cytochrome c [80].

The rearrangement of actin after the activation of Bcl-2 seems to play a role in the translocation of pro- and anti-apoptotic proteins from the cytoplasm to organelles, or vice versa [82]. In the intrinsic mitochondrial apoptosis, Bax activation and its translocation to mitochondrion cause cytochrome c release and caspases activation [83], in particular caspase 9 (Figure 5.a) which in turn triggers the apoptotic caspase cascade [84]. Our recent studies have shown that cisPt (40 μM for 48 h) induces both caspase-dependent and -independent apoptosis through caspase activation and AIF translocation, respectively [85]. Furthermore, after cisPt treatment also the ER appears alterated, too; this event leads off the activation of caspase 12 and caspase 3 (Figure 5.b, c), consequently [86]. In conclusion, the drug is able to affect different subcellular components damaging the different organelles and causing the re-location of several proteins on the base of their functionality. These processes end with the cellular death by means of apoptosis.

CONCLUDING REMARKS

This review provides our latest information on cisPt neurotoxicity *in vivo* and *in vitro*. In the CNS, neurotoxicity appears to be ascribable to cell death of proliferating cells or degeneration of differentiating neurons in rat developing cerebellum and hippocampus.

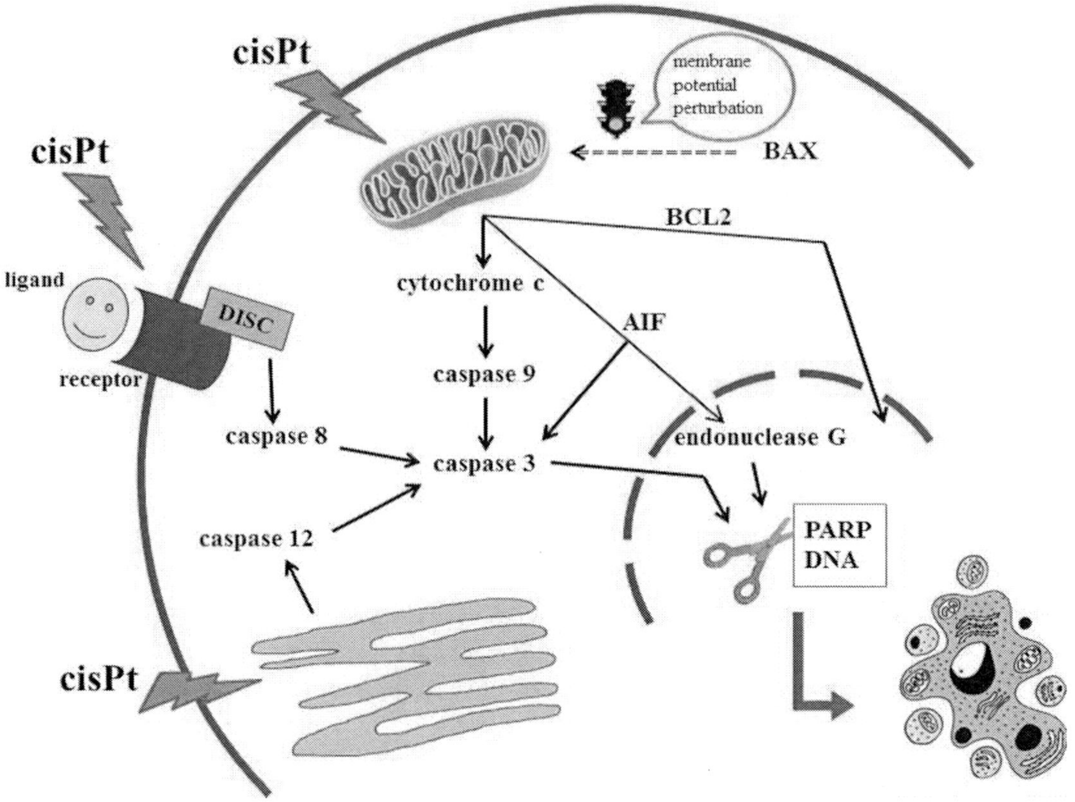

Figure 6. *Apoptosis cisPt-induced through different pathways.* CisPt treatment triggers the activation of regulatory pro-apoptotic cytosolic protein Bax, that moves to the mitochondrial outer membrane when induces the potential perturbation. The consequent formation of pore leads off the expulsion of cytochrome c, AIF and Bcl-2 into the cytosol. Cytochrome c induces the activation of caspase 9, which in turn activates effector caspase 3; AIF, as well as the indirect cooperation with caspase 3, goes to the nucleus where it cooperates with endonuclease G; Bcl-2 moves into the nucleus also, but losing its ability of cellular protection from cell death. CisPt stimulates the ligand/receptor binding with a signalling cascade that lead to the activation of caspase 8 which in turn activates the effector caspase 3. At ER level, the cisPt treatment causes a dysfunction of UPR functionality with the activation of caspase 12 and , also in this case, of caspase 3. The result of the whole process is the cleavage of the PARP and the fragmentation of chromatin DNA with the consequent induction of apoptosis.

Generally, injured neurons and altered neuroarchitecture involve the balance between Bax and Bcl-2 proteins [15]; the increased immunocytochemical expression of Bax and the unchanged or decreased immunopositivity for Bcl-2 leads to cell damage or death.

Instead, high labelling intensity for the anti-apoptotic protein preserves neurons and CNS morphology. The involvement of apoptotic proteins and the mechanism in which cisPt has a role are summarized in Figure 6. Particularly, the data obtained on neuroblastoma rat cells show that cisPt treatment induces different apoptotic patterns: Bax and Bcl-2 proteins regulate a caspase-dependent pathway, causing changes in mitochondrial (release of cytocrome c and caspase 9 activation) and in cytoskeleton organization [76]; moreover, mitochondrial changes start a caspase-independent apoptosis mediated by AIF protein. Caspase 8 is activated after a receptor signaling cascade, while an ER stress condition activates caspase 12 [86]. Caspases 8, 9 and 12 are initiator caspases and so they lead to the activation of effector caspase 3, this process leads off the execution phase of apoptosis in which the different subcellular targets are affected. These results show that cisPt may have important direct interactions, not only with DNA, but also with organelles, which can induce apoptosis or cell damages and may account for a significant part of the clinical activity associated with this drug, including CNS injury.

ACKNOWLEDGEMENTS

The research was supported by the following Italian Institutions: Fondazione Banca del Monte di Lombardia and University of Pavia (FAR - Fondi di Ateneo per la Ricerca, 2010). Santin G. is supported by funding from "Superpig Program", project co-financed by Lombardy Region through the "Fund for promoting institutional agreements"

REFERENCES

[1] McWhinney, SR; Goldberg, RM and McLeod, HL. Platinum neurotoxicity harmacogenetics. *Molecular Cancer Therapeutics* 2009, 8, 10–16.

[2] Prestayko, AW; D'Aoust, JC; Issell, BF and Crooke, ST. Cisplatin (cis-diamminedichloroplatinum II). *Cancer Treatment Reviews* 1979, 6, 17–39.

[3] English, MW; Skinner, R; Pearson, ADJ; Price, L; Wyllie, R and Craft AW. Dose-related nephrotoxicity of carboplatin in children. *Brit. J Cancer* 1999, 81, 336–341.

[4] Pearson, AD; Pinkerton, CR; Lewis, IJ; Imeson, J; Ellershaw, C; Machin, D. European Neuroblastoma Study Group; Children's Cancer and Leukaemia Group. High-dose rapid and standard induction chemotherapy for patients aged over 1 year with stage 4 neuroblastoma: a randomised trial. *Lancet Oncol.* 2008, 9, 247-256.

[5] Andre, T; Boni, C; Mounedji-Boudiaf, L; Navarro, M; Tabernero, J; Hickish, T; Topham, C; Zaninelli, M; Clingan, P; Bridgewater, J; Tabah-Fisch, I and de Gramont, A. Oxaliplatin, fluorouracil, and leucovorin as adjuvant treatment for colon cancer, *N. Engl. J. Med.* 2004, 350, 2343–2351.

[6] Eastman, A. Analysis and quantitation of the DNA damage produced in cells by the cisplatin analog cis-[3H]dichloro(ethylenediamine)platinum. *Anal. Biochem.* 1991, 197, 311–315.

[7] Ahmad, S. Platinum-DNA interactions and subsequent cellular processes controlling sensitivity to anticancer platinum complexes. *Chem. Biodivers.* 2010, 7, 543-566.

[8] Qin, LF and Ng, IO. Induction of apoptosis by cisplatin and its effect on cell cycle-related proteins and cell cycle changes in hepatoma cells, *Cancer Lett.* 2002, 175, 27–38.

[9] Mandic, A; Hansson, J; Linder S and Shoshan, MC. Cisplatin induces endoplasmic reticulum stress and nucleus-independent apoptotic signaling, *J. Biol. Chem.* 2003, 278, 9100–9106.

[10] Jamieson, ER; Lippard, SJ. Structure, Recognition, and Processing of Cisplatin-DNA Adducts. *Chem. Rev.* 1999, 99, 2467-2498.

[11] Ishida, S; Lee, J; Thiele, DJ; Herskowitz, I. Uptake of the anticancer drug cisplatin mediated by the copper transporter Ctr1 in yeast and mammals. *Proc. Natl. Acad. Sci. U S A* 2002, 99, 14298-14302.

[12] Zwelling, LA; Filipski, J; Kohn, KW. Effect of thiourea on survival and DNA cross-link formation in cells treated with platinum(II) complexes, L-phenylalanine mustard, and bis(2-chloroethyl)methylamine. *Cancer Res.* 1979, 39, 4989-4995.

[13] Zhu, C; Raber, J; Eriksson, LA. Hydrolysis process of the second generation platinum-based anticancer drug cis-amminedichlorocyclohexylamineplatinum(II). *J. Phys. Chem. B.* 2005, 109, 12195-12205.

[14] McWhinney, SR; Goldberg, RM; McLeod, HL. Platinum neurotoxicity pharmacogenetics. *Mol. Cancer Ther.* 2009, 8, 10-16.

[15] Bernocchi, G; Bottone, MG; Piccolini,VM; Dal Bo, V; Santin, G;. De Pascali, SA; Migoni, D; Fanizzi, FP. Developing central nervous systemand vulnerability to platinum compounds. *Chemotherapy Research and Practice* 2011, 1-14.

[16] McKeage, MJ; Hsu, T; Screnci, D Haddad, G; Baguley, BC. Nucleolar damage correlates with neurotoxicity induced by different platinum drugs. *Br. J. Cancer* 2001, 85, 1219-1225.

[17] Kostova, I. Platinum complexes as anticancer agents. *Recent Pat. Anticancer Drug Discov.* 2006, 1, 1-22.

[18] Wang, G; Reed, E; Li; QQ. Molecular basis of cellular response to cisplatin chemotherapy in non-small cell lung cancer (Review). *Oncol. Rep.* 2004, 12, 955-965.

[19] Scherini, E and Bernocchi, G. CisDDP treatment and development of the rat cerebellum," *Progress in Neurobiology* 1994, 42, 161–196.

[20] Pisu, MB; Guioli, S; Conforti, E and Bernocchi, G. Signal molecules and receptors in the differential development of cerebellum lobules. Acute effects of cisplatin on nitric oxide and glutamate systems in Purkinje cell population. *Developmental Brain Research* 2003,145, 229–240.

[21] Pisu, MB; Roda, E; Avella, D and Bernocchi, G. "Developmental plasticity of rat cerebellar cortex after cisplatin injury: inhibitory synapses and differentiating Purkinje neurons. *Neuroscience* 2004, 129, 655–664.

[22] Pisu, MB; Roda, E; Guioli, S; Avella, D; Bottone, MG and Bernocchi, G. Proliferation and migration of granule cells in the developing rat cerebellum: cisplatin effects. *The Anatomical. Record. Part A* 2005, 287, 1226–1235.

[23] Avella, D; Pisu, MB; Roda, E; Gravati, M and Bernocchi, G. Reorganization of the rat cerebellar cortex during postnatal development following cisplatin treatment," *Experimental Neurology* 2006, 201, 131–143.

[24] Roda, E; Avella, D; Pisu, MB and Bernocchi, G. "Monoamine receptors and immature cerebellum cytoarchitecture after cisplatin injury," *Journal of Chemical Neuroanatomy* 2007, 33, 42–52.

[25] Piccolini, VM; Cerri, S; Romanelli, E; Bernocchi, G. Interactions of some neurotransmitter systems during postata development of rat hippocampal formation: effects of cisplatin treatment. *Submitted to Exp. Neurol.* 2011.

[26] Ureña-Guerrero, ME; Orozco-Suárez, S; López-Pérez, SJ; Flores-Soto, ME; Beas-Zárate, C. Excitotoxic neonatal damage induced by monosodium glutamate reduces several GABAergic markers in the cerebral cortex and hippocampus in adulthood. *Int. J. Dev. Neurosci.* 2009, 27, 845-855.

[27] Hanahan, D; Weinberg, R.A. The hallmarks of cancer. *Cell* 200, 100, 57–70.
[28] Kerr, JF; Wyllie, AH; Currie, AR. Apoptosis: a basic biological phenomenon with wide-ranging implications in tissue kinetics, *Br. J. Cancer* 1972, 26, 239–257.
[29] Scaffidi, C; Fulda, S; Srinivasan, A; Friesen, C; Li, F; Tomaselli, KJ; Debatin, K;. Krammer, PH; Peter, ME. Two CD95 (APO-1/Fas) signaling pathways, *EMBO J.* 1998, 17, 1675–1687.
[30] Hengartner, MO. The biochemistry of apoptosis, *Nature* 2000, 407, 770–777.
[31] Jourdain, A; Martinou, J.C. Mitochondrial outer-membrane permeabilization and remodelling in apoptosis, *Int. J. Biochem. Cell Biol.* 2009, 41, 1884–1889.
[32] Daugas, E; Susin, SA; Zamzami, N; Ferri, KF; Irinopoulou, T; Larochette, N; Prévost, MC; Leber, B; Andrews, D; Penninger, J; Kroemer, G. Mitochondrio-nuclear translocation of AIF in apoptosis and necrosis. *FASEB J.* 2000, 14, 729-739.
[33] Kopito, RR. Aggresomes, inclusion bodies and protein aggregation. *Trends Cell Biol.* 2000, 10, 524-530.
[34] Szegezdi, E; Logue, SE; Gorman, AM; Samali, A. Madiators of endoplasmic reticlum stress-induced apoptosis. *EMBO Rep.* 2006, 7, 880-885.
[35] Bredesen, DE; Rao, RV and Mehlen, P. Cell death in the nervous system. *Nature* 2006, 443, 796–802.
[36] Yuan, J and Yankner, BA. Apoptosis in the nervous system. *Nature* 2000, 407, 802–809.
[37] Akhtar, RS; Ness, JM and Roth, KA. Bcl-2 family regulation of neuronal development and neurodegeneration," *Biochimica et Biophysica Acta* 2004, 1644, 189–203.
[38] Nakka, VP; Gusain, A; Mehta, SL and R. Raghubir, Molecular mechanisms of apoptosis in cerebral ischemia: multiple neuroprotective opportunities," *Molecular Neurobiology* 2007, 37, 7–32.
[39] Kroemer, G; Reed J. Mitochondrial control of cell death. *Nat. Med.* 2000, 6, 513-519.
[40] Portier, BP; Taglialatela, G. Bcl-2 localized at the nuclear compartment induces apoptosis after transient overexpression. *J. Biol. Chem.* 2006, 281, 40493-40502.
[41] D'Alessio, M; De Nicola, M; Coppola, S; Gualandi, G; Pugliese, S; Cerella, C; Cristofanon, S, Civitareale, P; Ciriolo, MR; Bergamaschi, A; Magrini, A; Ghibelli, L. Oxidative Bax dimerization promotes its translocation to mitochondria independently of apoptosis. *FASEB J.* 2005, 19, 1504-1506.
[42] Gregg, RW; Molepo, JM; Monpetit, VJ; Mikael, NZ; Redmond, D; Gadia, M and Stewart, DJ. Cisplatin neurotoxicity: the relationship between dosage, time, and platinum concentration in neurologic tissues, and morphologic evidence of toxicity. *Journal of Clinical Oncology* 1992, 105, 795–803.
[43] Troy, L; McFarland, K; Littman-Power, S; Kelly, BJ; Walpole, ET; Wyld, D; Thomson, D. Cisplatin based therapy: a neurological and neuropsychological review. *Psycho-Oncology* 2000, 9, 129-139.
[44] Stillman, M and Cata, JP. Management of chemotherapyinduced peripheral neuropathy," *Current Pain and Headache Reports* 2006, 10, 279–287.
[45] Dunlap, B and Paice, JA. Chemotherapy-induces peripheral neuropathy: a need for standardization in measurement. *The Journal of Supportive Oncology* 2006, 4, 398–399.
[46] Sul, JK and De Angelis, LM. Neurologic complications of cancer chemotherapy. *Seminars in Oncology* 2006, 33, 324–332.

[47] Albers, JW; Chaudhry, V; Cavaletti, G; Donehower, RC. Interventions for preventing neuropathy caused by cisplatin and related compounds. *Cochrane Database Syst. Rev*. 2011, 2.

[48] Juillerat-Jeanneret, L. The targeted delivery of cancer drugs across the blood-brain barrier: chemical modifications of drugs or drug-nanoparticles? *Drug Discov. Today*. 2008, 13, 1099-1106.

[49] Namikawa, K; Asakura, M; Minami, T; Okazaki, Y; Kadota, E; Hashimoto S. Toxicity of cisplatin to the central nervous system of male rabbits. *Biol. Trace Elem. Res*. 2000, 74, 223-235.

[50] Rodier PM. Vulnerable periods and processes during central nervous system development. *Environ Health Perspect*. 1994, 2, 121-124.

[51] Rodier PM. Environmental causes of central nervous system maldevelopment. *Pediatrics*. 2004, 113, 1076-1083.

[52] Sugimoto, S. Yamamoto, Y. L. Nagahiro, S and Diksic, M. Permeability change and brain tissue damage after intracarotid administration of cisplatin studied by double-tracer autoradiography in rats. *Journal of Neuro-Oncology*, 1995, 229–240.

[53] Wick, A; Wick, W. Hirrlinger J. Gerhardt, E; Dringen, R; Dichgans, J; Weller, M; and Schulz JB. Chemotherapy-induced cell death in primary cerebellar granule neurons but not in astrocytes: in vitro paradigm of differential neurotoxicity. *Journal of Neurochemistry* 2004, 91, 1067–1074.

[54] Rzeski, W; Pruskil, S; Macke, A; Felderhoff-Mser, U; Reiher, AK; Hoerster, F; Jansma, C; Jarosz, B; Stefovska, V; Bittigau, P; Ikonomidou, C; Anticancers agents are potent neurotoxins in vitro and in vivo," *Annals of Neurology* 2004, 56, 351–360.

[55] Costa, LG; Aschner, M; Vitalone, A; Syversen, T; Soldin, OP; Developmental neuropathology of environmental agents. *Annu. Rev. Pharmacol. Toxicol*. 2004; 44, 87-110.

[56] Kleshcheva, RP. The development of components of the blood-brain barrier in the neocortex of the white rat. *Arkh. Anat. Gistol. Embriol*. 1998, 95, 22–26.

[57] Clark, J.B; Bates, T.E; Cullingford, T. and Land, JM. Development of enzymes of energy metabolism in the neonatal mammalian brain. *Dev. Neurosci*. 1993, 15, 174–180.

[58] Groothuis, DR; Vriesendorp, FJ; Kupfer, B; Warnke, PC; Lapin, GD; Kuruvilla, A; Vick, NA; Mikhael, MA; Patlak, CS. Quantitative measurements of capillary transport in human brain tumors by computed tomography. *Ann. Neurol*. 1991, 30, 581-588.

[59] Ballabh, P; Braun, A; Nedergaard, M. The blood-brain barrier: an overview: structure, regulation, and clinical implications. *Neurobiol. Dis*. 2004, 16, 1-13.

[60] Rodier, PM.; Chronology of neuron development: animal studies and their clinical implications. *Developmental Medicine and Child Neurology* 1980, 22, 525–545.

[61] Altman, J. Morphological development of the rat cerebellum and some of its mechanisms. The Cerebellum. Springer 1982, 8–49.

[62] Oppenheim, RW. Cell death during development of the nervous system. *Annual Review of Neuroscience* 1991, 14, 453–501.

[63] Lossi, L; Mioletti, S and Merighi, A. Synapse-independent and synapse-dependent apoptosis of cerebellar granule cells in postnatal rabbits occur at two subsequent but partly overlapping developmental stages. *Neuroscience* 2002, 112, 509–523.

[64] Zhang, L; and Goldman, JE. Generation of cerebellar interneurons from dividing progenitors in white matter. *Neuron* 1996, 16, 47–54.

[65] Altman, J. Postnatal development of the cerebellar cortex in the rat. II. Phases in the maturation of Purkinje cells and of the molecular layer. *J Comp Neurol.* 1972, 145, 399-463.

[66] Cerri, S; Piccolini, VM; Santin, G; Bottone, MG; De Pascali, SA; Migoni, D; Iadarola, P; Fanizzi, FP; Bernocchi, G. The developmental neurotoxicity study of platinum compounds. Effects of cisplatin versus a novel Pt(II) complex on rat cerebellum. *Neurotoxicol Teratol.* 2011, 33, 273-281.

[67] Altman, J; Bayer, AS. Mosaic organization of the hippocampal neuroepithelium and the multiple germinal sources of dentate granule cells. *J. Comp. Neurol.* 1990a, 301, 325-342.

[68] Altman, J; Bayer, AS. Prolonged sojourn of developing pyramidal cells in the intermediate zone of the hippocampus and their settling in the stratum pyramidale. *J. Comp. Neurol.* 1990b, 124, 319-336.

[69] Altman, J; Bayer, AS. Migration and distribution of two populations of hippocampal granule cell precursors during the perinatal and postnatal periods. *J. Comp. Neurol.* 1990c, 301, 365-381.

[70] Danglot, L; Triller, A; Marty, S. The development of hippocampal interneurons in rodents. *Hippocampus*. 2006, 16, 1032-1060.

[71] Bayer, SA. Development of the hippocampal region in the rat I. Neurogenesis examined with [3H] thymidine autoradiography. *J. Comp. Neurol.* 1980a, 190, 87-114.

[72] Bayer, SA. Development of the hippocampal region in the rat II. Morphogenesis during embryonic and early postnatal life. *J. Comp. Neurol.* 1980b, 190, 115-134.

[73] Fisher, DE. Apoptosis in cancer therapy: Crossing the threshold. *Cell* 1994, 78, 539-542.

[74] Park, MS; De Leon, M and Devarajan, P. Cisplatin induces apoptosis in LLC-PK1 cells via activation of mitochondrial pathways. *J. Am. Soc. Nephrol.* 2002,13, 858-865.

[75] Kim, JS.; Lee, JM.; Chwae, YJ; Kim, Y.H; Lee, JH; Kim, K; Lee, T.H; Kim, SJ and Park JH. Cisplatin-induced apoptosis in Hep3B cells: mitochondria-dependent and independent pathways. *Biochem. Pharmacol.* 2003, 67, 1459-1468.

[76] Bottone, MG; Soldani, C; Veneroni, P; Avella, D; Pisu, M; Bernocchi, G. Cell proliferation, apoptosis and mitochondrial damage in rat B50 neuronal cells after cisplatin treatment. *Cell Prolif.* 2008, 41, 506-520.

[77] Chang, DT; Reynolds, IJ. Mitochondrial trafficking and morphology in healthy and injured neurons. *Prog. Neurobiol.* 2006, 80, 241–268.

[78] Foster, KA; Galeffi, F; Gerich, FJ; Turner, DA; Muller, M. Optical and pharmacological tools to investigate the role of mitochondria during oxidative stress and neurodegeneration. *Prog. Neurobiol.* 2006, 79, 136–171.

[79] Bedner, E; Li, X; Kunicki, J; Darzynkiewicz, Z. Translocation of Bax to mitochondria during apoptosis measured by laser scanning cytometry. *Cytometry* 2000, 41, 83–88.

[80] Yang, J; Liu, X; Bhalla, K; Kim, CN; Ibrado, AM; Cai, J; Peng TI; Jones, DP; Wang, X. Prevention of apoptosis by Bcl-2: release of cytochrome c from mitochondria blocked. *Science* 1997, 275, 1129–1132.

[81] Srinivasula, SM; Ahmad, M; Fernandes-Alnemri, T; Alnemri, ES. Autoactivation of procaspase-9 by Apaf-1-mediated oligomerization. *Mol. Cell* 1998, 1, 949–957.

[82] Thomas, SG; Hwang, S; Li, S; Straiger, CJ; Franklin-Tong, VE. Actin depolymerization is sufficient to induce programmed cell death in self-incompatible pollen. *JCB* 2007, 174, 221–229.

[83] Jurgensmeier, JM; Xie, Z; Deveraux, Q; Ellerby, L; Bredesen, D; Reed, JC. Bax directly induces release of cytochrome c from isolated mitochondria. *Proc. Natl. Acad. Sci. USA* 1998, 95, 4997–5002.

[84] Costantini, P; Bruey, JM; Castedo, M; Metivier, D; Loeffler, M; Susin, SA; Ravagnan, L; Zamzami, N; Garrido, C; Kroemer, G. Pre-processed caspase-9 contained in mitochondria participates in apoptosis. *Cell Death Differ*. 2002, 9, 82–88.

[85] Bottone, MG; Giansanti, V; Veneroni,P; Scovassi, AI; Bernocchi, G; Pellicciari, C. The Apoptosis-Inducing Factor (AIF) Moves from Mitochondria to the Nucleus and Back to the Cytoplasm, during Apoptosis. Mitochondria: Structure, Functions and Dysfunctions, Nova Publishers, 2011, 913-926.

[86] Santin, G; Piccolini, VM; Veneroni, P; Barni, S; Bernocchi, G; Bottone MG. Different patterns of apoptosis in response to cisplatin in B50 neuroblastoma rat cells. *Histol. Histopathol.* 2011, 26, 831-842.

In: Cisplatin: Pharmacology, Clinical Uses and Adverse Effects ISBN: 978-1-61942-359-6
Editors: Toshiko Kojima and Yoko Morita

Chapter VII

THERMAL PROPERTIES OF CISPLATIN

***Márta Juhász*[1,*]*, Sundaram Arulmozhiraja*[2,†]**
***and Toshihiro Fujii*[3,‡]**

[1]University of Szeged, Institute of Pharmaceutical Chemistry,
Szeged, Eötvös u. 6., Hungary
[2]Australian National University, Research School of Chemistry,
Canberra, ACT, Australia
[3]Meisei University, Department of Chemistry,
Faculty of Sciences and Engineering, Hodokubo 2-1-1, Hino, Tokyo

ABSTRACT

This article focuses primarly on the thermal properties of the anti-cancer drug cisplatin and shows that information on its thermal properties provide positive impact in a broad range of applications in addition to extending our understanding of the basic science of coordination chemistry and pharmaceutical chemistry. Studies on the thermal properties of cisplatin include: i) The bond energies (Pt–NH_3, Pt–Cl) and proton affinity of cisplatin are calculated by means of the density functional theory. Comparison of the calculated bond energies with the experimental values that are derived from enthalpy changes are also given. ii) Temperature-resolved thermal analysis with the use of evolved gas analysis-electron impact ionization mass spectrometry (EGA-EIMS) and ion attachment mass spectrometry (IAMS) techniques. iii) Thermal decomposition kinetics for cisplatin in nitrogen by using EGA-IAMS. Activation energy and pre-exponential factor of cisplatin obtained via EGA-IAMS are reported. iv) Mass spectrometric analysis of cisplatin by the conventional EIMS and the newly developed novel Li^+-IAMS in connection with a quadrupole mass analyzer are also described.

* Dr. Márta Juhász E-mail: jmarta@chem.meisei-u.ac.jp; Postal address: University of Szeged, Institute of Pharmaceutical Chemistry, Szeged, Eötvös u. 6., Hungary.
† Dr. Sundaram Arulmozhiraja E-mail: raja@rsc.anu.edu.au; Postal address: Australian National University, Research School of Chemistry, Canberra ACT 0200, Australia.
‡ Prof. Dr. Toshihiro Fujii is the Corresponding author. E-mail: fujii@chem.meisei-u.ac.jp; Postal address: Meisei University, Department of Chemistry, Faculty of Sciences and Engineering, Hodokubo 2-1-1, Hino, Tokyo 191-8506, JAPAN; Tel. and Fax.: +81-42-591-5595.

INTRODUCTION

The platinum anti-cancer drug cisplatin (*cis*-$Pt(NH_3)_2Cl_2$) is successfully used for the treatment of various solid tumors including testicular and ovarian cancer tumors. Because of its importance in the cancer chemotherapy, cisplatin is still one of the most widely studied drugs in the theoretical and experimental fields of chemistry. However, its action-mechanism, monitoring and characterization still provide challenges to scientists. In addition – similar to other drugs – the pharmaceutical nature of cisplatin is not free from side effects. Therefore, the development of cisplatin analogues with lower toxicity and increased effectiveness becomes important [1–5].

In pharmaceutical research, data about the fundamental physical and chemical properties of target molecules, such as their geometrical structure, bond energies, thermal decomposition and decomposition kinetics, is meaningful. In that sense, studying the fundamental properties of cisplatin can be expected to provide valuable information about the chemistry of this important drug candidate under physiological conditions, which, in turn, would be useful for designing novel metal-based anti-cancer agents.

Cisplatin has already been studied by means of various analytical techniques [6–9]. However, due to its thermal instability, non-volatility, its determination and characterization provides difficulties. Furthermore, neither the absence nor the existence of biotransformation products in plasma or urine collected from patients receiving cisplatin have been proved unambiguously because of the lack of analytical techniques capable of determining these species at low concentration levels [10].

In the following sections, we describe the most important fundamental thermal properties of cisplatin recently studied in our laboratory [11–13]. As one can see, these characteristics can help us have a better knowledge of cisplatin's properties in gas phase in terms of decomposition and kinetics. Also, the results of these studies could improve cisplatin-characterization and contribute to the development of new cisplatin-analogs.

1. BOND ENERGIES (PT-NH_3, PT-CL) AND PROTON AFFINITY

Bond energy is defined as the amount of energy required to break one mole of bonds of a particular type between the atoms of a molecule in the gaseous state and is expressed in terms of kcal mol^{-1} or kJ mol^{-1}. The knowledge of Pt–ligand bond energies in various platinum complexes is essential because of their involvement in processes of industrial and biological interest [14]. As cisplatin plays an important role in pharmacology as well as in various processes in the fields of catalysts and biology, knowing its Pt–NH_3 and Pt–Cl bond strengths is important. It should be mentioned however, that accurate bond energies of cisplatin has not been studied before though there were a few indirect studies on bond energies. Skinner et al. [8,15] made micro-calorimetric measurements to determine the thermal decomposition enthalpy of cisplatin. From the thermal decomposition data, the formation enthalpy of cisplatin could be calculated and the strengths of Pt–ligand bonds could be deduced [14]. In this way, the Pt–Cl bond energy in cisplatin was obtained to be 69.31 kcal mol^{-1}. Kappes and Staley [16] made ion-cyclotron studies on gaseous NiL_2^+ ions (where L = ammonia, amines, pyridine) and established a relative order of Ni^+–L bond dissociation energies. It has been found in the study that the Ni^+–NH_3 bond has the smallest dissociation energy, which is 5.98 kcal mol^{-1} lower than the Ni^+–pyridine bond dissociation energy [16]. Accepting that the same tendency is valid for the bond energies in amine–$PtCl_2$ complexes and using the bond energy value of 69.31 kcal mol^{-1} determined for Pt–Cl bond, the energy of the Pt–NH_3 bond was calculated to be 37.28 kcal mol^{-1} [14].

Though cisplatin is one of the most widely studied drugs in computational chemistry [17–20], its Pt–NH_3 and Pt–Cl bond energies have not been computed. Recently, by using density functional theory (DFT), we obtained bond energies for the Pt–Cl and Pt–NH_3 bonds of cisplatin and also studied the gas-phase reactivity of cisplatin with H^+ ion [11]. It has been proved through many studies that the bond energies and ion affinites calculated using DFT methods are highly reliable [21–24]. DFT has been shown to be reliable to calculate cation affinity values for various compounds [25–30]. For example, highly reliable gas-phase proton, sodium, and lithium ion affinities of *n*-alkyl fluorides [25], β-dicarbonyl compounds [26], perfluorocarbons [27], pyridine derivatives [28], C_{60} fullerene [29], and Cu(hfac)(tmvs) [30] were obtained using density fucntional theories. DFT methods were also used to study the molecular properties of cisplatin and its related compounds and also to study the chemical reactions of these compounds with water and DNA [18–20,31–33]. The results derived in those studies were in good agreement with the experimental results. By considering all of these facts, our calculated bond energies and proton affinity of cisplatin should be highly reliable.

All calculations were performed using Gaussian 03 revision D. 01 [34]. Popular B3LYP density functional [35–38] was utilized throughout the theoretical study. We employed a variety of basis sets including the split valence-type 6-311+G(*d,p*) for the H, N, and Cl atoms and an effective core potential (ECP) included SDD (Stuttgart/Dresden) basis set for Pt atom. We optimized the cisplatin [*cis*-$Pt(NH_3)_2Cl_2$] structure using B3LYP functional with different basis sets as mentioned above. We also performed separate optimizations to obtain the structures and total energies for $Pt(NH_3)_2$, $PtCl_2$, NH_3, and Cl fragments. Vibrational frequency calculations were made for all of the optimized structures to characterize them as minimum energy structures on their respective potential energy surfaces. Bond energies were obtained from the energies of the individual species: $\Delta E[Pt–NH_3] = ½\{E[PtCl_2] + 2E[NH_3] – E[Pt(NH_3)_2Cl_2]\}$, and $\Delta E[Pt–Cl] = ½\{E[Pt(NH_3)_2] + 2E[Cl] – E[Pt(NH_3)_2Cl_2]\}$. Here, for example, $\Delta E[Pt–NH_3]$ represents the Pt–NH_3 bond energy and $E[PtCl_2]$ is the total energy of the fragment $PtCl_2$. Zero-point energies and thermal energy corrections at room temperature were included in the bond energies. The Pt–Cl and Pt–NH_3 bond energies calculated with various basis sets were listed in Table 1 along with the experimental values available in the literature [14]. The results show that, independent of the basis sets used, the Pt–Cl bond energy is almost double that of Pt–NH_3 bond energy, which is consistent with the literature values and they reveal that the covalent Pt–Cl bond is stronger than the dative bond between Pt and NH_3.

The calculated bond energies (Table 1) correlates well with the experimentally derived bond energies. The calculated Pt–NH_3 bond energy (37.38 kcal mol^{-1}) was almost equal to the experimental value (37.28 kcal mol^{-1}), and the calculated Pt–Cl bond energy was around 5 kcal mol^{-1} smaller than the experimental value. These results show that reliable bond energies could be derived by using a triple-zeta basis set augmented with polarization functions and diffuse functions for heavy atoms and augmented with the SDD ECP basis set for the Pt atom.

Table 1. Calculated bond energies (ΔE, kcal mol^{-1}) at 298.15 K

method	ΔE[Pt–NH_3]	ΔE[Pt–Cl]
SDD[a]	46.96	63.02
6-31+G(*d*) + SDD[b]	38.86	64.32
6-311+G(*d*,*p*) + SDD[b]	37.38	64.35
Experimental values from Ref. 15.	37.28	69.31

[a] SDD ECP basis sets for all atoms.

[b] 6-31+G(*d*) or 6-31s1+G(*d*,*p*) basis set for nonmetal atoms; SDD ECP basis set for Pt.

We also studied the proton affinity of cisplatin by considering the fact that the knowledge of a molecule's proton affinity, which is a fundamental property of the molecule, is required for understanding proton transfer reactions. Also, it is a measure of the gas-phase basicity of an anion, neutral atom, or molecule that accepts a proton. The proton affinity of cisplatin has neither been determined experimentally or calculated theoretically.

Starting from the global energy minimum structure of cisplatin, we searched the possible site in the cisplatin molecule for the formation H^+ adduct. The possible structures of the complexes were optimized, and then frequency calculations were used to find the global energy minimum structure for the protonated complex. The Cl atoms in the cisplatin molecule are the most basic center for proton attachment. Therefore, in the protonated complex, H^+ was connected to one of the Cl atoms, which resulted in a 60° rotation of the amine group from its orientation in the cisplatin monomer; the orientation of the other amine group was unchanged (Figure 1). The global energy minimum structure of protonated cisplatin has C_s symmetry while cisplatin has a C_{2v} symmetry.

Figure 1b shows the optimized structure and important geometrical parameters of protonated cisplatin complex. For comparison, the structure for the global energy minimum of the monomer cisplatin along with its structural parameters are also shown in Figure 1 (1a). As seen in the Figure, in the protonated cisplatin complex, the Pt–Cl (attached to H^+) and the Pt–N (oriented in the same side of protonated Pt–Cl bond) bonds were elongated (2.430 Å) relative to the corresponding bonds in cisplatin, whereas the other Pt–Cl and Pt–N bonds were shorter (2.317 Å and 2.066 Å, respectively). The lengthening of former Pt–Cl and the Pt–N bonds indicates that electron-density is shifted through the N–Pt and the Pt–Cl bonds toward the H^+. Due to the abovementioned 60° rotation of NH_3 group eventuated in the protonated complex, H•••H repulsions are less significant, forcing the closure of the N–Pt–N bond angle and increasing both the Cl–Pt–N bond angles. Like in the Cl–Pt–N bond angle, a remarkable change was also observed in the Cl–Pt–Cl bond angle. While the Cl–Pt–N bond angle is increased, the Cl–Pt–Cl bond angle is substantially decreased. The big changes detected in these bonds are thanks to the attached H^+, which may be somehow better attracted by the Cl than by the completely saturated N.

The proton affinity was calculated according to the following equation: $\Delta H_{298K} = \Delta E_0 + \Delta E_{thermal} + \Delta(pV)$, where ΔE_0 is interaction energy between the cisplatin and the H^+ ion, *i.e.* the difference in energy between the sum of the isolated monomers and the protonated cisplatin complex. $\Delta E_{thermal}$ is the thermal energy correction to the room temperature enthalpy, while $\Delta(pV)$ accounts for the translational energy of the cation as well as the $\Delta(nRT)$ term.

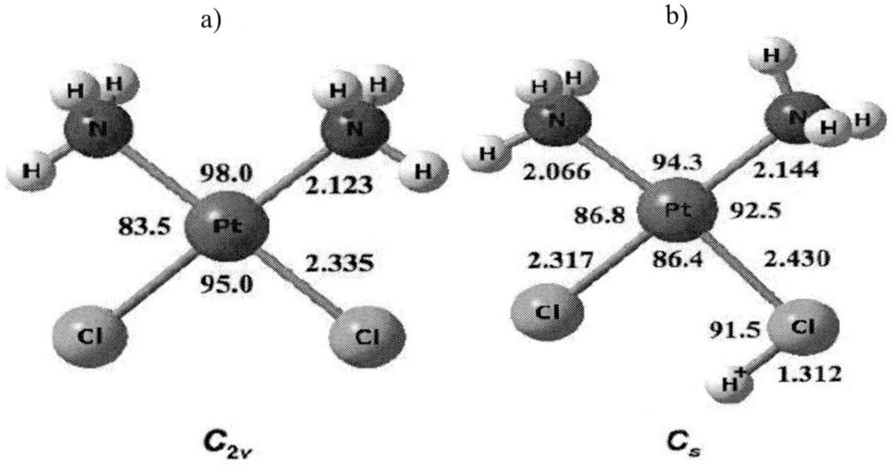

Figure 1. Structures optimized with the B3LYP functional and the combination of the 6-311+G(*d,p*) and ECP included SDD basis sets of (a) cisplatin and (b) protonated cisplatin. Bond lengths are given in Angstrøms (Å), and the bond angles are in Degrees (°).

The calculated proton affinity for cisplatin is 198.71 kcal mol^{-1} in gas phase. This indicates that H^+ is strongly bound to cisplatin which may be noteworthy among physical and synthetic chemists. The high proton affinity for cisplatin suggests that protonated cisplatin could be formed and detected easily in chemical ionization–mass spectrometry systems. Furthermore, under electrospray ionization–mass spectrometry conditions, the large proton affinity can be expected to assist the easier detection of cisplatin samples because protonated cisplatin adducts would form readily.

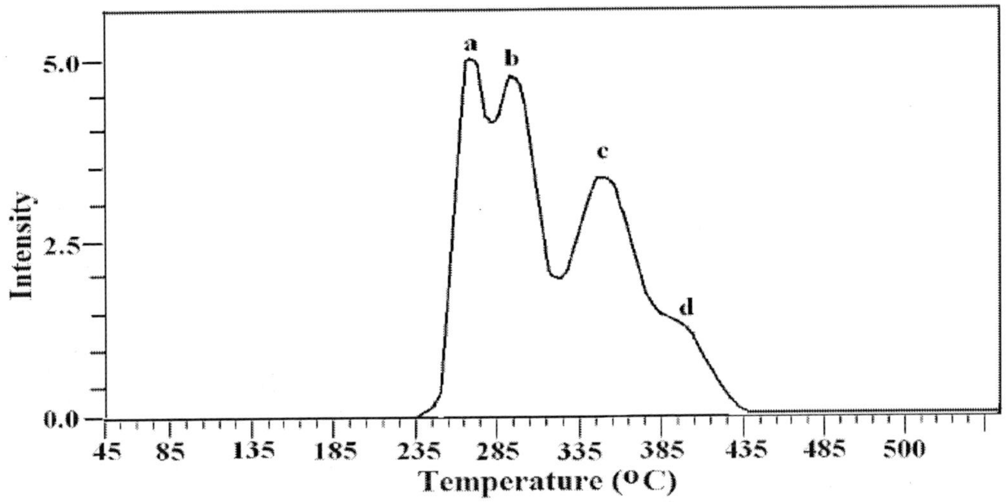

Figure 2. Total ion chromatogram (TIC) of cisplatin obtained in total ion monitoring mode at a heating rate of 20°C min^{-1} in the temperature range of 45 to 500°C. Four peaks labeled a, b, c, and d exist in TIC. Mass spectra belonging to these peaks are discussed below.

It should be mentioned here that the cisplatin–H^+ complex can exist only in gas phase because bonding of the H^+ to Cl implies that HCl will dissociate in solution and it will be replaced by a water molecule. As it is known [39–41], under physiological conditions, both Cl are substituted by water molecules, and becomes *cis*-$[Pt(NH_3)_2(H_2O)_2]^{2+}$, an anti-cancer form of cisplatin.

2. Thermal Analysis

As noted earlier, cisplatin is a thermally labile, non-volatile, and highly insoluble drug molecule. Various analytical methods have been utilized in the past to make thermal analysis studies of cisplatin and other platinum complexes. For example, flame atomic absorption spectrophotometry has been utilized to estimate the thermal stability of cisplatin, along with the stabilities of other platinum complexes [6,7]. Micro-calorimetry at 590 and 615 K temperature argon atmosphere and in vacuo has been applied for thermal decomposition studies of cisplatin [42] . Solution calorimetry technique has been used to determine the formation enthalpy of cisplatin [8]. The thermal breakdown of cisplatin solution during atomization in a carbon furnace atomic absorption system has also been discussed [9].

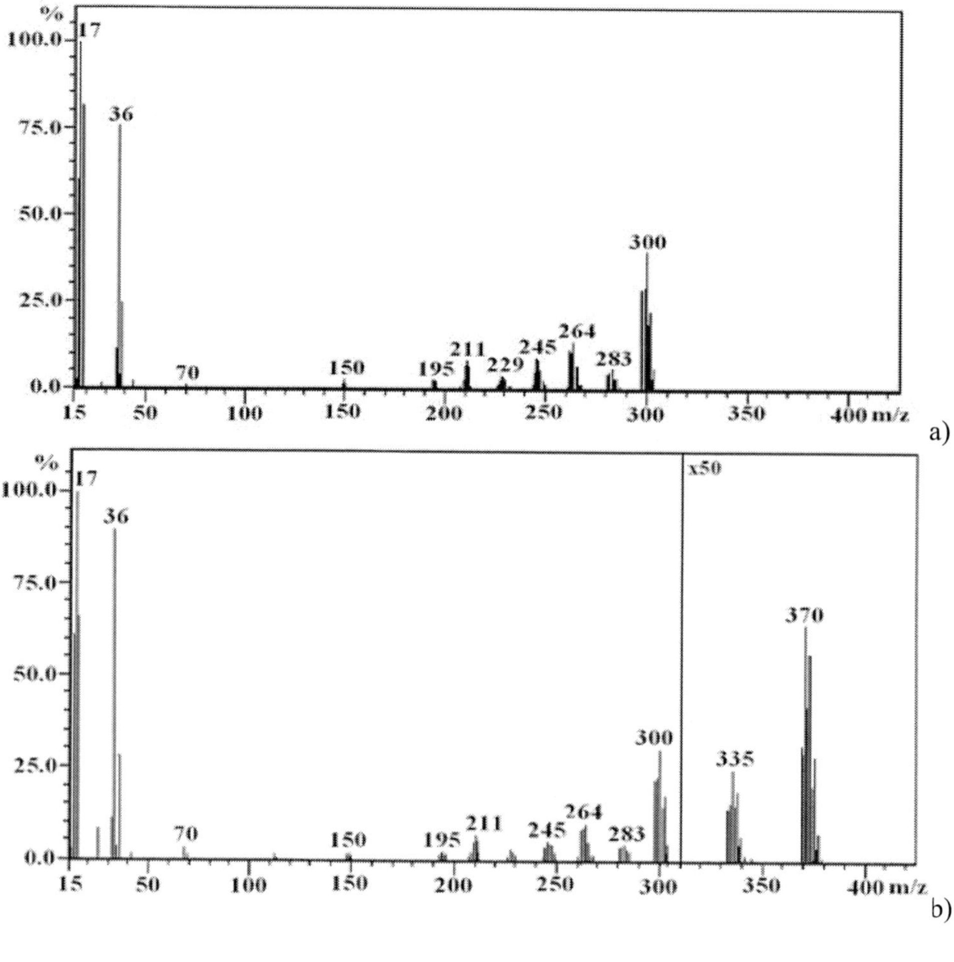

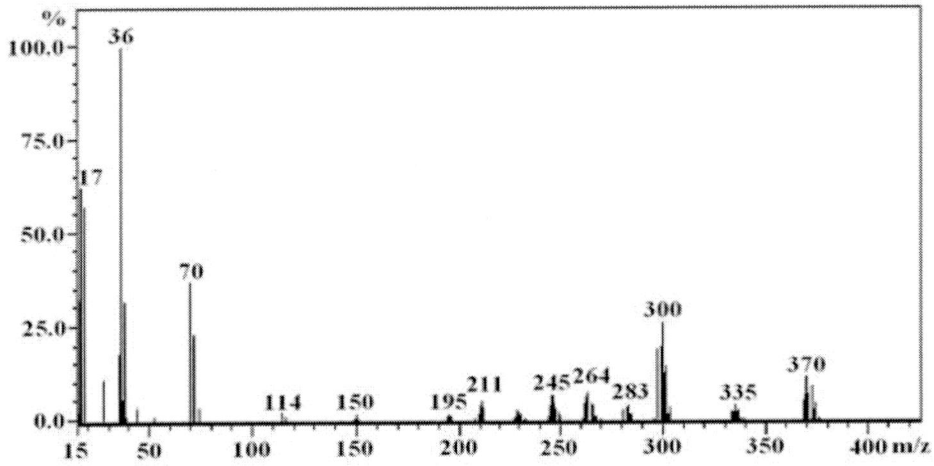

c)

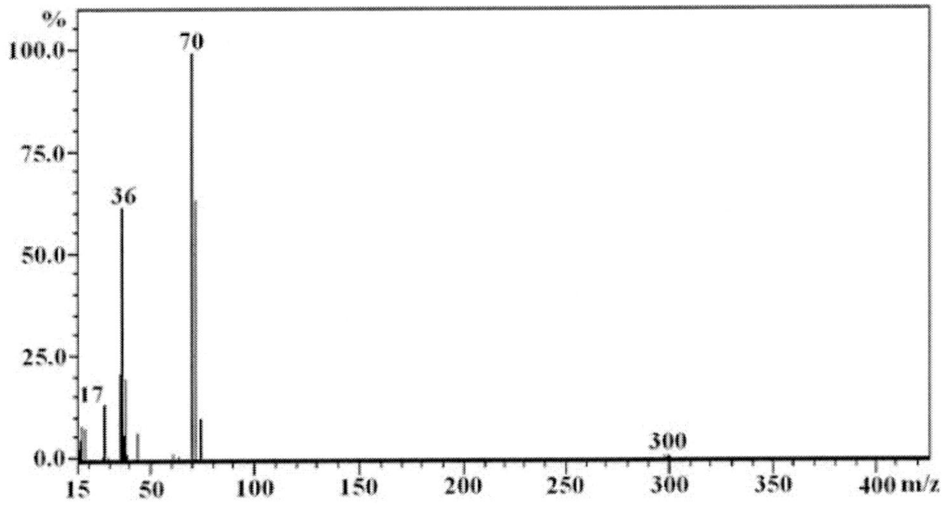

d)

Figure 3. (a) EI mass spectrum for the peak of the TIC of cisplatin (b) EI mass spectrum for the peak of the TIC of cisplatin. For better visualization, the peaks with *m/z* values greater than 310 are magnified by a factor of 50. (c) EI mass spectrum for the peak of the TIC of cisplatin. (d) EI mass spectrum for the peak of the TIC of cisplatin.

Evolved gas analysis mass spectrometry (EGA-MS) is a powerful technique that is widely used in various research areas such as pharmaceutical research, environmental science, forensic science, and catalysis [43]. It has also been used to study the temperature programmed decomposition of polymers and inorganic materials [16], to characterize the molecular properties of materials under thermal degradation conditions, to analyze an unknown gas mixture, and to study gas–solid interactions [43,44].

In our study, we used EGA in conjunction with EI ionization quadrupole MS to investigate the thermal behavior of cisplatin. EGA-MS analysis was carried out with 1 mg of the sample, which was heated from 25°C to 500°C with a heating rate of 20°C min^{-1}. From the total ion chromatogram (TIC) obtained in total ion monitoring mode at a heating rate of 20°C min^{-1} in the temperature range of 45°C to 500°C (Figure 2), we observed that the cisplatin samples yielded the bulk of gaseous emissions within the temperature range of 235°C to

435ºC. In addition, four peaks, labeled a, b, c, and d, appeared after the EGA probe temperature reached 235°C.

The mass spectra recorded for the four peaks are shown in Figures 3a–d.

The mass spectra recorded for all of the four peaks are shown in Figure 3. As evidence from the Figure, the mass spectra of peaks (a) and (b) (Figures 3a and 3b) were almost the same. Hence, although two peaks were observed in the TIC, we could not distinguish between them based on their mass spectra. Both spectra contained molecular ion ($M^{+\bullet}$) of cisplatin at *m/z* 300 and several other ions coming from thermal decomposition of cisplatin and/or fragmentation of ionized cisplatin. In mass spectrum of peak (c), besides the ions observed in mass spectra of peak (a) and peak (b), intense cluster ions at *m/z* 335 and 370 were also detected. These ions may correspond to *cis*-$[Pt(NH_3)_2Cl_3]^+$ and *cis*-$[Pt(NH_3)_2Cl_4]^+$, respectively. The peak at *m/z* 370 also appeared in the spectrum of peak (b), although at a lower intensity. In the mass spectrum of peak (c), the intensity of peak at *m/z* 70 (Cl_2^+) substantially increased comparing to same peak in Figures 3a and b. Furthermore, in the mass spectrum of peak (c), the peak at *m/z* 70 (Cl_2^+) differs very much in intensity from the corresponding peaks detected in Figures 3a and b. In the spectrum of peak (c), the intensity of peak for Cl_2^+ substantially increased, and in the spectrum of peak (d) (Figure 3d), this peak provided the base peak.

On the other hand, Li^+ ion attachment mass spectrometry (Li^+IAMS) proposed and developed by Fujii [45–49] is a novel technique that employs soft ionization. Unlike the well-known EI-MS, the ion attachment process in IAMS is non-dissociative and generates the ions that do not fragment. This technique has been extensively tested, optimized, and shown to have high efficacy and sensitivity [30,50–53]. Recently, we also used infrared image furnace-ion attachment mass spectrometry (IIF-IAMS) system to study thermal decomposition of cisplatin [12]. Also, we recently coupled the EGA system with the Li^+IAMS technique (EGA-IAMS) to study involatile, untreated, and complex samples, such as polyethylene polymers [47]. It has been shown that by using the EGA-IAMS technique, temperature-programmed decomposition of a number of solid materials can be studied in detail by directly detecting any chemical species in real-time and in situ.

In the IIF-IAMS study on cisplatin, we observed the formation of NH_3Li^+ and $HClLi^+$ adducts from NH_3 and HCl that are produced by the thermal decomposition of cisplatin, at 220–370°C and 270–380°C, respectively [12]. The features of the IIF-IAMS technique such as its specificity, high sensitivity, rapid response ensures almost exclusively that the primary thermal decomposition products formed from the target molecule are detected. Therefore, the observed NH_3^+ and HCl^+ at *m/z* 17 and *m/z* 36 in the EGA-EIMS experiment should be at least partly due to the thermal decomposition products of cisplatin. It should be noted that the evolution of substantial amounts of NH_3 occurred at 235°C, and a substantial loss of HCl occurred at the same time.

3. Thermal Stability

Understanding the thermal stability of a chemical compound is important for many known reasons and the results obtained from thermal decomposition kinetic studies may lead to improve the stability of the formulations of many pharmaceutical and food products.

Hence, knowledge of cisplatin thermal decomposition kinetics is essential for the preparation and preservation of cisplatin and cisplatin-containing pharmaceutical forms.

We used IIF-IAMS to study cisplatin's decomposition kinetics. Assuming a first-order reaction, the ionic signal acquired from real-time total-ion monitoring of chemicals released from a thermally decomposing specimen was used to obtain the functional forms of the following kinetic rate equation:

$$d\alpha/dT = (A/\beta)e^{-(E_a/RT)}(1 - \alpha) \quad (1)$$

where α is the degree of yield of the decomposed specimen, T is the temperature, β is the heating rate, A is the pre-exponential factor, E_a is the activation energy, and R is the universal gas constant.

Mathematically this equation can not be solved easily. To overcome this problem, Knümann et al. [54] applied multiple linear regression analysis to the logarithmic form of eqn (1):

$$\ln(d\alpha/dT) = \ln(A/\beta) - E_a/RT + \ln(1 - \alpha) \quad (2)$$

A pyrogram obtained from the EGA-IAMS provides the relative number of decomposition product molecules, thus indicating the decomposition rate. The degree of conversion (α) at any temperature (T) is equal to the integrated area under the pyrogram curve between the temperature at the signal start (T_0) and T. The ionic signal (i) acquired from real-time, multiple-ion detection of chemicals released from thermally decomposed specimens has been used to obtain the functional form of kinetic rate expressions [54]. Activation energy and pre-exponential factor can be determined from plots of $\ln[(d\alpha/dT)/(1 - \alpha)]$ versus $1/T$.

In order to obtain the rate expressions for cisplatin decomposition, the intensities of NH_3 signals at m/z 24 was investigated in a temperature range of 220–370°C.

We investigated the decomposition kinetics over the 225°C to 249°C temperature to obtain rate expressions for cisplatin decomposition. The slope of the plot of temperature versus NH_3 signal intensity in this limited region was constant (Figure 4). Activation energy (E_a = 38.0 kcal mol^{-1}) and pre-exponential factor ($A = 2.2 \times 10^{12}$) were calculated from this plot.

Because pyrolysis is initiated by bond breakage, the experimentally determined energy of decomposition (apparent activation energy, E_a) of cisplatin into $PtCl_2$ and NH_3 was expected to be associated with the energy of the Pt–NH_3 bond. Indeed, the obtained E_a value of 38.0 kcal mol^{-1} for the decomposition of cisplatin into NH_3 and $PtCl_2$ is in good agreement with the bond energy for Pt–NH_3 determined in DFT calculations [12].

From this kinetic data (E_a and A), we calculated a shelf life for powder cisplatin in a nitrogen atmosphere. Shelf life is generally defined as the time required for a target molecule to decompose up to 90%. For a first-order reaction at 25°C, $t_{90\%}$ is given with the following equation [55]:

$$t_{90\%,25°C} = 0.105/k_{25°C} \quad (3)$$

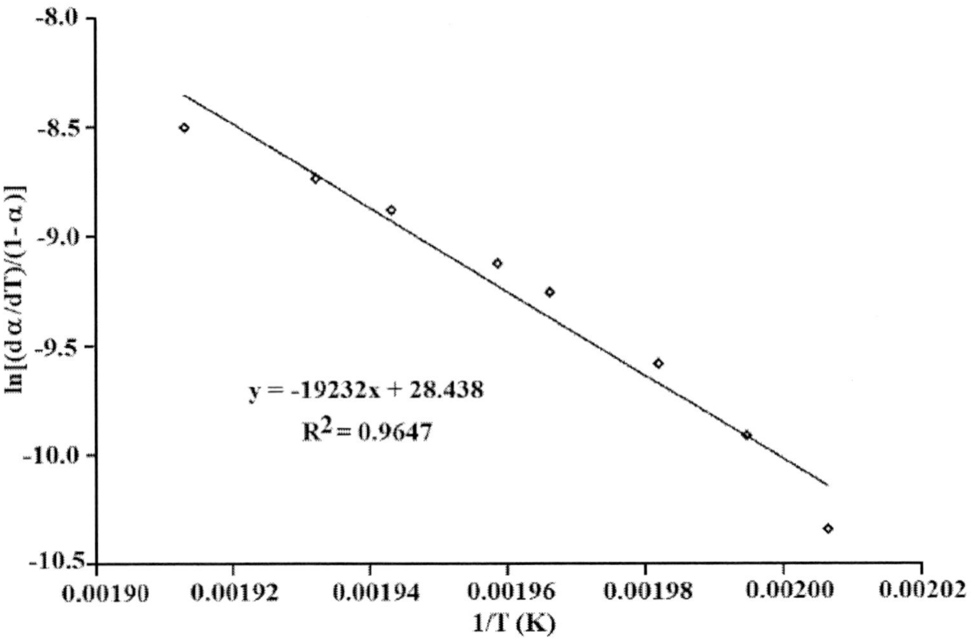

Figure 4. Arrhenius plot for data calculated from the NH_3 curve of cisplatin decomposition in temperature range from 225°C to 249°C.

where $t_{90\%,25°C}$ is the shelf life of the target molecule at a 10% decomposition level and at 25°C, and $k_{25°C}$ is the degradation rate constant at 25°C.

In a nitrogen atmosphere, $t_{90\%,25°C}$ of cisplatin determined by using EGA-IAMS was 9.2×10^8 years.

4. Mass Spectrometry

Cisplatin and its derivatives have been studied by MS with various ionization techniques, such as electrospray ionization, fast atom bombarment, desorption chemical ionization and field desorption.

Conventional MS can not provide useful information for the determination and characterization of platinum-containing drugs because they have low volatility and readily decompose at moderate temperatures [56]. Only one report of the EI spectra of cisplatin and its various derivatives have been published, and Fourier transform and solid sample techniques were used to obtain these spectra [57]. However, FT-MS is a complex and expensive method, and therefore obtaining a mass spectrum of cisplatin by means of a simpler, cheaper technique is highly desirable.

We recorded both the EI and Li^+ ion attachment mass spectra of the cisplatin sample. For comparison, both mass spectra were acquired with the DIP at the same 270°C, a temperature low enough to allow ionization of cisplatin complex without severe thermal decomposition.

In EI-MS measuring of cisplatin, 1mg sample amount was investigated with a quadrupole mass spectrometer (GCMS-QP2010 Series, Shimadzu Corporation, Japan). In the 70 eV-EI mass spectrum recorded, cisplatin was detected in molecular ion form and a cluster of peaks corresponding to $M^{+\bullet}$ containing various platinum and chlorine isotopes were observed (Figure 5, right inset). The eight peaks at *m/z* 298, 299, 300, 301, 302, 303, 304, and 306 corresponded to combinations of ^{194}Pt, ^{195}Pt, ^{196}Pt, and ^{198}Pt and ^{35}Cl and ^{37}Cl isotopes. The calculated peak intensities show that the ratios of the cluster peaks were as expected from the natural abundances of the isotopes.

In addition to $M^{+\bullet}$, EI ionization provided several other types of ions, such as the doubly charged molecular ion (M^{2+}). This ion is formed by the loss of two electrons and presents at one-half the molecular mass of the target compound.

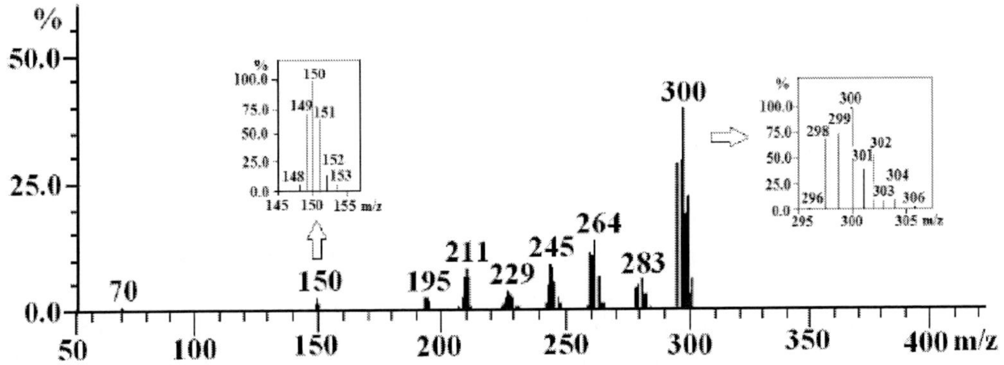

Figure 5. EI mass spectrum of cisplatin sample heated to 270°C. The insets show expansions of the peak clusters at *m/z* 300 and 150 enlarged to 100% for *m/z* 300 and 150, respectively. The theoretical peak intensities calculated for the peaks in the $M^{+\bullet}$ ($[(NH_3)_2PtCl_2]^{+\bullet}$) cluster at *m/z* 298, 299, 300, 301, 302, 303, 304, and 306 were 73, 74, 100, 47, 56, 8, 15, and 2%, respectively.

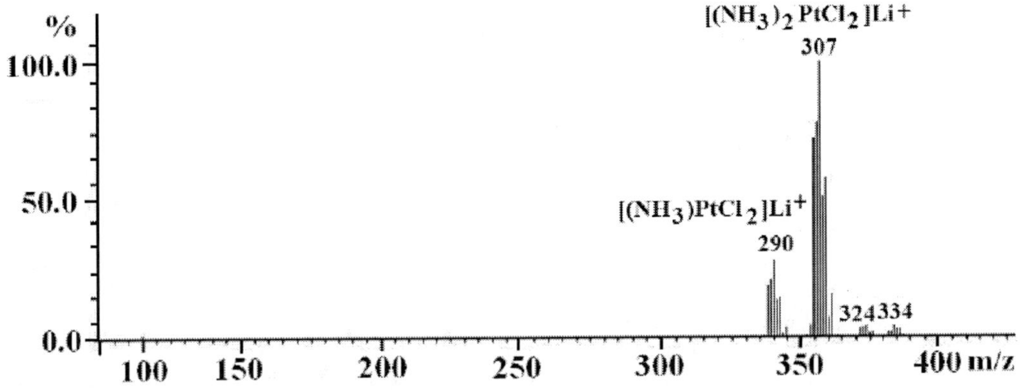

Figure 6. An ion attachment mass spectrum of cisplatin sample heated to 270°C. The theoretical peak intensities calculated for the peaks in the MLi^+ ($[(NH_3)_2PtCl_2]Li^+$) cluster at *m/z* 305, 306, 307, 308, 309, 310, and 311 were 74, 78, 100, 49, 56, 8, and 15%, respectively.

Usually, the chance of M^{2+} formation is less than the chance of $M^{+\bullet}$ formation. The calculated peak intensities of the peaks at *m/z* 149, 150, 151, 152, and 153 were 69, 100, 56, 14, and 1.5% respectively, and these peaks corresponded to the peaks at *m/z* 298, 300, 302, 304, and 306 for $M^{+\bullet}$. The peaks at *m/z* 149.5, 150.5, and 151.5 corresponding to half the *m/z* values of the peaks at *m/z* 299, 301, 303, and 305 for $M^{+\bullet}$, were not reported on the mass scale, because data-treatment software ignored them.

Since the isotopic pattern of the cluster at *m/z* 150 was the same as the pattern of the $M^{+\bullet}$ cluster, the peak at *m/z* 150 should correspond to M^{2+}, with an elemental composition of $[Pt(NH_3)_2Cl_2]^{2+}$.

Our EI mass spectrum was consistent with the mass spectrum obtained in Riley's Fourier-transform-MS study [44], though we successfully detected and identified some ions for the first time, like $Pt(NH_3)NH_2Cl^+$ at *m/z* 264, $Pt(NH_2)_2^+$ at *m/z* 228 or the double-charged ion $[Pt(NH_3)_2Cl_2]^{2+}$ at *m/z* 150. The detected new ions in our study may be due to the higher electron ionization used. We applied 70 eV ionization energy [13], while Riley used 50 eV ionization energy in their experimental work [57].

Since the simplicity of the IA spectrum permits the analysis of compounds whose spectra are difficult to interpret using the electron impact (EI) mode of operation, we recorded ion attachment mass spectrum for cisplatin also. 10 μg of cisplatin sample amount was inserted into the sample holder of the direct probe (DIP) of the quadrupole Li Ion Attachment Mass Spectrometer system (Canon ANELVA Corporation, Kanagawa, Japan) and was heated up to 270°C. The obtained ion attachment mass spectrum for cisplatin sample is shown in Figure 6.

This ion attachment mass spectrum was completely different from the electron ionization (EI) mass spectra. According to our and Riley's MS works, both the 70-eV and 50-eV EI mass spectra of cisplatin provides many fragment ions which are attributed to extensive ligand cleavage occurring under harsh EI conditions [13,57]. In the ion attachment mass spectrum, the Li^+ adduct molecular ion without fragmentation was observed [12].

A cluster of peaks corresponding to molecular ions containing various platinum and chlorine isotopes were observed for Li^+ adduct molecular ions. The eight peaks at *m/z* 305, 306, 307, 308, 309, 310, 311, and 313 included among others ^{194}Pt, ^{195}Pt, ^{196}Pt, and ^{198}Pt and ^{35}Cl and ^{37}Cl isotopes. The calculated peak intensities show that the ratios of the cluster peaks were as expected from the natural abundances of the isotopes. The obtained cisplatin molecular Li^+ ion adduct suggests that continuous monitoring of cisplatin in patients is possible.

Among H^+ affinity, Li^+ ion affinity is also an important molecular property of compounds. For example, the ionization efficiency in $(M + Li)^+$ ion formation mainly depends on the Li^+ ion affinity of the molecule M, which can reach approximately 70 kcal mol^{-1}. Unfortunately, for many molecules, especially for the metal complex systems, Li^+ ion affinity values were not yet reported. However, theory is an effective tool to determine accurate ion affinities that are useful indicative for which molecule can be detected at low concentrations as lithiated complex [48–53]. As an example, the calculated 50.75 kcal mol^{-1} Li^+ ion affinity for a transition metal complex Cu(hfac)(tmvs) was large enough to have been detected successfully by Li^+ ion attachment mass spectrometer [30]. Cispaltin's gas-phase reactivity with Li^+ ion was also studied theoretically. Upon the Li^+ ion attachment, both Cl atoms share the interaction with the Li^+ ion symmetrically, which is evidenced by the equal Cl–Li bond lengths (2.249 Å) and Li–Cl–Pt bond angles (85.3°). Since, in the lithiated cisplatin, the Pt–Cl bond lengths become longer and the Cl–Pt–Cl bond angle reduces significantly due to the charge transfer ($0.3e^-$ moved from the cisplatin to Li^+), Pt–NH_3 bond lengths decreased slightly. These observations suggest that Li^+ ion interactes with the cisplatin ligand easily and strongly. This assumption was supported by the Li^+ ion affinity value of 70.32 kcal mol^{-1} calculated for cisplatin. The large Li^+ ion affinity obtained for the cisplatin indicates that cisplatin can react with Li^+ ions easily and hence it can be detected by LiAMS still in small amounts. Indeed, cisplatin-Li^+ complex could be observed in the IAMS mass spectrum.

In comparison, under FAB and ESI conditions, the structurally relevant fragment ions of cisplatin were absent and only the collision-induced dissociation technique applied for the molecular ion-like species could provide structural information for the cisplatin [58,59]. The ESI spectrum of ciplatin gave peaks which correspond to the cisplatin-sodium and to the cisplatin-potassium adduct ions [59], while the FAB spectrum of cisplatin gave adducts with both the ionized glycerol matrix sample and the ionized DMSO solvent [58]. In the HPLC-electrospray mass spectrum [59,60] of cisplatin, $[M - H_2O]^+$, $[M + H]^+$, and $[M - H_2O + MeCN]^+$ clusters beginning at *m/z* 263, 281, and 304, respectively, were observed. In addition, a Na^+ adduct ion of cisplatin was also observed when acetonitrile was used in the HPLC solvent mixture.

Conclusion

Thermal properties of the thermally labile, non-volatile, and insoluble compound cisplatin, were studied. Reliable bond energies for Pt–NH_3 and Pt–Cl in cisplatin were obtained by using the density functional theory with the B3LYP functional and various basis sets. The knowledges of the bond energies and the proton affinity contribute for designing and developing new Pt-complex pharmaceuticals and catalytic systems. Furthermore, the high proton affinity value (198.71 kcal mol^{-1}) ensures the easier detection and characterization of cisplatin by various ionization techniques such as chemical ionization, electrospray ionization modes. Also, the calculated large value (70.32 kcal mol^{-1}) for cispaltin's Li^+ affinity-assisted cisplatin detection by Li^+IAMS system which promises the continous monitoring of cisplatin in patients. The temperature-programmed decomposition of cisplatin under IIF-IAMS conditions showed evidently that HCl and NH_3 were evolved from the cisplatin sample as thermal decompostion products. The EI and Li^+IA mass spectra of cisplatin differed very much and indicated that under harsh EI conditions, extensive bond-cleavages of the cisplatin molecule occurred. In contrary, under the soft technique, Li^+IA, the only molecular ion in lithiated adduct form and a few decomposition products were formed.

Acknowledgement

M. Juhász sincerely thanks the Japan Society for the Promotion of Science (JSPS) for the award of a JSPS Fellowship (Code No. P09706).

References

[1] Rosenberg, B., Van Camp, L., Krigas, T. Inhibition of cell division in Escherichia coli by electrolysis products from a platinum electrode. *Nature*, 1965 205, 698–699.

[2] Borch, R. F. In: Powis, G., Prough, R. A., editors. Metabolism and Action of Anti-cancer Drugs. London: *Taylor and Francis*; 1987; 163–193.

[3] Loehrer, P. J. Einhorn, L. H. Cisplatin. *Ann. Intern. Med.,* 1984 100, 704–713.

[4] De Lena, M., Lorusso, V., Paradiso, A., Tommasi, S. Therapeutic efficacy of various dosages and modalities of administration. *Inorg. Chim. Acta,* 1987 137, 91–97.

[5] Reedijk, J. The mechanism of action of platinum anti-tumor drugs. *Pure Appl. Chem.*, 1987 59, 181–192.

[6] Macquet, J. P., Hubert, J., Theophanides, T. Dosage du platine par spectrométrie d'absorption atomique : Partie I. Mise au point d'une méthode d'analyse dans les complexes organométalliques et de coordination. *Anal. Chim. Acta,* 1974 72, 251–259.

[7] Macquet, J. P., Theophanides, T. Dosage du platine par spectrométrie d'absorption atomique: Partie II. Résultats analytiques sur les complexes or-ganométalliques d'intérêt biologique: effet cis-trans. *Anal. Chim. Acta*, 1974 72, 261–267.

[8] Al-Takhin, G., Skinner, H. A., Zaki, A. A. Micro-calorimetric studies of the thermal decomposition of ammonia–halide and amine–halide complexes of platinum(II), $[Pt(NH_2R)_2X_2]$. *J. Chem. Soc. Dalton.*, 1983 2323–2328.

[9] Jelas Haron, M. D., Wan M. D., Yunus, Z. W. The differences in the thermal breakdown of H_2PtCl_6 and *cis*-$Pt(NH_3)_2Cl_2$ in carbon furnace atomic absorption. *Pertanika*, 1989 12, 79–82.

[10] De Waal, W. A. J., Maessen, F. J. M. J., Kraak, J. C. Analytical methodologies for the quantitation of platinum anti-cancer drugs and related compounds in biological media. *J. Pharmaceut. Biomed. Anal.*, 1990 8, 1–30.

[11] Juhász, M., Takahashi, S., Arulmozhiraja, S., Fujii, T. Bond energies (Pt-NH_3, Pt-Cl) and proton affinity of cisplatin: a density functional theory approach. *J. Struct. Chem.*, 2011 [In press].

[12] Takahashi, S., Kitahara, Y., Nakamura, M., Shiokawa, Y., Fujii, T. Temperature-resolved thermal analysis of cisplatin by means of Li^+ ion attachment mass spectrometry. *Phys. Chem. Chem. Phys.*, 2010 12, 3910–3913.

[13] Juhász, M., Takahashi, S., Fujii, T. Temperature-resolved thermal analysis of cisplatin by evolved gas analysis-mass spectrometry. *J. Anal. Appl. Pyrol.*, 2011 91, 114–118.

[14] Mortimer, C.,T. Platinum–ligand and palladium–ligand bond energies. *Rev. Inorg. Chem.*, 1984 6, 233–257.

[15] Al-Takhin, G., Skinner, H. A. Zaki, A. A. Micro-calorimetric studies on the thermal decomposition of platinum and palladium complexes containing phosphine or diene ligands. *J. Chem. Soc. Dalton.*, 1984 371-378.

[16] Kappes, M. M., Staley, R. H. Relative bond dissociation energies for two-ligand complexes of nickel(+) with organic molecules in the gas phase.*J. Am. Chem. Soc.,* 1982. 104, 1813–1819.

[17] Lopes, J. F., Rocha, W. R. Dos Santos, H. F. De Almeida, W. B. Theoretical study of the potential energy surface for the interaction of cisplatin and their aquated species with water. *J. Chem. Phys.*, 2008 128, 165103–165116.

[18] Dans, P. D., Crespo, A., Estrin, D. A. Coitiño, E. L. Structural and energetic study of cisplatin and derivatives: comparison of the performance of density functional theory implementations. *J. Chem. Theory. Comput.*, 2008 4, 740–750.

[19] Da Silva, V. J., Costa, L. A. S., Dos Santos, H. F. Ab initio reaction path for cisplatin interaction with L-cysteine and L-methionine. *Int. J. Quant. Chem.,* 2008 108, 401–414.

[20] Amado, A. M., Fiuza, S. M., Marques, P. M., Batista de Carvalho, L. A. E. Conformational and vibrational study of platinum(II) anti-cancer drugs: *cis*-diamminedichloroplatinum (II) as a case study. *J. Chem. Phys*., 2007 127, 185104–185113.

[21] Fitzgerald, G., Andzelm, J. Chemical applications of density functional theory: comparison to experiment, Hartree-Fock, and perturbation theory. *J. Phys. Chem*., 1991 95, 10531–10534.

[22] Khlestov, N. M., Shendrik, A. N. Quantum-chemical DFT calculations of the energies of the O–H bond of phenols. *Theoretical and Experimental Chemistry,* 2010 46, 279–283.

[23] Jursic, B. S. The evaluation of nitrogen-containing bond dissociation energies using the ab initio and density functional methods. *J. Mol. Struc*., 1996 366, 103–108.

[24] Wang, H. J., Fu, Y. Designing new free-radical reducing reagents: Theoretical study on Si–H bond dissociation energies of organic silanes. *J. Mol. Struc*., 2009 893, 67–72.

[25] Zhang, K. C., Fan, J. M., Liu, L., Guo, Q. X. Quantitative structure-activity relationships in the lithium and sodium affinitites of *n*-alkyl fluorides. *Chin. Chem. Lett*., 2002 13, 41–44.

[26] Burk, P., Taul, K. Tammiku-Taul, J. Proton and lithium cation binding to some β-dicarbonyl compounds. A theoretical study. *Croat. Chem. Acta*, 2009 82, 71–77.

[27] Arulmozhiraja, S., Fujii, T. Li^+ ion affinities of global-warming perfluorocarbons. *J. Phys. Chem*. A, 2000 104, 9613–9618.

[28] Hwang, S., Jang, Y. H., Chung, D. S. Gas phase proton affinity, basicity, and pK_a values for nitrogen-containing heterocyclic aromatic compounds. *Bull. Korean Chem. Soc.,* 2005 26, 585–588.

[29] Šala, M., Hodošček, M., Arulmozhiraja, S., Fujii, T. Complete set of critical points on the $C_{60}H^+$ potential energy surface. *J. Phys. Chem. A*, 2009 113, 3223–3226.

[30] Fujii, T., Arulmozhiraja, S., Nakamura, M., Shiokawa, Y. Detection of Cu(hfac)(tmvs) by Li^+ ion attachment mass spectrometry. *Chem. Phys. Lett*. 2006 425, 134–137.

[31] Chval, Z., Sip, M. Pentacoordinated transition states of cisplatin hydrolysis – ab initio study. *J. Mol. Struc*., 2000 532, 59–68.

[32] Carloni, P., Andreoni, W., Hutter, J., Curioni, A.,Giannozzi, P., Parrinello, M. Structure and bonding in cispaltin and other Pt(II) complexes. *Chem. Phys. Lett.* 1995 234, 50–56.

[33] Lucas, M. F. A. Pavelka, M., Alberto, M. E., Russo, N. Neutral and acidic hydrolysis reactions of the third generation anti-cancer drug oxaliplatin. *J. Phys. Chem. B*, 2009 113, 831–838.

[34] Frisch, M. J., Trucks, G. W., Schegel, H. B., Scuseria, G. E., Robb M. A., Cheeseman J. R., Montgomery Jr, J. A., Vreven, T., Kudin, K. N. Burant J. C., Millam, J. M., Iyengar, S. S., Tomasi, J., Barone, V., Mennucci, B., Cossi M., Scalmani, G., Rega, N., Petersson, G. A., Nakatsuji, H., Hada, M., Ehara, M., Toyota, K., Fukuda, R., Hasegawa, J., Ishida, M., Nakajima, T., Honda, Y., Kitao, O., Nakai, H., Klene, M., Li, X., Knox, J. E., Hratchian, H. P., Cross, J. B., Bakken, V. Adamo, C., Jaramillo, J., Gomperts, R., Stratmann, R. E., Yrazyev, O., Austin, A. J., Cammi, R., Pomelli, C.,

Ochterski, J. W., Ayala, P. Y., Morokuma, K., Voth, G. A. Salvador, P.; Dannenberg, J. J., Zakrzewski; V. G. Dapprich, S. Daniels, A. D., Strain, M. C., Farkas, O., Malick, D. K., Rabuck, A. D. Raghavachari, K., Foresman, J. B., Ortiz, J. V., Cui, Q., Baboul, A. G., Clifford, S., Cioslowski, J., Stefanov, B. B., Liu, G., Liashenko, A., Piskorz, P., Komaromi, I., Martin, R. L., Fox, D. J., Keith, T., Al-Laham, M. A., Peng, C. Y., Nanayakkara, A., Challacombe, M., Gill, P. M. W., Johnson, B., Chen, W., Wong, M. W., Gonzalez, C., Pople, J. A. Gaussian 03, Revision D.01–Gaussian, Inc., Wallingford CT, 2004.

[35] Parr, R. G., Yang, W. Density-Functional *Theory of Atoms and Molecules.*–UK, Oxford: University Press, 1989.

[36] Becke, A. D. Density-functional exchange-energy approximation with correct asymptotic behavior. *Phys. Rev. A,* 1988 38, 3098–3100.

[37] Becke, A. D. Density-functional thermochemistry. III. The role of exact exchange. *J. Chem. Phys.*, 1993. 98, 5648–5652.

[38] Lee, C., Yang, W., Parr, R. G. Development of the Colle-Salvetti correlation-energy formula into a functional of the electron density. *Phys. Rev. B*, 1988 37, 785–789.

[39] Bamcroft, D. P., Lepre, C. A., Lippard, S. J. Nucleic acids and molecular biology. Berlin: *Springer;* 1990.

[40] Miller, S. E., House, D. A. The hydrolysis products of *cis*-dichlorodiammineplatinum(II) 2. The kinetics of formation and anation of the *cis*-diamminedi(aqua)platinum(II) cation. *Inorg. Chim. Acta*, 1989 166, 189–197.

[41] Carloni, P., Andreoni, W., Hutter, J., Curioni, A., Giannozzi, P., Parrinello, M. Structure and bonding in cisplatin and other Pt(II) complexes. *Chem. Phys. Lett.*, 1995 234, 50–56.

[42] Al Takhin, G., Skinner, H. A., Zaki, A. A. Micro-calorimetric studies of the thermal decomposition of ammonia–halide and amine–halide complexes of platinum (II), [Pt $(NH_2R)_2X_2$]. *J. Chem. Soc. Dalton Trans.*, 1983, 2323–2328.

[43] Kamruddin, M., Ajikumar, P. K., Dash, S., Tyagi, A. K., Raj, B. Thermogravimetry-evolved gas analysis-mass spectrometry system for materials research. *Bull. Mater. Sci.,* 2003 26, 449–460 and references therein.

[44] Materazzi, S., Gentili, A., Curini, R. Applications of evolved gas analysis Part 2: EGA by mass spectrometry. *Talanta,* 2006 69, 781–794 and references therein.

[45] Fujii, T. Ionization methods: ion attachment mass spectrometry. In: Gross, L. M., Caprioli, R. M., editors. Encyclopedia of Mass Spectrometry. Amsterdam: *American Society for Mass Spectrometry/Elsevier*; 2007; 327–334.

[46] Fujii T. A novel method for detection of radical species in the gas phase: usage of Li^+ ion attachment to chemical species. *Chem Phys Lett.* 1992; 191: 162–168.

[47] Takahashi, S., Tsukagoshi, M., Kitahara, Y., Juhász, M., Fujii, T. Design and performance of an evolved gas analysis ion attachment mass spectrometer. *Rapid Commun. Mass Spectrom.*, 2010 24, 2625–2630.

[48] Fujii, T. Quadrupole mass spectrometry in combination with lithium ion attachment for sampling at atmospheric pressure: possible coupling to supercritical fluid chromatography. *Anal. Chem.*, 1992 64, 775–778.

[49] Fujii, T. A novel method for detection of radical species in the gas phase; usage of Li^+ ion attachment to chemical spcies. *Chem. Phys. Lett.* 1992 191, 162–168.

[50] Sablier, M., Fujii, T. Mass spectrometry of free radicals. *Chem. Rev.*, 102 2002, 2855–2924.

[51] Fujii, T. Neutral product analysis of the microwave C_2H_2 plasma: C_n, C_nH_2, C_nH_3, C_nH_4, C_nH_5, and larger species. *J. Appl. Phys.*, 1997 82, 2056–2059.

[52] Fujii, T., Syouji, K. Mass spectrometic detection of neutral radicals in a CH_4 microwave discharge by use of Li^+ ion attachment techniques. *J. Appl. Phys.* 1993 74, 3009–3012.

[53] Fujii, T., Syouji, K. Mass spectrometric studies of the neutral and ionic products in a methane/oxygen microwave discharge plasma. *J. Phys. Chem.* 1993 97, 11380–11384.

[54] Knümann, R., Bockhorn, H. Investigation of the kinetics of pyrolysis of PVC by TG-MS-analysis. *Combust. Sci. Technol.*, 1994 101, 285–299.

[55] Florence, A. T. Attwood, D. Drug stability/Stability testing and prediction of shelf life. In: Florence, AT; Attwood D., editors. Physicochemical principles of pharmacy. London: Pharmaceutical Press, *Royal Pharmaceutical Society of Great Britain;* 2006; 127–136.

[56] Claereboudt, J., De Spiegeleer, B., De Bruijn, E. A., Gijbels, R., Claeys, M. Structural characterization of cisplatin analogues by fast atom bombardment (FAB) and laser microprobe mass spectrometry (LAMMA). *J. Pharm. Biomed. Anal.,* 1989 7, 1599–1610.

[57] Weller, R. R., Eyler, J. R., Riley, C. M. Fourier transform mass spectrometry of cisplatin and analogues. *J. Pharmaceut. Biomed. Anal.*, 1985 3, 87–94.

[58] Claereboudt, J., De Spiegeleer, B., Lippert, B., De Bruijn, E. A., Claeys, M. Fast atom bombardment and tandem mass spectrometry for the structural characterization of cisplatin analogs and bis-nucleobase adducts with cisplatin. Spectrosc. *Int. J.,* 1989 7, 91–112.

[59] Ehrsson, H. C., Wallin, I. B., Andersson, A. S., Edlund, P. O. Cisplatin, transplatin, and their hydrated complexes: separation and identification using porous graphitic carbon and electrospray ionization mass spectrometry. *Anal. Chem.*, 1995 67, 3608–3611.

[60] Cui, M., Mester, Z. Electrospray ionization mass spectrometry coupled to liquid chromatography for detection of cisplatin and its hydrated complexes. *Rapid Commun. Mass Spectrom.*, 2003 17, 1517–1527.

In: Cisplatin: Pharmacology, Clinical Uses and Adverse Effects ISBN: 978-1-61942-359-6
Editors: Toshiko Kojima and Yoko Morita

Chapter VIII

CISPLATIN: PHARMACOLOGY, CLINICAL USES AND ADVERSE EFFECTS

Ana Lopez-Gonzalez, Patricia Ibeas Millan and Mariano Provencio
Medical Oncology, Hospital Universitario Puerta de Hierro-Majadahonda
Madrid, Spain

1. PHARMACOLOGY

1.1. Introduction

The discovery of cisplatin can be traced back to the 1960s, when a physical chemist named Rosenberg discovered it while working in a small laboratory in Michigan. He noted that when an electric current passed between two platinum electrodes within a bacterial culture, the growth of Escherichia coli was inhibited due to the formation of inorganic platinum compounds, provided that ammonium and chloride ions were present. This was due to the action of a compound in the environment, Peyronie´s chloride, which was described in 1845 as cis-diaminocloroplatinum.

It was not until 1969, when Rosenberg discovered that this compound inhibits tumor cell growth in culture, that his results were published in Nature [1].

At first, this discovery was not disseminated throughout the scientific community because the compound contained heavy metals that are highly toxic to humans. However, shortly thereafter, several phase 1 studies were conducted that showed great activity against ovarian and testicular tumors.

Additionally, during these studies, the first side effects were observed. The compound cis-diaminocloroplatinum was very emetic, with severe kidney toxicity and tubular necrosis; therefore, the trials were discontinued. In 1977, Dr. Cvitkovic added cisplatin to mannitol along with massive hydration and administered the combination to a dog to achieve greater clearance, to lower renal toxicity, and to prevent tubular damage [2]. After this success, cisplatin began to be used in humans because efficacy in several solid tumors was shown in addition to acceptable toxicity.

1.2. Cisplatin as a Chemical Element

Cis-diamino-dichloro-platinum II (cisplatin) is an inorganic heavy metal formed by a platinum atom that is covalently bonded to two chlorine atoms in a cis arrangement and two amine groups. The valency of platinum is indicated by II.

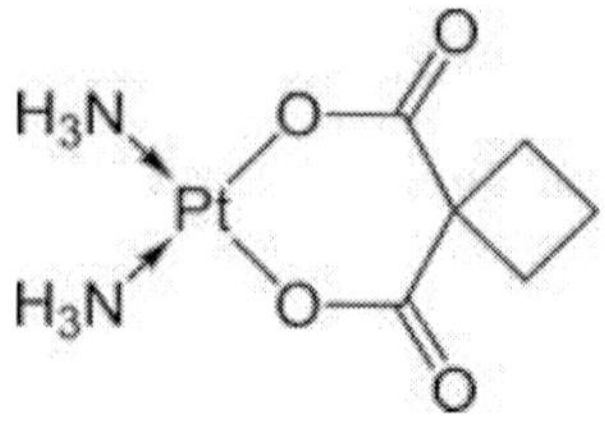

Cisplatin behaves as an alkylating agent, and its activity is highest within resting cells. In addition to the direct DNA damage it causes, it binds to proteins by altering the transmembrane transport of essential amino acids via calcium channels. Cisplatin enters cells by diffusion. Chloride atoms can be moved directly by a reaction with nucleophiles, such as thiols, and chloride hydrolysis may be responsible for the activated forms of the drug that act against nucleic acids and proteins.

When low concentrations of chloride are present, hydrolysis is favored, whereas high concentrations inhibit the stimulation of the drug.

Although its mechanism of action is not completely clear, it is believed that the cytotoxicity of cisplatin is primarily due to the development of DNA adducts. Cisplatin interacts mainly with the nitrogen of guanines and adenines and produces joints between different bases of the DNA chain. Its toxic effect can be attributed to the nuclear DNA damage it causes by forming of covalent bonds between the bases of these molecules, known as adducts [3]. Most of these adducts are between adjacent bases of the same strand (intrachain), although 5% are formed between bases on different strands (interchain), both of which appear to contribute to the cytotoxicity of the drug. It has also been observed that cisplatin is able to form bridges between nuclear proteins and DNA. The mechanism by which these adducts lead to cell death is still unknown, but there are three hypotheses that may explain the mechanism of action of cisplatin.

1. *Inhibition of DNA synthesis*. DNA synthesis has long been considered the cause of cell death due to cisplatin, which was noted when cells that were cultured with platinum inhibited DNA synthesis. Additionally, several cell types still die at lower doses than are required to inhibit DNA synthesis; thus, this hypothesis seems to be correct.
2. *Inhibition of RNA synthesis*. The same process that occurs in DNA also occurs with regard to RNA. Low concentrations do not inhibit the synthesis of RNA but do produce cell death. It is possible that this effect occurs temporarily by selectively inhibiting RNA because a rapid and selective repair of genes in cells has been shown.

3. *Induction of apoptotic death*. The concentration of cisplatin and the exposure time are critical factors involved in cisplatin-induced apoptosis. Cisplatin produces cell arrest in G2, prior to the induction of cell death.

The specificity of cisplatin with respect to the phase of the cell cycle seems to vary between different cell types, although the effects on cross-linkages are more pronounced in the S phase. In addition to its ability to react with DNA, cisplatin can also react with other nucleophiles, such as the sulfhydryl groups of proteins.

1.3. Mechanisms of Resistance

The following mechanisms of resistance are described:

1. Changes in the transmembrane transport of cisplatin.
2. Cellular inativation due to increased glutathione, matallothionein and sulfhydryl compounds.
3. Increased tolerance to platinum-DNA adducts and / or increased expression of DDH (dihydrodiol dehydrogenase) alters the expression of oncogenes, limits the formation of adducts and activates anti-apoptotic pathways, which prevent cell death.
4. Resistance to apoptosis may be due to a failure to activate caspase-9, a key enzyme in the initiation and progression of apoptosis, and also may be due to defects in p53 and bcl / abx.
5. Increased repair of DNA damage due to an increase in repair enzymes, such as ERCC-1 and NER (nucleotide excision repair); failure of MMR systems (mismatch repair), which include MHL 1 and MSH2; or increased expression of genes that act during DNA damage, such as c-fos/AP1 or AP2.

Certain genes have been associated with a resistance to platinum, such as ABCC5 (also known as MRP5) and XPA.

Experimental results suggest that increased expression of ABCC5 is associated with exposure to platinum drugs, and increased resistance to platinum drugs may be due to increased outflow through the glutathione S-platinum complex.

XPA and ERCC2 are components of the nucleotide excision repair (NER) mechanism that is generally recognized as the main repair response to DNA damage caused by chemotherapeutic agents, such as cisplatin.

In NER, XPA is the primary recognition protein of lesions in the DNA. Increased expression of NER genes is a major cause of the resistance to cisplatin. [4] ERCC2 (or XPD) is essential for helicase activity and has been shown to interact specifically with GTF2H2 (or p44). This interaction results in the stimulation of helicase activity.

XRCC1 is a key component of base excision repair (BER). The NER pathway is the main repair mechanism for DNA adducts produced by cisplatin.

1.4. Pharmacokinetics

Cisplatin is an inactive agent; it can be administered intravenously, intra-arterially and intraperitoneally. It is not recommended without a fluid therapy infusion because of the side effects it produces.

It is ineffective when used orally. After intravenous administration at standard doses, the drug has an initial life of 25 to 50 minutes in plasma; subsequently, concentrations decline with a half-life of 58 to 73 hours, which is greater if the dose is higer.

The recommended infusion rate is 1 mg per minute. Cisplatin must be diluted in saline because it is unstable in solutions containing glucose. Contact with aluminium must be avoided because it may precipitate and lose efficacy.

Cisplatin is unstable in biological matrices because it contains chlorine atoms, which are susceptible to nucleophilic substitution reactions (such as water or sulfydryl groups of proteins). Ninety percent of cisplatin binds to proteins, such as albumin, transferrin or gammaglobulin. The other 10% is activated after entering the cell by passive diffusion and the hydrolysis of chloride ions has occurred.

In organs such as the kidney, testis, liver or intestine, higher concentrations of cisplatin are detected. However, concentrations are lower in the central nervous system.

Cisplatin has a triphasic pattern of elimination, 30 minutes, one hour and 24 hours, respectively. At a dose of 50 mg/m2, approximately 13 to 27% of the drug is eliminated in the urine in the first hour after administration. After 5 days, the amount that can be collected in the urine is 43% of the drug administered [5]. The clearance of cisplatin exceeds the creatinine clearance, indicating that these molecules are actively excreted by the kidney. For its elimination, cisplatin undergoes enzymatic biotransformation, in which chloride ligands are displaced by water and form a platinum complex, which is positively charged and which reacts with nucleophiles, such as the sulfhydryl group in glutathione. Ninety percent of cisplatin is excreted by the kidneys by glomerular filtration, and 10% is excreted through the biliary tract. Cisplatin can undergo enterohepatic circulation.

1.5. Pharmacodynamics

Cisplatin should be used cautiously with other drugs that are eliminated via the urine, such as ifosfamide, bleomycin, methotrexate, or other nephrotoxic drugs, including aminoglycosides, tacrolimus, rituximab, amphotericin, diuretics or ifosfamide. Aminoglycosides and furosemide increase ototoxicity, while antihistamines mask it.

Cisplatin increases the metabolism of phenytoin and carbamazepine, thereby decreasing its effectiveness. The pharmacokinetics of lithium is also altered. Probenecid decreases its clearance. As for other cytotoxic drugs, cisplatin decreases the clearance of etoposide and paclitaxel and increases docetaxel´s neurotoxicity. It also increases the myelotoxicity of vinorelbine and topotecan. The risk of developing leukemia increases when cisplatin is combined with adriamycin, and renal failure risk increases when it is combined with topotecan. Therefore, it is mandatory to lower the dose of the latter.

2. Indications and Clinical Uses

Due to its high chemotherapeutic activity, cisplatin is used in the treatment of lymphoma, melanoma, and ovarian, testicular, head and neck, lung, bladder, lymphoma, and cervical cancers.

- Metastatic testicular tumors: Cisplatin is used in combination with other cytotoxic agents.

The following schemes are used:

- BEP or EP without bleomycin: every 21 days, bleomycin 30 U IV or IM on days 1, 8 and 15, etoposide (VP16) 100 mg/m2 iv on days 1 to 5, and platinum 20 mg/m2 i.v. on days 1 to 5.
- VIP: every 21 days, etoposide 75 mg/m2 i.v. on days 1 to 5, ifosfamide 1200 mg/m2 i.v. on days 1 to 5, and platinum 20 mg/m2 on days 1 to 5.
- VeIP scheme: similar to above but with vinblastine 0.11 mg/kg iv on days 1 and 2 instead of etoposide.

- Metastatic ovarian tumors: In combination with other drugs. Monotherapy is indicated in refractory patients and those who have not received cisplatin.

Cisplatin has been substituted by carboplatin and paclitaxel because this scheme was not inferior when compared with cisplatin and paclitaxel.

- Tumors of the ENT area (Al-Sarraf scheme) and the esophagus and stomach, where the classic association of cisplatin and fluorouracil (cisplatin 100 mg/m2 iv on day 1 + 5-FU 1000 mg/m2 by continuous infusion on days 1 to 5, out of 28 days) has been replaced by docetaxel (DCF scheme: docetaxel 75 mg/m2 iv on day 1 + cisplatin 75 mg/m2 iv on day 1 + 5FU 570 mg/m2 iv by continuous infusion on days 1 through 5, over 21 days). This is an aggressive combination that requires treatment with colony-stimulating factors and should only be used in patients in excellent physical condition.
- Bladder cancer: cisplatin associated with gemcitabine (cisplatin 75 mg/m2 iv on day 1 and gemcitabine 1250 mg/m2 iv on days 1 and 8, every 21 days).
- Lung cancer: associated with gemcitabine (same pattern as in the bladder), with vinorelbine (cisplatin 75 mg/m2 iv on day 1 and vinorelbine 30 mg/m2 on days 1 and 8, every 21 days) or in combination with docetaxel (cisplatin 75 mg/m2 iv on day 1 and docetaxel 75 mg/m2 iv on day 1, every 21 days).
- Cervical cancer: cisplatin is the standard of treatment. In advanced stages, it is used with the following scheme: cisplatin 50 mg/m2 iv on day 1 + topotecan 0.75 mg/m2 on days 1 to 3, every 21 days with prophylaxis of neutropenia.
- Osteosarcoma, retinoblastoma and neuroblastoma.
- Tumors of the biliary tract: cisplatin 75 mg/m2 and gemcitabine 1250 mg/m2 on days 1 and 8, every 21 days.

- Hodgkin´s lymphoma: ESHAP scheme (cisplatin 25 mg/m2 by continuous infusion on days 1 through 4, etoposide 40 mg/m2 on days 1 through 4, methylprednisolone 500 mg iv on days 1 to 4, and cytarabine 2000 mg/m2 on day 5 after end cisplatin and etoposide.
- Malignant mesothelioma: cisplatin 75 mg/m2 on day 1 and pemetrexed 500 mg/m2 on day 1, every 21 days, premedicated with folic acid and vitamin B12.

In conclusion, with the exception of colorectal tumors and brain tumors, cisplatin is a drug with a high antitumor capacity.

It is also used concomitantly with radiotherapy, especially in the ENT, lung and cervix. In standard doses, cycles should not be administered before 3 to 4 weeks. No further doses should be administered if kidney, hematological and ontological function are recovered.

Other ways to administer cisplatin:

- Intra-arterially: doses of 75 to 150 mg/m2. Cisplatin is used in regional neoplasms, such as advanced bladder cancer, advanced melanoma or ontogenetic sarcoma.
- Intraperitoneally: when the tumor is confined to the peritoneal cavity or malignant ascites exists, cisplatin can be administered intraperitoneally. The doses are usually 60 to 90 mg/m2 with intravenous sodium thiosulfate, every 3 weeks.

One of the most frequent problems with chemotherapeutic agents is to know the dose and schedule recommended in clinical practice. It has been demonstrated in several studies that higher doses, weekly treatment or continuous infusion does not increase efficacy.[6]

The best therapeutic index is achieved with doses of 25 mg/m2 weekly; therefore, cisplatin could be administered at 25 mg/m2 weekly, 50 mg/m2 every 2 weeks, 75 mg/m2 every 3 weeks or 100 mg/m2 every month and could be administered in single dose on day 1 or spread over several days.

3. Adverse Effects

Most of the adverse effects of the administration of cisplatin are dose-dependent, and they can be cumulative. The adverse reactions most frequently noticed are hematological, gastrointestinal, auditive, and/or renal disorders and fever.

1. Hematological disorders. Leukopenia, thrombocytopenia and anemia have been observed (all are dose-dependent, cumulative and reversible most of the time) in up to 25% of the patients treated with cisplatin (37). Leukopenia is usually observed between days 18 to 23 after administration (less than 1.5 x 10^9/liter in 5% of the patients). Thrombocytopenia is usually observed at approximately 21 days after administration because the recovery period is approximately 39 days (less than 10% of the patients have less than 50.000 platelets). Anemia can occur often (larger decreases with 2g of hemoglobin), but in general, anemia occurs after leukopenia and thrombocytopenia. Hematological disorders are usually more important with doses higher than 50 mg/m2.

Uncommonly, hemolytic anemia has been described, with a positive Coombs test, but it is reversible when cisplatin is stopped. After a high dose of cisplatin, severe bone marrow depression can occur (including agranulocytosis and/or aplastic anemia)

2. Gastrointestinal disorders. These are very common and may occur after the first hour of the infusion. The most characteristic disorders are nausea, vomiting, anorexia and diarrhea. Less frequently, metallic coloration of the gums and stomatitis can be observed.

3. Hearing disorders. Hearing loss has been documented in up to 30% of patients treated with cisplatin 50 mg/m2. The defect is cumulative and may be irreversible. It can affect one or both ears and is attributed to the toxicity of the outer hair cells of the organ of Corti and the epithelium of the lateral wall of the cochlea. Ototoxicity is manifested as tinnitus and / or hearing loss at high frequencies (4000-8000 Hz). Hearing loss at frequencies of 250-2000 Hz (normal hearing limits) was observed in 10-15% of patients.

Prior or simultaneous cranial irradiation increases the risk of hearing loss [7]. The cisplatin-induced auditory toxicity may be severe in children and the elderly. [8]

4. Kidney disorders. Nephrotoxicity is cumulative and may occur within 2-3 days after infusion and up to two weeks later. Moderate and reversible renal dysfunction can be observed after a single administration of an intermediate dose (of 20 mg/m2 to <50 mg/m2). The administration of a single high dose (50-120 mg/m2) or repeated daily use of cisplatin may cause renal failure with renal tubular necrosis manifested as uremia or anuria. Renal failure can be irreversible.

There are multiple mechanisms contributing to renal dysfunction by cisplatin, including toxicity on renal tubular epithelial cells, vasoconstriction of the renal microvasculature, and proinflammatory effects.

Over 50% of cisplatin is excreted in urine 24 hours after administration, reaching the renal cortex at a higher concentration than in plasma and other organs.

Renal tubule cells are selectively damaged by cisplatin, as manifested by necrosis and apoptosis [9]. One hypothesis is that cisplatin is involved in the decreased expression and function of amino acid and glucose-dependent sodium channels [10], decreased expression and function of magnesium and water channels [11], the metabolism of cisplatin in glutathione and cysteinyl-glycine and the generation of conjugates and reactive oxygen species [12].

Other hypotheses are the following:

- Inhibition of mitochondrial F1F0-ATPase and reduction of mitochondrial oxidative phosphorylation, which are two of the intracellular effects preceding the release of cytochrome c and apoptosis [13].
- Induction of hyperlipidemia and accumulation of triglycerides and fatty acids in the kidney tissue, probably due to the inhibition of fatty acid oxidation in the proximal tubules [14]
- Significant reduction in mitochondrial RNA levels and activity of the enzyme acyl-CoA dehydrogenase
- Possible direct effect on the inhibition of peroxisome proliferator-activated receptor alpha (PPAR-alpha) activity in renal epithelial cells. This may decrease the expression of PPAR-regulated genes, including those encoding potentially protective fatty acid binding proteins [15]

Vasoconstriction in the renal microvasculature appears to contribute to the decrease in renal blood flow at an early stage after the administration of cisplatin [16].

The proinflammatory effects are as follows: cisplatin increases the expression of cytokines, such as TNF-alpha, IL-6, IFN-gamma and caspase, which promotes the differentiation, maturation and activation of neutrophils, T cells and other components of the inflammatory process. Experimental models of acute renal failure induced by cisplatin showed an increased expression of endothelial adhesion molecules and subsequent infiltration of leukocytes and T cells into kidney tissue. Mice with defects in these inflammatory pathways suffered less severe acute kidney injury induced by cisplatin [17]

The clinical manifestations of nephrotoxicity are as follows:

1. *Renal failure*. The incidence of renal failure varies depending on the dose and frequency of drug administration and the criteria used to define nephrotoxicity. Prior to the use of hyperhydration regimens, nephrotoxicity was described in more than 50% of cases [18]. In cases with progressive renal failure, treatment with cisplatin should be discontinued.
2. *Thrombotic microangiopathy* (hemolytic uremic syndrome or thrombotic thrombocytopenic purpura). This other form of renal failure is described with the use of cisplatin combined with bleomycin or with gemcitabine [19]. Thrombotic microangiopathy should be suspected when renal failure is associated with hemolytic anemia and thrombocytopenia.
3. *Hypomagnesemia.* This is seen in more than half of the cases of nephrotoxicity secondary to cisplatin due to the loss of magnesium in the urine. [20]
4. *Fanconi-like syndrome*. This is characterized by urinary loss of glucose and amino acids, such as alanine, valine, leucine and methionine, and the presence of metabolites of tricarboxylic acid (lactate and pyruvate in the urine) [21].
5. *Salt-wasting syndrome* [22].
6. *Anemia*. In addition to myelotoxicity, anemia can be observed with erythropoietin deficiency that is secondary to renal tubular damage [23].

There are several risk factors that may predict renal failure by cisplatin:

- Pre-treatment with cisplatin [24].
- Previous kidney failure, primarily due to decreased renal clearance of cisplatin. There is no consensus about the maximum allowed amount of creatinine with respect to cisplatin, but it is generally contraindicated with greater than 1.5 mg/dl creatinine or a glomerular filtration rate less than 50 ml/min. Most trials excluded patients with a creatinine > 1.5 mg/dl (G Kemp 1996).
- Concomitant treatment with other neurotoxic drugs, such as aminoglycosides and amphotericin.
- Other factors, including in older women, smoking, hypoalbuminemia and paclitaxel co-administration [25].

There are several ways to prevent cisplatin-induced nephrotoxicity:

1. *Lower doses of cisplatin*: After the development of new chemotherapeutic regimens, the association of several drugs that allow the use of lower doses of cisplatin have been developed. This management has decreased the incidence of nephrotoxicity without reducing its effectiveness.
2. *Administration of saline intravenously.* In the first phase I and phase II trials, nephrotoxicity was described in more than 50% of cases. These numbers declined dramatically with the administration of intravenous saline (even reaching 0% in some small trials). The amount of saline to administer is not clear because there have been no prospective studies. [26]
3. *Analogues of cisplatin.* In some treatment regimens, cisplatin has been replaced by carboplatin.
4. *Amifostina.* This is an agent that has shown a triphosphate decrease in cisplatin-induced nephrotoxicity in animal models and in preliminary clinical studies [27].
5. *Other agents:* N-acetylcysteine, theophylline, glycine [28].

5. Nervous system disorders. Cisplatin causes a predominantly sensory axonal neuropathy [29]. The dorsal root ganglion is the first place affected, but peripheral nerves may also be affected. The effect is typically bilateral. [30] The clinical manifestations are paresthesias and occasionally pain, beginning in the fingers and toes and extending proximally to the legs and arms. It can sometimes be confused with hand-foot syndrome (erythema acro), which has also described with cisplatin. Rarely, this neuropathy can present as a loss of taste, touch, or retrobulbar optic neuritis with decreased visual acuity and cerebral dysfunction (confusion, dysarthria, individual cases of cortical blindness, memory loss). This is described as Lhermitte's syndrome (autonomic neuropathy and myelopathy the spinal cord). Very often, cerebral arteritis, encephalitis, acute stroke and seizures are also described.

Neuropathy usually develops after a cumulative dose of 300 mg/m2; however, there is a wide inter-individual variation [29]. There should be a differential diagnosis with paraneoplastic neuropathies and autoimmune disorders, which must be distinguished from the metabolic imbalance secondary to tetany and secondary to cisplatin (hypocalcemia, hypomagnesemia). Once established, there is no effective treatment except for reducing the dose or replacing with a less neurotoxic agent, such as carboplatin. Even after the drug has been discontinued, cisplatin neurotoxicity may continue to worsen in 30% of patients [31].

Several agents have been tested to prevent the neurotoxicity of cisplatin, such as vitamin E, amifostine or L-acetyl-carnitine, with little success [24. 32, 33]. There are several ongoing trials with new agents, such as nerve growth factor, neurotrophin-3 or glial growth factor-2.

6. Cardiovascular disorders. Cardiac arrhythmias are described as changes in the ST segment, particularly when cisplatin is used in combination with other cytotoxics drugs. Infrequently, cisplatin can cause hypertension and myocardial infarction [34].

Intravenous administration of cisplatin can cause phlebitis and peripheral circulation disorders, such as Raynaud's syndrome.

7. Hepatobiliary disorders. Treatment with cisplatin can cause the elevation of transaminases and bilirubin in blood, which are usually reversible. Hypoalbuminemia has also been described.

8. Endocrine and metabolic disorders. Very often the inappropriate secretion of antidiuretic hormone can occur [35]. Hypomagnesemia, hypocalcemia, hyponatremia, hypophosphatemia and hypokalemia may also occur as a result of kidney injury by cisplatin by reducing the tubular reabsorption of cations. It can cause high cholesterol and high blood amylase.

9. Immune system disorders. Rarely, hypersensitivity reactions, such as rashes, hives or anaphylactic reactions, have been observed [36].

10. Others. Skin changes are rare and can include erythema at the site of infusion and alopecia. Abnormal spermatogenesis and ovulation and painful gynecomastia are also described. Cisplatin increases the risk of secondary leukemia, which is dose dependent and not related to age and sex.

References

[1] Calabresi P, Chabner B. Agentes antineoplásicos. En: Capítulo 51. Goodman y Gilman. Las bases farmacológicas de la terapéutica. *Editorial panamericana.* 1991: 1209-11.

[2] Cvitkovic E, Spaulding J, Bethune V et al. Improvement of cis-dichlorodiammineplatinum (NSC 119875): therapeutic index in an animal model. *Cancer* 1977; 39: 1357-1361.

[3] Meléndez J, Maldonado V. Cisplatino: avances recientes en el estudio de su mecanismo de acción. *Rev. Inst. Nal. Cancerol* (Mex) 1998: 44(1): 28-34.

[4] Weaver AD, Crawford EL, Warner KA, Elkhairi F, Khuder SA, Willey JC. ABCC5, ERCC2, XPA and XRCC1 transcript abundance levels correlate with cisplatin chemoresistance in non-small lung cancer cell lines. *Mol. Cancer* 2005 May 9; 4(1):18.

[5] Santos Garza F, González Álvarez EK, Gerardo Molina J. Ototoxicidad por cisplatino. Medicina Universitaria. Volumen 4, número 17. 2002.

[6] Livingston RB. Cisplatin in the treatment of solid tumors: Effect of dose and Schedule. *J. Natl. Cancer Inst.* 1989; 81 (10): 724-725.

[7] Low WK, Toh ST, Wee J, et al. sensorineural hearing loss after radiotherapy and chemoradiotherapy: a single, blinded, randomized study. *J. Clin. Oncol.* 2006; 24:1904.

[8] Kolinsky DC, Hayashi SS, Karzon R, et al. Late onset hearing loss: a significant complication of cancer survivors treated with cisplatin containing chemotherapy regimens. *J. Pediatr. Hematol. Oncol.* 2010;32:119.

[9] Portilla D, Kaushal GP, Basnakian AG. Recent progress in the pathopsysiology of acture renal failure. Principles of Molecular Medicine 2nd ed, *Runge MS and Patterson.* Ed Humana Press. NJ 2006. pp 643-649.

[10] XU EY, Perlina A, Vu H, et al. integrated pathway analysis of rat urine metabolic profiles and kidney transcriptomic profiles to elucidate the systems toxicology of model nephrotoxicants. *Chem. Res. Toxicol.* 2008;21:1548.

[11] Litterst CL, Torres IJ, Guarino AM et al. Plasma levels and organ distribution of platinum in the rat, dog, and dog fish following intravenous administration of cis-DDP. *J. Clin. Hematol. Oncol.* 1977;7:169.

[12] Townsed DM, Deng M, Zhang L, et al. Metabolism of Cisplaatin to a nephrotoxin in proximal tubule cells. *J. Am. Soc. Nephrol.* 2003;14:1.

[13] Nowak G. Protein kinase C-alpha and ERK1/2 mediate mitochondrial dysfunction, decreases in active Na+ transport, and cisplatin-induced apoptosis in renal cells. *J. boil. Chem.* 2002;227:4337.

[14] Portilla D, Li S, Nagothu KK, et al. Metabolomic study of cisplatin-induced nephrotoxicity. *Kidney Int* 2006;69:2194.

[15] Li S, Wu P, Yarlagadda P, et al. PPAR alpha ligand protects during cisplatin-induced acute renal failure by preventing inhibition of renal FAO and PDC activity. *Am. J. Physiol. Renal. Physiol.* 2004;286:F572.

[16] Luke DR, Vadie K, Lopez-Berestein G. Role of vascular congestion in cisplatin-induced acute renal failure in the rat. *Nephrol. Dial Transplant* 1992;7:1.

[17] Ramesh G, Reeves WB. TNF-alpha mediates chemokine and cytokine expression and renal injury in cisplatin nephrotoxicity. *J. Clin. Invest* 2002;110:835.

[18] Cvitkovic E, Spaulding J, Bethune V et al. Improvement of cis-dichlorodiammineplatinum (NSC 119875): therapeutic index in an animal model. *Cancer* 1977;39:1357.

[19] Jackson AM, Rose BD, Graff LG et al. Thrombotic microangiopathy and renal failure associated with antineoplastic chemotherapy. *Ann. Intern. Med.* 1984; 101:41.

[20] Schilsky RL, Anderson T. Hypomagnesemia and renal magnesium wasting in patients receiving cisplatin. *Ann. Intern. Med.* 1979;90:929.

[21] Hutchison FN, Perez EA, Gandara DR, et al. Renal SALT wasting in patients treated with cisplatin. *Ann. Intern Med.* 1988;108-21.

[22] Wood PA, Hrushesky WJ. Cisplatin-associated anemia: an erythropoietin deficiency syndrome. *J. Clin. Invest* 1995;95-1650.

[23] Siegert W, Beyer J, Strohscheer I et al. High dose treatment with carboplatin, etoposide, and ifosfamide followed by autologous stem-cell transplantation in relapsed or refractory germ cell cancer: a phase I/II study. The German Testicular Cancer Cooperative Study Group. *J. Clin. Oncol.* 1994;12:1223.

[24] Kemp G, Rose P, Lurain J, et al. Amifostine pre-treatment for protection against cyclophosphamide-induced and cisplatin-induced toxicities: results of a randomized control trial in patients with advanced ovarian cancer. *J. Clin. Oncol.* 1996;14:2101.

[25] De Jongh FE, van Veen RN, Veltman SJ, et al. Weekly high-dose cisplatin is a feasible treatment option: analysis on prognostic factors for toxicity in 400 patients. *Br. J. Cancer* 2003;88:1199.

[26] Stark JJ, Howel SB. Nephrotoxicity of cis-platinum (II) dichlorodiammine. *Clin. Pharmacol. Ther.* 1978;23:461.

[27] Capizzi RL. Amifostine reduces the incidence of cumulative nephrotoxicity from cisplatin: laboratory and clinical aspects. *Semin Oncol.* 1999;26:72.

[28] Wu YJ, Muldoon LL, Neuwelt EA. The chemoprotective agent N-acetylcysteine blocks cisplatin-induced apoptosis through caspase signalling pathway. *J. Pharmacol.* 1989;97:313.

[29] Van der Hoop RG, Vecht CJ, van der Burg ME, et al. Prevention of cisplatin neurotoxicity with and ACTH analogue in patients with ovarian cancer. *N. Engl. J. Med.* 1990;332:89.

[30] Krarup-Hansen A, Helweg-Larsen S, Schmalbruch H, et al. Neuronal involvement in cisplatin neuropathy: prospective clinical and neurophysiological studies. *Brain* 2007;130:1076.

[31] Siegal T, Haim N. Cisplatin-induced peripheral neuropathy. Frequent off-therapy deterioration, demyelinating syndromes, and muscle cramps. *Cancer* 1990;66-1117.

[32] Pace A, Savarese A, Picardo M, et al. Neuroprotective effect of vitamin E supplementation in patients treated with cisplatin chemotherapy. *J. Clin. Oncol.* 2003;21:927.

[33] Kanat O, Evrensel T, Baran I, et al. Protective effect of amifostine against toxicity of paclitaxel and carboplatin in non-small cell lung cancer: a single center randomized study. *Med. Oncol.* 2003;20-237.

[34] Keller GA, Ponte ML, Di Girolamo G. Other drugs acting on nervous system associated with QT-interval prolongation. *Curr. Drug Saf.* 2010 Jan;5(1):105-11. Review.

[35] Brown KR, Leitao MM Jr. Cisplatin-induced syndrome of inappropriate antidiuretic hormone (SIADH) in a patient with neuroendocrine tumor of the cervix: a case report and review of the literature. *Eur. J. Gynaecol* Oncol. 2010;31(1):107-8.

[36] Basu R, Rajkumar A, Datta NR. Anaphylaxis to cisplatin following nine previous uncomplicated cycles. *Int.J. Clin. Oncol.* 2002 Dec;7(6):365-7.

[37] https://sinaem4.agemed.es/consaem/especialidad.do?metodo=verFichaWordPdfandcodigo=64569andformato=pdfandformulario=FICHAS.

In: Cisplatin: Pharmacology, Clinical Uses and Adverse Effects ISBN: 978-1-61942-359-6
Editors: Toshiko Kojima and Yoko Morita

Chapter IX

MOLECULAR CHAPERONE HSP90 AS A CISPLATIN-SPECIFIC BINDING PROTEIN

***Hideaki Itoh*[*,1], *Ryuichi Ishida*[1], *Atsushi Komatsuda*[2] and *Hideki Wakui*[2]**

[1]Department of Life Science, Graduate School and Faculty of Engineering and Resource Science, Akita University, Japan
[2]Third Department of Internal Medicine, Akita University School of Medicine, Akita City, Akita, Japan

MOLECULAR CHAPERONES

The environment of the earth has changed consistently since primitive life was born on the earth hundreds of millions of years before 40. The change of the external environment for hundreds of millions of years brought the evolution of the creature, and the straight foundation that was not able to support a change of the external environment perished.

On the other hand, the creature coped by a cell defense mechanism called the heat shock response mechanism for a change of the sudden external environment of the unit at the time by temperature, the water pressure and atmospheric pressure, metal ions, oxygen, the certain inorganic compound or organic compound. Because a heat shock response mechanism is confirmed to all existing creatures, the straight foundation that was able to live underwater in the ancient times when it is thought that the most initial stage of the evolution of the creature, namely primitive life, was born acquires the heat shock response mechanism, and it is thought with the physiological reaction during the evolution.

There is "heat shock" in the representative stress of the change of sudden external environments. For example, change the growth temperature of the cultured cells such as HeLa cells into 42°C of the temperature of the sub-causing death from 37°C, and the normal protein synthesis is suppressed under these conditions, but some of the proteins, so-called "Heat Shock Proteins, (HSP)" are induced. Under heat shocked conditions, as for the existing protein in the cell, a part of the secondary structure is destroyed, and a physiological function

[*] 1-1 Tegata-Gakuen Town, Akita 010-8502 Japan; Tel & Fax: +81-18-889-3041; E-mail: itohh@ipc.akita-u.ac.jp.

of those proteins are remarkably reduced, and will make a aggregation composed from denatured protein and falls into the state that is extremely harmful to the cell.

The HSP is combined with protein destroyed partly of such a high level structure selectively and revives a physiological function by returning the protein of the combination partner to the high level structure of the original peculiarity by using energy, hydrolysis of the ATP. In addition, it is thought to be that the aggregation formation by proteins to each other is unstable, and the inhibition of the denatured protein defends the living body for life function maintenance.

Therefore, the HSP was called "heat shock protein" at first and "the stress protein", but named the "molecular chaperon" in particular from the latter half of the 1990's. By the way, with "a chaperon" of French "Chaperone" : it means a helper person.Almost all molecular chaperones usually constitutively exist in some amount in a cell, and HSPs are quickly and remarkably induced under various stress conditions.

The molecular chaperone usually has various physiological functions under normal- or heat-shocked conditions cells, such as folding of the newly synthesized protein, also in the cell defense reaction within a cell corresponding to a rapid change of growth environment.

Structure and a Physiological Functions of HSP90

The 90-kDa Heat Shock Protein (HSP90) is a molecular chaperone highly conserved from prokaryotes to eukaryotes. In mammalian cells, HSP90 is the most abundant molecular chaperone in the cytosol and exerts a variety of essential functions. These functions include aggregation prevention, maintenance, transport, assembly and degradation of client proteins and are performed through an ATP-dependent conformational change.

The HSP90 protein is modular with three well-defined domains, an N-terminal ATP binding domain, a middle domain that completes the ATPase site and binds to client proteins, and a C-terminal dimerization domain. During the ATPase cycle, the three domains of HSP90 move from an ATP-free “open” state to an ATP-bound “closed” state (Figure 1) [4]. Three main structural events can be observed when the chaperone changes from the open to the closed state. Two of these movements are around hinge regions, with the domains behaving as rigid bodies. One hinge is located at the interface of the dimerized C-terminal and the middle domains. This movement radically changes the orientation of the two subunits, leading to a stronger twisting and a narrowing of the distance between the two N-terminal domains. The other twist happens at the interface of the N-terminal domain and the middle domain. Here, each N-terminal domain rotates about 90° to orient to the new dimerization interface. Lastly, there is a strand exchange between the N-terminal domains, which leads to the functional assembly of the catalytic site after nucleotide binding.The HSP90 dimer which started from the C-terminus takes in the client protein, and it is to dissociate the protein of the client protein by ATP hydrolysis after the formation in a transient complex depending on the N domain aspect between each other that is common to these models. It is the HSP90 dimer formation by a C-terminus reported conventionally, and these models form dimer in the N terminal, and the protein of the client protein that is a substrate taken in close down space is released after an ATP hydrolysis reaction [5].

All major chaperones appear to bind their clients mainly via hydrophobic binding interfaces. An interesting aspect of the HSP90 structures is that hydrophobic loops at the inner side of the HSP90 dimer are exposed in the open states—one each in the middle and C-terminal domains. They point to the inner sphere of the HSP90 dimer and would be favorably positioned to transmit nucleotide induced conformational changes of the HSP90 dimer onto a bound client.

Both of the loops in the middle and C-terminal domains change positions relative to each other. However, whether they are truly involved in client binding remains to be shown. The first glimpse of HSP90 in a complex with a client protein is that of HSP90 bound to a kinase together with the kinase-specific co-chaperone Cdc37.

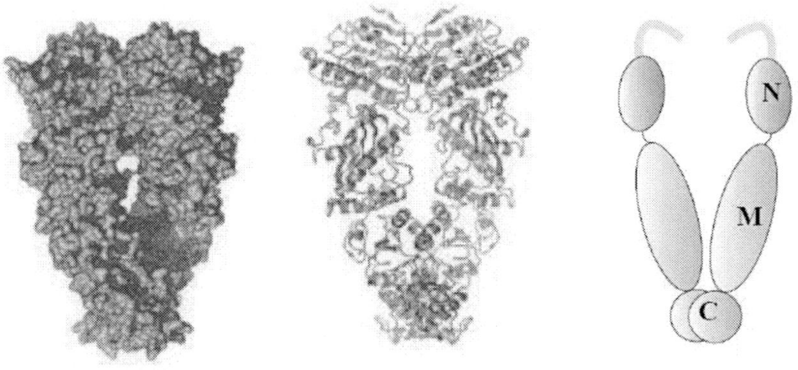

Figure 1. Current Model of HSP90.

Reconstructions based on electron micrographs showed that the complexes are asymmetric with respect to the binding of the kinase and the co-chaperone. Within the limits of the resolution of electron microscopy, this data suggests that client interactions are formed simultaneously by the N-terminal and middle domains of one HSP90 monomer. One Cdc37 molecule binds to the N-terminal domain of the other HSP90 subunit. Interestingly, these interactions seem to occur on the outside of the molecule. Given the wide range of client proteins that are unrelated in the structure and sequence, it is possible that there are several ways for them to interact with HSP90. This would be facilitated by flexible interaction sites on the surface of the HSP90 molecule.

It is known that HSP90 binds to a variety of target proteins, among them, many steroid hormone receptors and kinases. The number of client proteins identified for HSP90 has been growing steadily. Because of its many target proteins, HSP90 is considered a promising target for cancer therapy. The recent HSP90 structures will further stimulate the search for novel therapeutic interventions that affect HSP90 function.

Many HSP90 client proteins are known to be associated with cancer phenotypes. For example, akt, src, raf-1, bcr-abl, and are HSP90-dependent protein kinases that are involved in signal transduction pathways required for abnormal cancer cell growth by self-sufficient signals. HSP90 regulates the activity of the tumor suppressor protein p53, and HSP90 regulates the degradation of hypoxia-inducible factor 1, a transcription factor important for tumor cell survival under hypoxic conditions. These observations indicate that HSP90 plays crucial roles in cancer cell growth and survival by molecular chaperone tumorigenic proteins.

As shown above, it has been reported that HSP90 has been dissected by proteolysis into three domains; an N-terminal, a middle and a C-terminal domain. HSP90 is the cellular target protein of geldanamycin (GA), a novel anti-tumor drug and a specific inhibitor of HSP90-mediated protein folding [6]. The crystal structure of the N-terminal fragment of HSP90 (about 25 kDa) has recently been reported. This domain contains a unique site for the high affinity binding of GA, and this site is the same domain for the binding of ATP, suggesting that GA is an inhibitor of ATP binding to HSP90. GA also prevents p23 binding to HSP90 and inhibits the proper folding of the steroid hormone receptor. Inhibition of HSP90 activity by GA or their analogue 17-allylaminogeldanamycin (17-AAG) abrogates the maturation process, which results in the degradation of the client proteins. These observations are consistent with the fact that 17-AAGis a useful drug to treat cancers [7].It has been reported that HSP90 formed complexes with HOP and p23 in tumor tissues and that the complex forming HSP90 showed a very high affinity to 17-AAG. These observations suggest that the HSP90-containing chaperone complex is a potential target for anti-cancer therapies.

Multi-Chaperone Complex in the Cancer Cells

Co-chaperone Hop (HSP70 and HSP90 organizing protein) has three TPR (tetratricopeptide repeat) domains, and two DP domains. The C-terminus of HSP90 is MEEVD sequence, and, on the other hand, the C-terminus of HSP70 has PTIEEVD sequence. HSP90 is combined with TPR2a domain of the Hop central part. Met-5 of C-terminal MEEVD of HSP90 is combined with the 236th tyrosine (Y236) of Hop TPR2a by channeling interaction, and Asp -1 is connected by the 229th lysin (K229) of Hop TPR2a, the 301st lysin (K301) and the 305th arginine (R305) and electrostatic interaction.

On the other hand, HSP70 is combined with the TPR1 domain of the Hop N terminus end. Isoleucine (I-5) of -5 joints of C-terminal PTIEEVD of HSP70 is combined with the 49th alanyl (A49) of Hop TPR1 by channeling interaction, and aspartic acid (D-1) of -1 joint is connected by the 73rd lysin (K73) of Hop TPR1 and the 77th (R77) and electrostatic interaction. In addition, it is thought that combination to Hop TPR1 of HSP70 is higher in selectivity than a combination of Hop TPR2a of HSP90.

We analyzed 19 normal parts of a colon cancer patient and the increase and decrease of the molecular chaperone in the cancer lesion and having molecular chaperone complex or not. As a result, in approximately 70% of cancer lesions, molecular chaperone (HSP90, HSP70, HOP) increased. In addition, as a result of immunoprecipitation using the HOP antibody, a molecular chaperone complex was detected in a cancer lesion and was not able to confirm it in the normal part. Furthermore, as a result of organization dyeing of the cancer lesion, it was recognized that HOP specifically gathered to a cancer lesion part. As a cell cancerated, as for this result, composition of the molecular chaperone was derived, and it was suggested that formed a molecular chaperone complex. As a result of study using 19 operation grafts of a colon cancer patient, the legitimacy of the molecular chaperone complexation hypothesis with the cell canceration that writers drew up was proved [8].

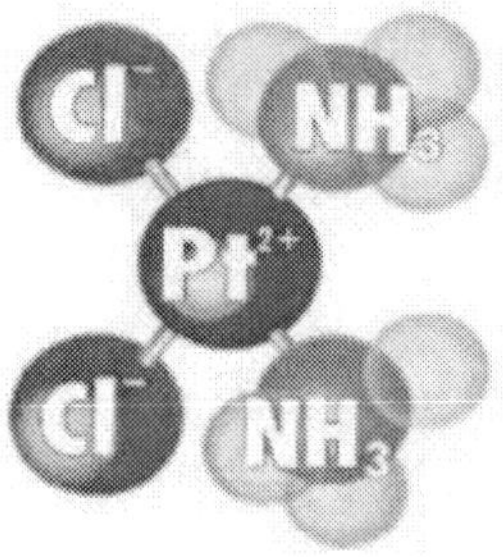

Cisplatin

CDDP: cis-diamminedichloroplatinum (II)

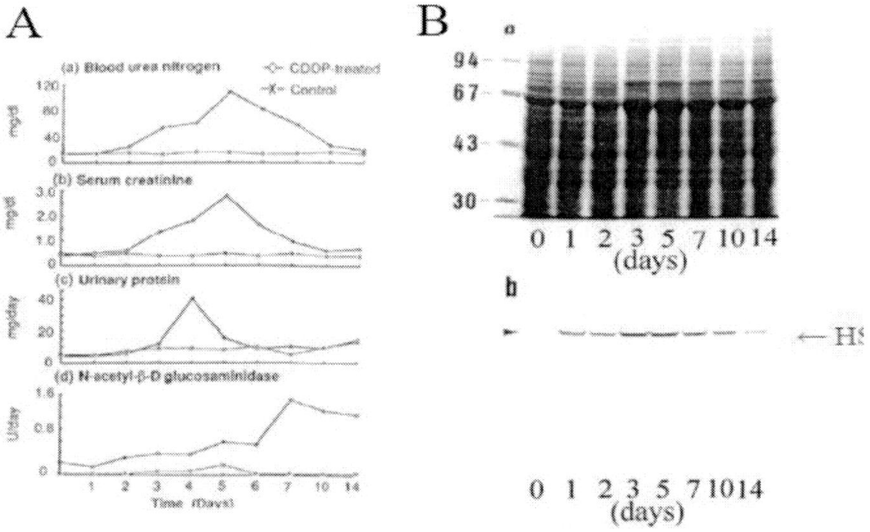

Figure 2.A. Time Course of Levels of Blood Urea Nitrogen, Serum Creatinine, Urinary Protein, andUrinary N-acetyl-β-D-glucosaminidase in Rats with Cisplatin-induced Acute Tubular Injury.Profilesof the level of blood urea nitrogen (a),serum creatinine (b), urinary protein (c), and urinaryN-acetyl-β-D-glucosaminidase (d) are shown. Values shown in (a-d) are means of data from 3 cisplatin-treatedrats and from 3 control rats at various time periods. B. Serial immunoblot analysis of Tris-HCl, pH 7.4 buffered-saline extracts obtained from cisplatin-treated rat kidneys. (a) SDS-PAGE (9% gel) stained with Coomassie brilliant blueR-250. Numbers on the left indicate molecular-mass standards (kDa). Immunoblot proved with rabbit antibody against HSP90 and with peroxidase-conjugated anti-rabbit IgG.Lanes 1, 2,3, 4, 5, 6, 7, and 8 are rat renal extracts at days 0, 1, 2 3, 5, 7, 10, and 14 after the cisplatinexposure, respectively.

HSP90IS INDUCED IN RAT KIDNEYS WITH CISPLATIN-INDUCED ACUTE RENAL FAILURE

We observed serial immunohistochemical localizations of HSP90 in rat kidneys with cisplatin-induced acute renal failure. In normal kidneys, HSP90 was mainly localized in the cytoplasm of distal tubules and collecting ducts. Twenty four hours after the cisplatin exposure, a rapid inducton of HSP90 was observed in the cytoplasm of epithelial cells in the Henle's loops (especially at the luminal side), although there was little change in these cells on light microscopy. Degenerative changes of epithelial cells appeared in the S3 segment of proximal tubules on day 3, and epithelial cell regeneration in this portion was found from day 5. On day 5, HSP90 was markedly expressed in both the cytoplasm and the nucleus of epithelial cells in the S3 segment with a granular pattern. The induced HSP90 was then accumulated in the cytoplasm of these cells on day 7 and disappeared on day 14. Immunoblot analysis of isotonic buffer-extractable renal fractions showed that there was a rapid induction of HSP90 from day 1, and that the maximum induction of HSP90 in the extract at day 5 was 6-fold that of a control. These results suggest that HSP90 plays some role related 10 functional abnormalities of the Henle'sloops at the luminal side, and in the regeneration of damaged cells in the S3 segment of proximal tubules, during the course of cisplatin-induced acute tubular injury [9].

The levels of blood urea nitrogen, serum creatinine, urinary protein, and urinary NAG in rats in groups 1 and 2 are shown in Figure 2A. (a), (b), (c), and (d), respectively. The levels of blood urea nitrogen and serum creatinine in the experimental group (group 1) began to increase on day 3, reached a peak level on day 5, and decreased on day 10. The urinary protein level began to increase abruptly on day 3, reached a peak level on day 4, and decreased steeply on day 5. The urinary NAG level began to increase on day 2, reached a peak level on day 7, and was still considerably higher than that of the control group until day 14.

The intensity of immunoreactiveHSP90 in TBS (Tris-HCl, pH 7.4 buffered saline) extracts of whole rat kidneys increased steeply on day 1 after cisplatin exposure (Figure 2B). Quantitative densitometric measurements of these proteins bands showed that the maximal induction of HSP90 in the extract at day 5 was 6-fold that of a control.

Cisplatin Binding Proteins

We have previously reported that HSP90 is specifically induced in rat kidneys with cisplatin treatments. The physiological meaning of the protein induction by cisplatin has not yet been adequately understood. In the present study, we investigated the interaction between cisplatin and HSP90 *in vitro*. To determine whether cisplatin interacts with HSP90 directly, we observed the interaction between HSP90 and cisplatin using a cisplatin-affinity column. Bovine brain cytosols were applied to the affinity column and/or the control CH-activated Sepharose 4B column. To avoid non-specific binding proteins, those columns were washed thoroughly with a buffer containing 0.15 M NaCl. The proteins were eluted with a linear gradient of cisplatin and detected on SDS/PAGE. Although no proteins bands were detected in the elutants from the control column, the 90-kDa proteins were detected as major protein bands in the elutants from the cisplatin affinity column on silver-stained gels (Figure 3) [9]. We could not detect other proteins except for the 90-kDa protein in the elutants. We investigated whether the 90-kDa protein is HSP90. On immunoblotting using anti-HSP90 antibody, HSP90 was clearly detected in the eluted fractions from the affinity column with a linear gradient of cisplatin but not in the elutants from the control column. We could not find HSP70 in the elutants from the affinity column. These results indicated that HSP90, but not HSP70, in the cytosol can interact with cisplatin. In order to determine whether the association between HSP90 and cisplatin is direct or indirect (mediates other proteins), we analyzed the interaction using a purified HSP90 alone under the same conditions. On

SDS/PAGE, we could confirm that purified HSP90 was also able to bind to the cisplatin-affinity column and could be eluted by increasing the cisplatin concentration. Purified HSP90 and HSP90 in the cytosols were eluted from the column at the same cisplatin concentrations (about 0.5-2 mM). These results indicated that cisplatin has a high affinity for HSP90 and this affinity is highly specific.

We checked the binding of cisplatin to HSP90 and it was confirmed with a control experiment showing that transplatin, a geometric isomerof cisplatin, does not bind HSP90 (Fig. 4). These results confirmed that cisplatin specifically binds to HSP90.

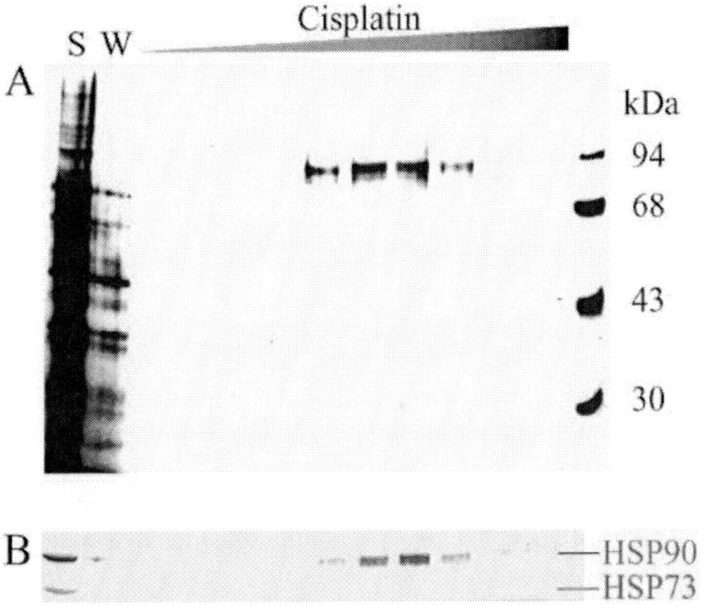

Figure 3. Cisplatin Affinity-Column Chromatography Using Cytosol. Bovine brain cytosols were applied to the control CH-activated Sepharose 4B column or the cisplatin-affinity column. After washing, the proteins were eluted with 3.33 mM cisplatin from the control column or eluted with a linear gradient of cisplatin (0-3.33 mM) from the affinity column. The elutants from those columns were electrophoresed on SDS/PAGE (9% gel) followed by staining with silver (*A*) or immunoblotting using anti-HSP90 antibody or anti-HSP70 antibody (*B*). *A* and *B*, cisplatin-affinity column chromatography. In *A*, S, W, and *M*r denote applied samples, washed proteins, eluted proteins with 3.33 μM cisplatin, and molecular standard proteins, respectively. In *B*, HSP90 and HSP70 are indicated, respectively.

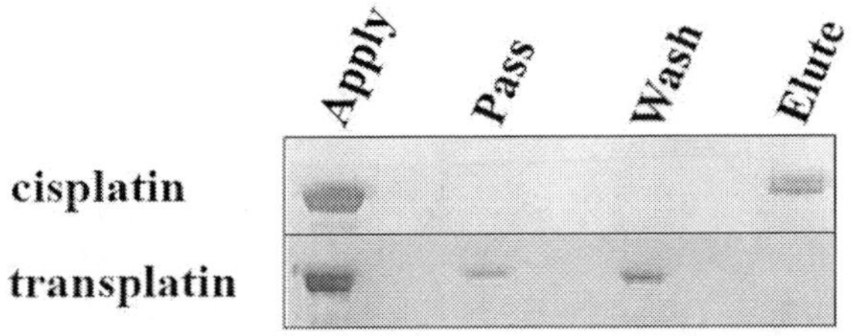

Figure 4. Transplatin does not interact with HSP90. The purified HSP90 was applied onto ciplatin-affinity column or transplatin-affinity column. After washing, the proteins were eluted with 3.33 mM cisplatin or transplatin from the column, respectively.

Conformational Change in HSP90 on Binding with Cisplatin

It has been reported that HSP90 has an average composition of 36% α-helix and 46% β-strand structure [34] under normal conditions. A conformational change in the protein has been caused by ATP with decreasing a-helix and increasing β-strand structure. Based on the available information, we analyszed whether cisplatin may give rise to a conformational change (secondary structure) in HSP90 using a far-UV CD spectrum. As shown in Figure 5, our data (HSP90 alone) was in good agreement with the CD spectrum data of HSP90. The binding of cisplatin to HSP90 resulted in the conformational changes in HSP90. By binding cisplatin to HSP90, decreasing of the mean residue ellipticity [θ] near 208 nm and increasing of [θ] near 218 nm indicated the decreasing α-helix and increasing β-strand structure of HSP90, respectively, in the CD spectrum. These results indicate that the binding of cisplatin to HSP90 is not a transient association and may cause a conformational change in the protein with a significant meaning.

Measurement of Protein Aggregation

One of the characteristic features of molecular chaperones is their ability to suppress the aggregation of proteins under stressed conditions. To analyze the functional properties of HSP90, we studied its action in protein folding and unfolding reactions *in vitro*. As an assay system, the thermal unfolding and aggregation of mitochondrial citrate synthase (CS) was used, because CS is inactivated and aggregates rapidly upon incubation at 43°C. As shown in Figure 6, spontaneous aggregation of CS has been caused at 43 °C and the reaction reached a plateau at 60 min. Although there was no effect on the reaction in the presence of a 200-fold molar excess of albumin, an equimolar amount of HSP90 suppressed the reaction and a two-fold molar excess ofHSP90 inhibited the aggregation of CS almost completely. HSP90 apparently interacts transiently with these highly structured early unfolding intermediates. As a consequence, CS is effectively stabilized in the presence of HSP90. The spontaneous aggregation of CS was not affected in the presence of cisplatin itself, and also cisplatin did not cause any optical changes in HSP90 in the lightscattering analysis. Interestingly, cisplatin reduced the chaperone activity of HSP90 in a dose-dependent manner. Amolar ratio of 1:1 (HSP90:cisplatin) and 1:5 (HSP90:cisplatin) caused about 20 and 60% suppression of the chaperone activityof HSP90, respectively. The chaperone activity was suppressed almost completely at a molar ratio of 1:10 (HSP90:cisplatin). The cisplatin concentration (1.5 μM) is lower than that of the geldanamycin (GA) concentration (18 μM) which inhibits the ATPase activity of HSP90 almost completely.

Next, we investigated the influence of Mg/ATP on this assay system. The Mg/ATP has a slight influence on the suppression of CS aggregation by HSP90. An addition of Mg/ATP to a preformed HSP90/CS complex also partly affected the chaperone activity of HSP90. An addition of ATP to the HSP90/CS complex (after 30 min of thermal aggregation of CSand HSP90) shows little influence. These results were in good agreement with data from yeast HSP90. On the contrary, the chaperone activity of HSP90, which was suppressed completely by cisplatin, was slightly affected (about 20% of the chaperone activity of HSP90 was recovered) in the presence of Mg/ATP.

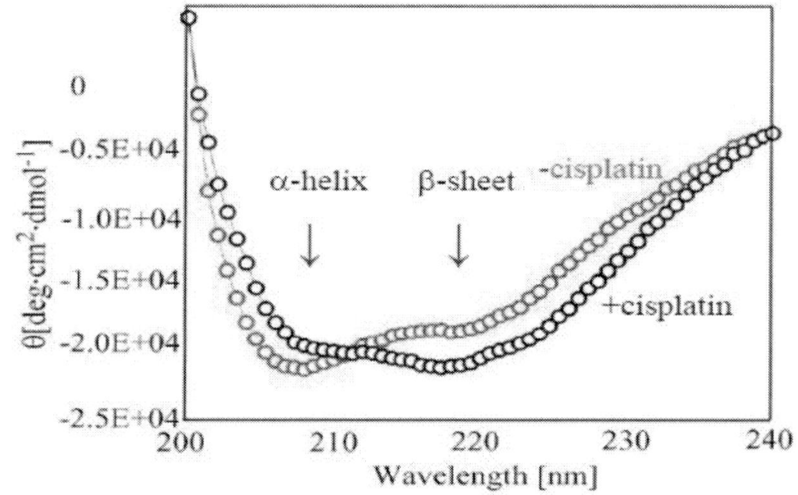

Figure 5. Effect of Cisplatin on the CD spectrum of HSP90. The CD spectrum of HSP90 was measured in the absence or presence of CISPLATIN as described in the methods section. θ denotes the mean residue ellipticity.

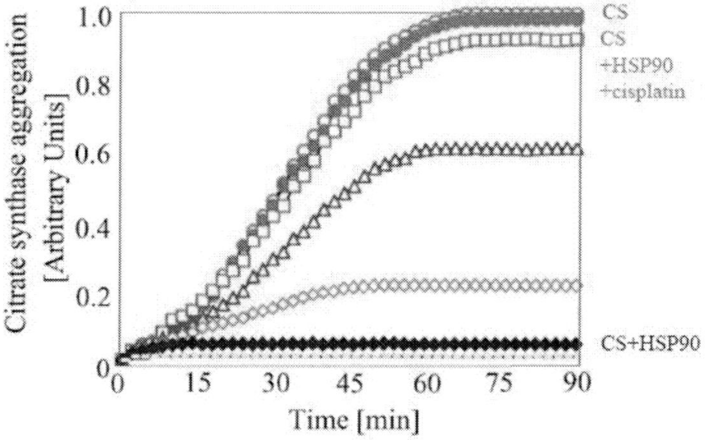

Figure 6. Effect of Cisplatin on the chaperone activity of HSP90. The effect of HSP90 and cisplatin on the thermal aggregation of CS was monitored as described (Materials and methods section). Thermal aggregation of 015 μM HSP90 in the presence of15 μM cisplatin (----).Thermal aggregation of CS (0.075 μM) in the presence of 15 μM cisplatin (closed circle) or 0.075 μM CS and 015 μM HSP90 in the presence of 0.15 μM cisplatin (open diamond), 0.75 μM cisplatin (open triangle), and 1.5 μM cisplatin (open square).Thermal aggregation of CS (0.075μM) in the absence of additional components (open circle), and a two-fold molar ratio of HSP90 (closed diamond) was monitored at 500 nm.

BINDING AND INFLUENCE OF CISPLATIN TO THE N- AND C-DOMAINS OF HSP90

We previously reported that the C-terminal tryptic fragment ofHSP90 could be purified by cisplatin affinity chromatography, suggesting the existence of a cisplatin binding site at the C terminus. To analyze whether cisplatin exclusively binds the Cterminal domain, we prepared recombinant HSP90N andHSP90C proteins (Figure 7) and carried out cisplatin column chromatography (Figure 8). The elution patterns indicated that cisplatin can bind both HSP90N and HSP90C, and suggested that cisplatin binds HSP90C, slightly more strongly than HSP90N [10-12].

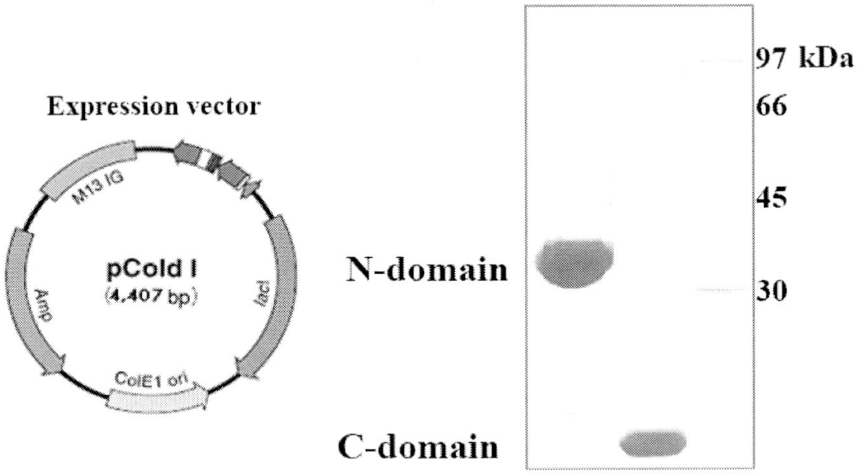

Figure 7. Construction and Purification of HSP90N- and HSP90C-domains.

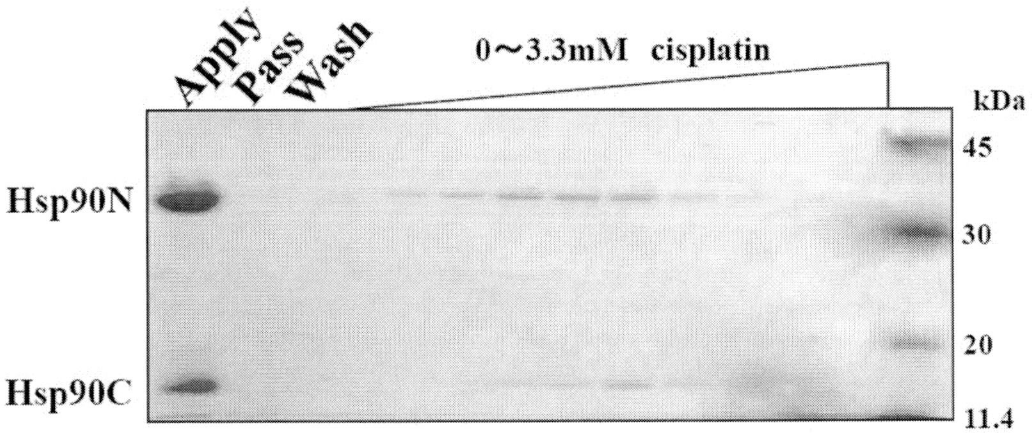

Figure 8. Cisplatin binds to HSP90C-domain rather than that of N-domain. Recombinant HSP90N- and C-domains were applied onto cisplatin-affinity column. After washing, proteins were eluted with a linear gradient of cisplatin (0-3.33mM). Fractions were analyzed by SDS/PAGE.

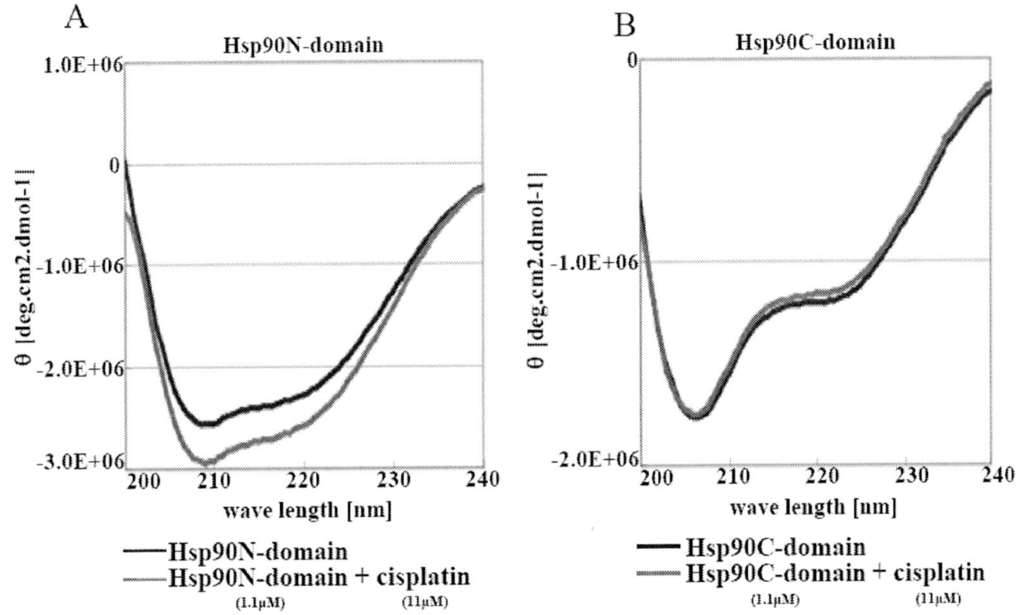

Figure 9. Cisplatin Alters Two-dimensional Structure of HSP90N, but not of HSP90C as determined by Far-UV CD spectrum.CD spectrum ofHSP90N (A) and HSP90C (B) were determined in the absence or presence of cisplatin. θ denotes mean residue ellipticity.

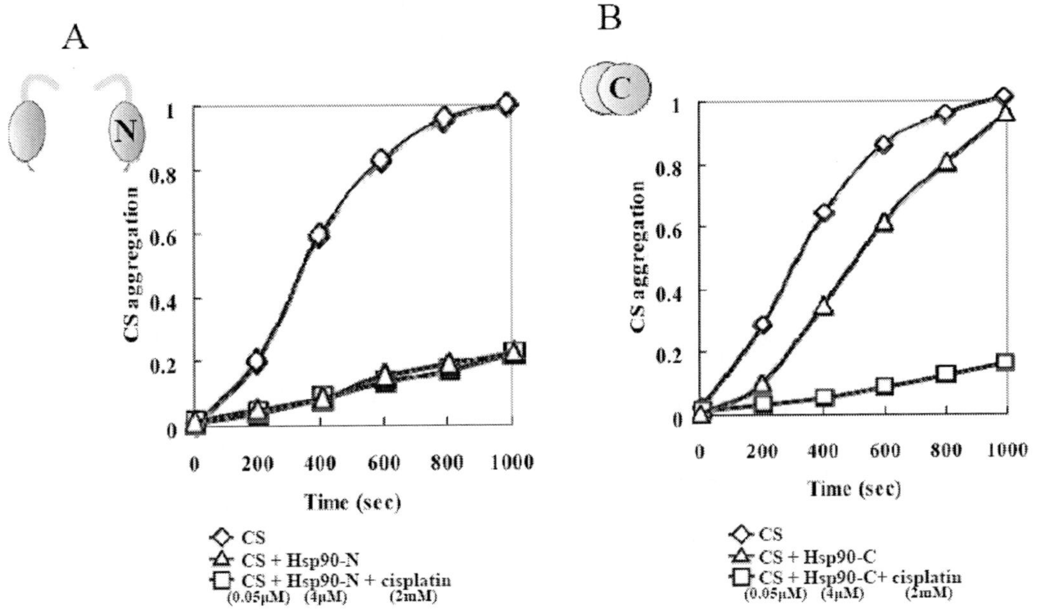

Figure 10. Cisplatin Strongly Inhibits Aggregation Prevention Activity of HSP90C, but not of HSP90N.Thermal aggregation of CS (0.05 μM) in the presence of 0.05 μM HSP90 (square), in the presence of 0.05 μMHSP90 and 2 mM cisplatin (triangle), or in the absence of both components (diamond) was monitored by optical density at 500 nm(mean with standard deviation of three independent experiments). (A)HSP90N. (B) HSP90C.

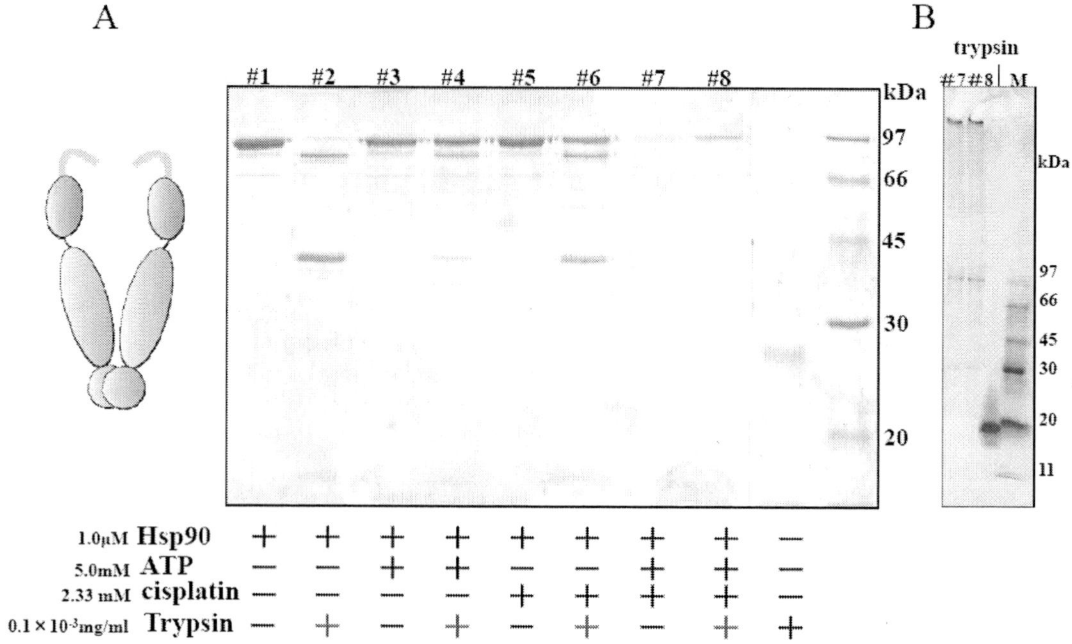

Figure 11. Tryptic Digestion of Full-length HSP90 is Prevented by the Presence of Cisplatin. (A) HSP90 was treated with trypsin in the presence of ATP and cisplatin. These samples were analyzed on SDS-PAGE (11% gel) and stained with Coomassie brilliant blue. (B) The same samples was used in the lanes 7, 8 of panel A were analyzed by SDS-PAGE using a 2-15% gradient gel. Note that large complexes of HSP90 are formed in the presence of ATP and cisplatin. Lane 9, trypsin.

We also previously reported that cisplatin induces changes in the secondary structures of the full-length HSP90 as determined by the CD spectrum. To analyze which domain is responsible for the conformational change, structural changes in the HSP90N and HSP90C were analyzed by CD measurements in the presence of cisplatin. Intriguingly, HSP90N, but not HSP90C, underwent structural changes in the presence of cisplatin (Figure 9). These results indicate that cisplatin affects the HSP90N and HSP90C differently.

HSP90 inhibits CS aggregation and cisplatin blocks the HSP90-dependent aggregation prevention. To determine which domain is affected by cisplatin, aggregation prevention by HSP90N or HSP90C against CS was tested in the presence of cisplatin. The CS aggregation was inhibited in the presence of HSP90C and this aggregation prevention effect was significantly reduced by the cisplatin (Figure 10) although the effect of cisplatin was slightly weaker than the case of the full-length HSP90. In contrast, the HSP90N-dependent aggregation prevention was not affected by the presence of cisplatin. These results appear to be consistent with the observation that cisplatin binds more strongly to HSP90C than HSP90N. Despite the fact that full-length HSP90 posses theHSP90N domain that is potentially unable to be inhibited by cisplatin for aggregation prevention activity, this drug did inhibit full-length HSP90. This may due to global conformational changes in full-length HSP90, because it induces the alteration of a secondary structure of HSP90N.

To examine whether the binding of cisplatin to HSP90N andHSP90C induces conformational changes, the protease resistance was analyzed in the presence and absence of cisplatin. We checked the effect of ATP for protease resistance and confirmed the ATP-dependent protection of the full-lengthHSP90 (Fig. 11), HSP90C (Figure 12) and HSP90N (Figure 13). It is notable that ATP protects the HSP90C dimerization domain as well as the HSP90N ATPase domain. This may be due to the ATP-binding activity of HSP90C as described by Soti etal. Under the same conditions, cisplatin stimulated the protease resistance of the full-length HSP90 and HSP90N,but not HSP90C (Figures 11-13, compare lanes 2 and 6). Although bands of the full-length HSP90 became weaker in the presence of both ATP and cisplatin (Figures 11-13, lanes 7 and 8, top), this is unlikely to be due to increased protease sensitivity because large complexes of HSP90 were detected using 2–15% gradient gel (Figure 11, right panel lanes 7 and 8, top). The formation of large complexes of HSP90 is also reported in the simultaneous presence of geldanamycin and cisplatin. Taken together, these observations are consistent with the results of the CD measurements, and confirmed that cisplatin induces conformational changes in HSP90N, but not HSP90C.

We observed the conformational changes of HSP90 by binding of cisplatin and/or ATP using an electron microscopy (Figure 14). We could find HSP90 as a dimer (in the presence of cisplatin and in the absence of ATP). On the contrary, HSP90 made an oligomer in the presence of both cisplatin and ATP. The current model of HSP90 and cisplatin are shown in Figure 15.

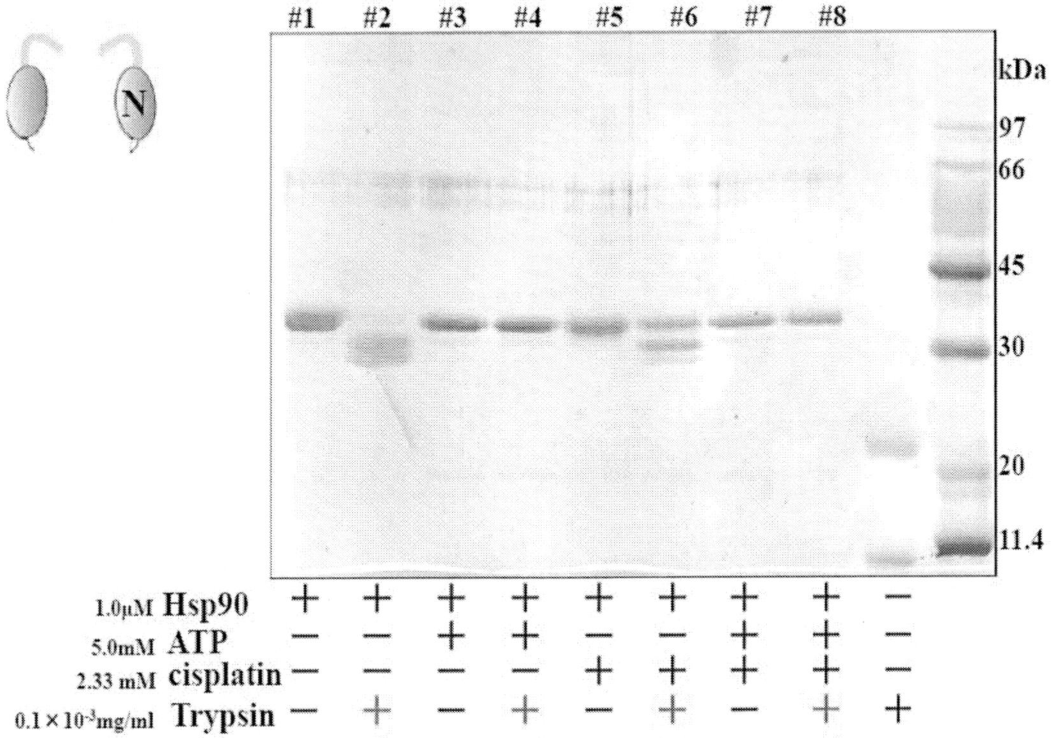

Figure 12. Tryptic Digestion of HSP90N is Prevented by the Presence of Cisplatin.

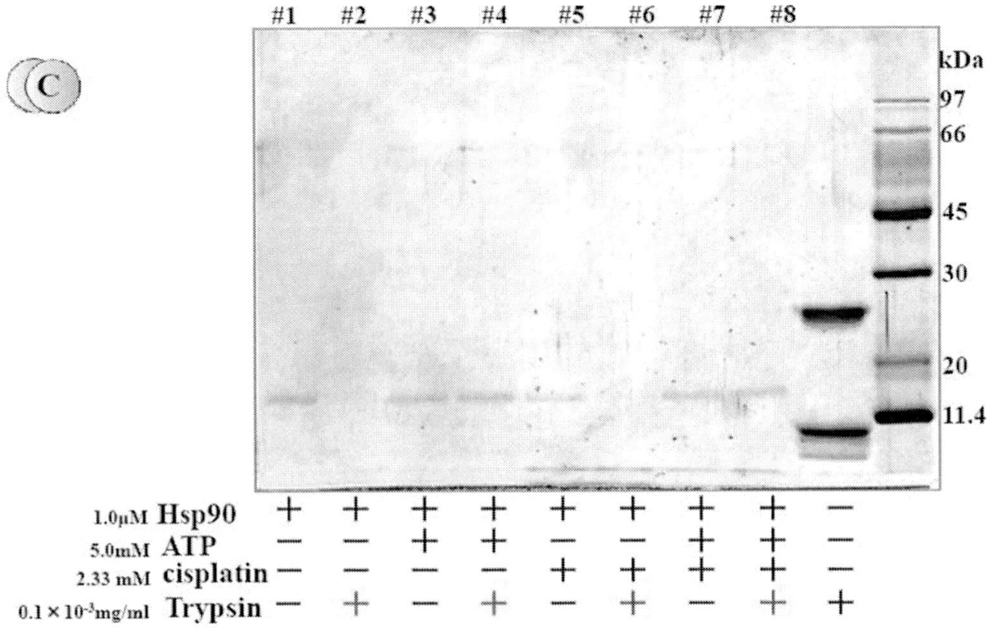

Figure 13. Tryptic Digestion of HSP90C is Prevented by the Presence of Cisplatin.

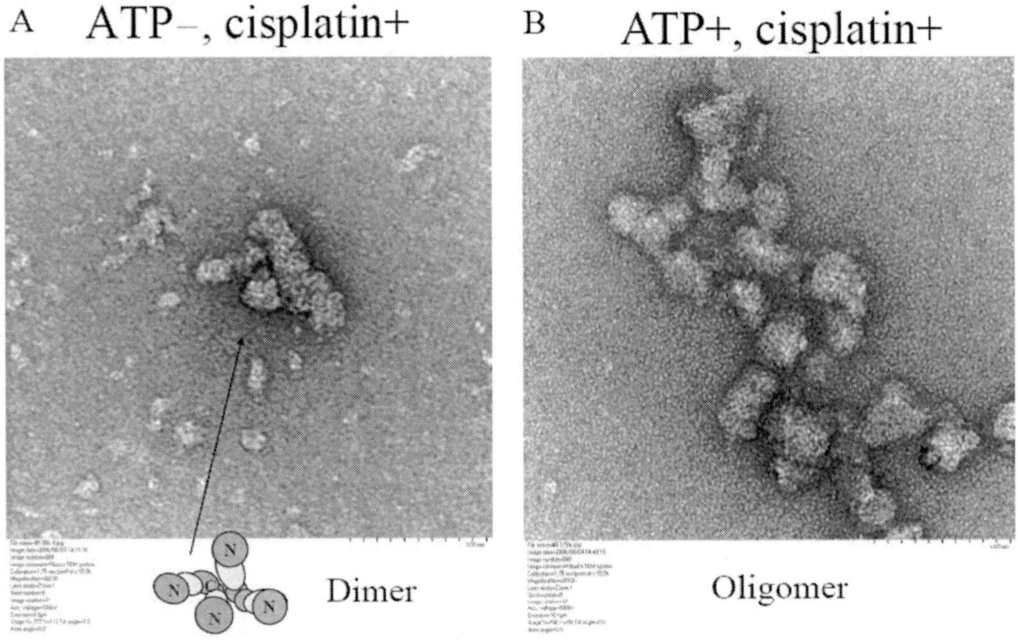

Figure 14. Electron-microsopy of HSP90. A) In the presence of cisplatin, but not ATP. (B) In the presence of both cisplatin and ATP.

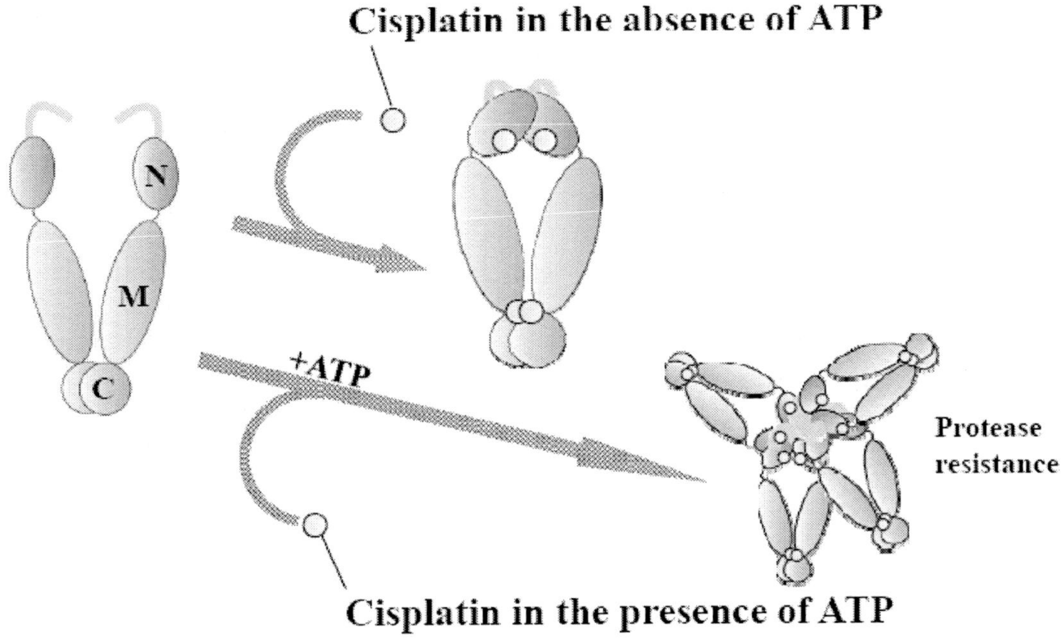

Figure 15. Influence of Cisplatin on HSP90 Conformation and Functions.

REFERENCES

[1] Hartl, FU., Hayer-Hartl, M.: Molecular chaperones in the cytosol: from nascent chain to folded protein. *Science*. 2002, 295(5561):1852-8.

[2] Hartl, FU., Bracher, A., Hayer-Hartl, M.: Molecular chaperones in protein-folding and proteostasis. *Nature*. 2011, 475(7356):324-32.

[3] Buchberger, A., Bukau, B., Sommer, T.: Protein quality control in the cytosol and the endoplasmic reticulum: brothers in arms. *Mol. Cell*. 2010, 40(2):238-52

[4] Ali, MM., Roe, SM., Vaughan, CK., Meyer, P., Panaretou, B., Piper, PW., Prodromou, C., Pearl, LH.: Crystal structure of an Hsp90-nucleotide-p23/Sba1 closed chaperone complex. *Nature*. 2006, 440(7087):1013-7.

[5] Young, JC., Schneider, C., Hartl, FU.: In vitro evidence that hsp90 contains two independent chaperone sites. *FEBS Lett.*1997, 418(1-2):139-43.

[6] Stebbins, CE., Russo, AA., Schneider, C., Rosen, N., Hartl, FU., Pavletich, NP.: Crystal structure of an Hsp90-geldanamycin complex: targeting of a protein chaperone by an anti-tumor agent. *Cell*. 1997,89(2):239-50.

[7] Kamal, A., Thao, L., Sensintaffar, J., Zhang,. L., Boehm, MF., Fritz, LC., Burrows, FJ.: A high-affinity conformation of Hsp90 confers tumor selectivity on Hsp90 inhibitors. *Nature.* 2003, 425(6956):407-10.

[8] Kubota, H., Yamamoto, S., Itoh, E., Abe, Y., Nakamura, A., Izumi, Y., Okada, H., Iida, M., Nanjo, H., Itoh, H., Yamamoto, Y.: Increased expression of co-chaperone HOP with HSP90 and HSC70 and complex formation in human colonic carcinoma. *Cell Stress Chaperones*. 2010, 15(6):1003-11.

[9] Satoh, K., Wakui, H., Komatsuda, A., Nakamoto, Y., Miura, AB., Itoh, H., Tashima, Y.: Induction and altered localization of 90-kDa heat-shock protein in rat kidneys with cisplatin-induced acute renal failure. *Ren. Fail.* 1994, 16(3):313-23.

[10] Itoh, H., Ogura, M., Komatsuda, A., Wakui, H., Miura, AB., Tashima, Y.: A novel chaperone-activity-reducing mechanism of the 90-kDa molecular chaperone HSP90. *Biochem J.* 1999, 343 Pt 3:697-703.

[11] Söti, C., Rácz, A., Csermely, P.: A nucleotide-dependent molecular switch controls ATP binding at the C-terminal domain of Hsp90. N-terminal nucleotide binding unmasks a C-terminal binding pocket. *J. Biol. Chem.* 2002, 277(9):7066-75.

[12] Ishida, R., Takaoka, Y., Yamamoto, S., Miyazaki, T., Otaka, M., Watanabe, S., Komatsuda, A., Wakui, H., Sawada, K., Kubota, H., Itoh, H.: Cisplatin differently affects amino terminal and carboxyl terminal domains of HSP90. *FEBS Lett.* 2008, 582(28):3879-83.

In: Cisplatin: Pharmacology, Clinical Uses and Adverse Effects ISBN: 978-1-61942-359-6
Editors: Toshiko Kojima and Yoko Morita

Chapter X

MULTIPLE BRAIN INFARCTION DUE TO GEMCITABINE-CISPLATIN THERAPY

Jessica Fernandez-Dominguez, Raquel Garcia-Rodriguez and Valentin Mateos
Servicio de Neurología, Centro Médico de Asturias, Oviedo, Asturias, Spain

INTRODUCTION

Neoplasm is a well-established risk factor for suffering a thrombotic vascular event. However, the relationship of chemotherapic agents with these events, particularly with cerebral infarction has not been well established yet. Some publications have related to cisplatin with a slight increase in the probability of suffering a stroke, but the underlying mechanism implicated remains still unknown.

CASE REPORT

52-year-old patient with a history of pulmonary embolism anticoagulated and large cell lung carcinoma,presente an ischemic stroke in the right middle cerebral artery territory days after the first dose of chemotherapy (cisplatin-gemcitabine). Additional studies documented a baseline hypercoagulable state. Fifteen days later, and again after administration of chemotherapic scheduled dose, undergoes a new event involving multiple ischemic areas.

CONCLUSIONS

Certain chemotherapeutic agents such as gemcitabine and cisplatin may be associated with stroke, especially in those patients in whom a prothrombotic state such as the existence of alterations in the hypercoagulability is present.

The relation between vascular event (VE) and cancer has been widely proved, being well known that the presence of a tumor increases the prothrombotic activity due to the release of strong pro-coagulant agents as tumoral necrosis factor and some interleukines (specially 6 and 1 IL1). Anyways, the relation between chemotherapy and VE, as stroke, is not well established. Some papers suggest that the use of chemotherapy agents is related with VE, even though its incidence is very low (in a 10,936 series of tumor patients receiving chemotherapy, there was only a 0,137% stroke incidence2), being cisplatine mostly mentioned as potentially involved in VE 2-5.

The reason why chemotherapy promotes VE is not well known. For cisplatin, there are several mechanisms hypothesized: apoptosis, direct vascular toxicity, endothelial disfunction, artherosclerosis, tumoral embolization, hipomagnesemia..., but none of them has fully explained the presence of those VE [4,5-8].

We present the case of a 58- year old man, with tobacco consume in his youth, who has the diagnostic of hemochromatosis treated with regular blood-letting. Some months before his first admission, he had an episode of deep vein thrombosis (DVT) with secondary pulmonary embolism (PET). By studying this event, a pulmonar mass was observed and was confirmed as a large cell lung carcinoma. Extension study showed the presence of bone metastasis. At that moment, a neuroimaging study (Craneal MRI) excluded cerebral extension (Picture 1-A). Based on these data, anticoagulant treatment with low-molecular weight heparine (LMWH), and chemotherapy with cisplatine + gemcitabine + biphosphonates were instaured. Two weeks after the first dose of chemotherapy, he was admitted at Neurology department for sudden dysarthria and facial palsy which lasted more than 24 hours. The cranial MRI performed showed an acute right insular stroke (Picture 1-B). Carotid and intracranial ultrasound study were performed without hemodynamically relevant data. A 48 hour-EKG monitor was also done, and showed no abnormalities. The hypercoagulability exam found out the presence of factor V Leiden mutation and also a resistance to the active C protein. Due to these findings, an increased in the anticoagulant dose was done. Fifteen days after this episode, he suffered a new stroke which coursed with consciousness impairment, seizures and loss of strength in the left arm. The neurological exam revealed bradipsiquia, left hemianopia, left central palsy and sensorial extinction in the left side (NIHSS: 4). A new Cranial MRI confirmed the presence of new acute ischemic lesions in both median cerebral arteries and right posterior cerebral artery (Picture 1-C). Cardiological and carotid ultrasounds were normal.

To date, the relation between cerebral ischemia and chemotherapy has not yet been elucidated, especially those patients with prior vascular risk factors, as procoagulant states (in this case, the factor V Leiden and the resistance to the active C protein). It is known for sure that some drugs, like cisplatine, increases the stroke incidence among those patients with any tumor. Cisplatine has also been related with a pro-coagulable state[1,3-4,8]. Gemcitabine implication in stroke is less known, but up to 1/6000 patients could suffer from thrombotic microangiopathy, which cause is still unknown. Gemcitabine also increases the procoagulant factors, reducing the anticoagulant factors, stimulating platelet aggregation and leading to endothelial damage[9-15].

In this patient, both stroke incidents happened at the same time that the patient was receiving intravenous chemotherapy (cisplatine plus gemcitabine): the first stroke occurred 17 days after the first chemoterapy cycle and the second one, coinciding exactly with the day of the second cycle. Thrombotic microangiopathy doesn't seem to be the cause of the stroke, as the patient didn't have renal disfunction, thrombopenia or anemia. Anyway, the temporal coincidence of the second ischemic event with the second course of cisplatine-gemcitabine leads us to reasonably think that in this particular case, gemcitabine has had an important role as those strokes related with cisplatine, mostly happened several days after cisplatine administration. On the other hand, we have to remark that, eventhough VE are rare in those patients under chemotherapy as it is suggested in the medical literature (some studies showed a 2-8% stroke incidence for diferente tumors and chemotherapeutic drugs[11,16]), when a VE happens, chemotherapy should be ended. Our decision of kept on going with the cisplatine-gemcitabine therapy drived our patient into a new stroke. Moreover, in this case the change of these drugs for other ones was not associated with a new VE.

So in conclusion, we think that the prior existence of vascular risk factors (as procoagulant states) has to be taken into account once we decide to use chemotherapy, looking forward the risk and benefice profile of the patient, and, in case a VE happens, the current chemotherapy regime should be stopped.

Picture 1: A: Cranial MRI with FLAIR secuence made previous the first VE. B: Cranial MRI, FLAIR secuences, done in the first admission, which showed a right MCA stroke. C: Cranial MRI, FLAIR secuences, done in the third admission.

REFERENCES

[1] Bick RL. Cancer-associated thrombosis. *N Engl J Med.* 2003; 349:109–111.

[2] Li SH, Chen WH, Tang Y, Rau KM, Chen YY, Huang TL, Liu JS, Huang CH: Incidence of ischemic stroke post-chemotherapy: A retrospective review of 10,963 patients. *Clin Neurol Neurosurg* 2006;108:150–156.

[3] Gamble GE, Tyrrell P. Acute stroke following cisplatin therapy. *Clin Oncol.* 1998; 10:274 –275.

[4] Czaykowski PM, Moore MK, Tannock IF. High risk of vascular events in patients with urothelial transitional cell carcinoma treated with cisplatin-based chemotherapy. *J Urol.* 1998;160:2021–2024.

[5] Etgen T, Weidenhöfer G, Kubin T. Cisplatin-associated occlusion of the internal carotid artery. *Onkologie* 2009; 32:754.757.

[6] Serrano-Castro PJ, Guardado-Santervas P, Olivares-Romero J. Ischemic stroke following cisplatin and 5-fluorouracil therapy: a transcranial Doppler study. *Eur Neurol.* 2000; 44: 63– 64.

[7] Dursun B, He Z, Somerset H, Oh DJ, Faubel S, Edelstein CL. Caspases and calpain are independent mediators of cisplatin-induced endothelial cell necrosis. *Am J Physiol Renal Physiol.* 2006; 291: F578 –F587.

[8] Pretnar-Oblak J, Zaletel M, Jagodic M, Zaletel M:Thrombosis of internal carotid artery after cisplatin-based chemotherapy. *Eur Neurol* 2007;57:109–110.

[9] Barcelo R, Munoz A, Lopez-Vivanco G. Prospective evaluation of major vascular events in patients with nonsmall cell lung carcinoma treated with cisplatin and gemcitabine. *Cancer* 2005;104:1110-1.

[10] Blaise S, Appeltants H, Carpentier PH, Debru JL. Digital ischaemia and gemcitabine. Two new cases. *J Mal Vasc* 2005;30:53-7.

[11] Numico G, Garrone O, Dongiovanni V, Silvestris N, Colantonio I, Di Costanzo G, et al. Prospective evaluation of major vascular events in patients with nonsmall cell lung carcinoma treated with cisplatin and gemcitabine. *Cancer* 2005;103:994-9.
[12] Humphreys BD, Sharman JP, Henderson JM, Clark JW, Marks PW, Rennke HG, et al. Gemcitabine-associated thrombotic microangiopathy. *Cancer* 2004;100:2664-70.
[13] Kuenen BC, Levi M, Meijers JC, van Hinsbergh VW, Berkhof J, Kakkar AK, et al. Potential role of platelets in endothelial damage observed during treatment with cisplatin, gemcitabine, and the angiogenesis inhibitor SU5416. *J Clin Oncol* 2003;21:2192-8.
[14] Teixeira L, Debourdeau P, Zammit C, Estival JL, Pavic M, Colle B. Gemcitabine-induced thrombotic microangiopathy. *Presse Med* 2002;31:740-2.
[15] Phelan PJ, Liew A, Magee C. A case of progressive hypertension preceding gemcitabine-associated thrombotic microangiopathy complicated by acute kidney injury and stroke. *Ren. Fail* 2009; 31(8):743-744.
[16] Goodnough LT, Saito H, Manni A, Jones PK, Pearson OH. Increased incidence of thromboembolism in Stage IV breast cancer treated with a five-drug chemotherapy regimen. *Cancer.* 1984; 54:1264–1268.

INDEX

B

C

F

I

J

K

L

Q

R

S

T

U

V

W

X

Y

Z